ENHANCING ATTACHMENT AND REFLECTIVE PARENTING IN CLINICAL PRACTICE

Enhancing Attachment and Reflective Parenting in Clinical Practice

A *Minding the Baby* Approach

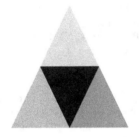

Arietta Slade

with Lois S. Sadler, Tanika Eaves,
and Denise L. Webb

THE GUILFORD PRESS
New York   London

It turns out that young people are incredibly resilient. It doesn't take that much.
All it takes is somebody to put a hand on them and say, "You know what?
You're important. And I'm listening to you."
—BARACK OBAMA

Slowly, I have come to see that asking, and listening,
and accepting are a profound form of doing.
—VINCENT J. FELITTI, MD

Copyright © 2023 The Guilford Press
A Division of Guilford Publications, Inc.
370 Seventh Avenue, Suite 1200, New York, NY 10001
www.guilford.com

Printed in the United States of America

This book is printed on acid-free paper.

Last digit is print number: 9 8 7 6 5 4 3 2 1

The authors have checked with sources believed to be reliable in their efforts to provide
information that is complete and generally in accord with the standards of practice
that are accepted at the time of publication. However, in view of the possibility of
human error or changes in behavioral, mental health, or medical sciences, neither the
authors, nor the editors and publisher, nor any other party who has been involved in the
preparation or publication of this work warrants that the information contained herein
is in every respect accurate or complete, and they are not responsible for any errors
or omissions or the results obtained from the use of such information. Readers are
encouraged to confirm the information contained in this book with other sources.

Library of Congress Cataloging-in-Publication data is available from the publisher.

ISBN 978-1-4625-5251-1 (cloth)

Minding the Baby™ is a registered trademark of Yale University. Used with permission.
All rights reserved.

We gratefully dedicate this book to the parents and children who moved us with their courage, their humanity, their resilience, and their willingness to bring us into their lives.

evaluation of specialized support programs for young parents and their children, and pediatric sleep. She has won numerous awards for her teaching and research and is a Fellow of the American Academy of Nursing.

Tanika Eaves, PhD, LCSW, IMH-E®, is a clinical social worker, Assistant Professor of Social Work at the Egan School of Nursing and Health Studies at Fairfield University, and an endorsed Infant Mental Health Specialist. Dr. Eaves joined the MTB team in 2009, where she worked with sites in the United States and Western Europe as both a clinician and training specialist. She helped develop an introductory training course on clinical approaches to enhancing reflective parenting that drew participants from around the world. She has published in the areas of reflective supervision and workforce well-being, culturally responsive parent–infant psychotherapeutic interventions, and equity in maternal–infant health and mental health outcomes. She has also worked to expand social work education competencies in infant/early childhood mental health and in promoting diversity, equity, and inclusion.

Denise L. Webb, MSN, APRN, PNP, IMH-E®, is a pediatric nurse practitioner and endorsed Infant Mental Health Mentor. She joined the MTB team at its inception, first as a clinician and later as a training specialist working with teams in the United States and Western Europe. She coined the term Reflective Nursing to describe the application of mentalization theory to nursing practice and played a pivotal role in developing an introductory training course on clinical approaches to enhancing reflective parenting that drew participants from around the world. Before completing her training as a nurse practitioner, Ms. Webb worked as an early childhood educator for many years.

Preface

The fields of infant and early childhood mental health and, more broadly, of relational health have blossomed over the course of the last decade. Its many practitioners include social workers, nurses, psychologists, family therapists, psychiatrists, occupational therapists, and educators, who work, variously, in homes and in community and clinic settings. The families seen in these settings are often coping with a wide range of challenges: poverty, discrimination, socioeconomic risk, limited access to health care, and early or ongoing adversity and trauma. Any or all of these can disrupt parenting and make it difficult for the parent to meet the child's needs for safety and security.

This book is written for the clinicians who work with these families and whose aim is to promote relational and physical health by helping parents become more reflective, able to "see" and "hear" their children in a variety of ways. Our twenty years' experience implementing *Minding the Baby*, an evidence-based, intensive, interdisciplinary, home-based reflective parenting intervention, served as the inspiration for our clinical approach— MTB-Parenting (MTB-P). Our clinical model unifies attachment, mentalization, and trauma theories, developmental research, and the scientific study of adversity to inform clinical practice, and as such it provides a broad and overarching framework for clinicians working across disciplines to help parents and their young children build strong and resilient relationships. MTB-P is unique in its emphasis on *first* establishing the foundations for reflection and *second* building parental capacities for reflection and mentalizing. Building these foundations is especially important for parents challenged by a range of historical, economic, familial, biological, and psychological adversities and who, as a consequence, often live in a constant state of threat. Despite clinicians' hunger for strategies to help parents become more reflective, we believe that beginning with safety, regulation, and trust are critical prerequisites to these efforts. The organization of the book reflects this, with capacities for reflection, insight, play, and exploration developed from the ground up.

The outline of the book is as follows. Chapter 1 introduces the book and the inspirations for our approach. Part I provides an overview of the theory and science that form the conceptual basis for our clinical approach. Chapters 2 and 3 summarize the critical contributions of attachment theory and research to our clinical model, and Chapters 4 and 5 provide an overview of mentalization theory and research, with particular attention to breakdowns or impairments in the development of reflective capacities as the sequelae of trauma and disrupted relationships. Chapter 6 summarizes contemporary developmental science and neuroscience on the multiple impacts of early adversity.

In Part II, we describe the first and core element of our clinical model: the relational foundations of reflection (RFR). These are the foundations upon which reflection and reflective parenting are built and rebuilt, namely, safety, regulation, and trust. It is a fundamental assumption of our approach that establishing these foundations is a necessary first step in working with parents and their young children. Their absence dramatically increases the likelihood of impaired mentalizing and disrupted parenting. Throughout the chapters in this section, we describe these foundations and the strategies clinicians can use to develop them. In Chapter 7, we describe the RFR model; in Chapter 8, we apply this model to the clinician's own safety, regulation, and openness to relationship; and in Chapter 9, we describe the development of these foundations in parents and children.

In Part III, we describe clinical approaches to enhancing reflective parenting once the relational foundations of reflection have been established. In Chapter 10, we describe a series of stepwise strategies for enhancing reflective parenting. In Chapter 11, we discuss the application of these principles to nursing practice. In Chapter 12, we consider some of the challenges of working with parents who are struggling with mental health difficulties. Finally, in Chapter 13, we discuss the clinical applications of two widely used parent interviews: the Pregnancy Interview (Slade, 2003) and the Parent Development Interview (Slade et al., 2004a). These interviews are also included in Appendices I and II. In Part IV, we describe the application of our clinical model to three cases. Case and interview material is also featured throughout the book, and most chapters close with a series of Questions for Clinicians to help concretize some of the theoretical and clinical approaches described throughout the book.

When we began writing this book, there was no novel coronavirus, and George Floyd, Rayshard Brooks, Breonna Taylor, and Ahmaud Arbery were still alive. But beginning in the winter of 2020, the pandemic ravaged cities and devastated marginalized and underresourced individuals nationwide. The burdens of the pandemic disproportionately affected communities of color, and their citizens suffered at three times the rate of resourced, largely White communities. Amidst this catastrophe came yet another spate of murders of unarmed Black men and women by the police, which—likely fueled by the disparities revealed by the coronavirus—led to an unparalleled eruption of rage, grief, and terror at the ubiquitous reality of systemic racism. It has been a perfect storm, a terrible storm, and one that has changed us all. These events, and all that came before them, demand deep reckoning, open conversations, and revolution.

Although we—and the majority of our colleagues in the field of perinatal and postnatal infant and parent health, infant mental health, and allied professions—have worked with families struggling with structural racism, historical trauma, and cultural oppression for decades, the dramatic events of the past 3 years affected us profoundly. We have seen health care, infant mental health, and educational practices change dramatically and overnight. Already-stressed parents have been thrown into the chaos of systems and economic collapse, and the vibrant power of the therapeutic relationship has been challenged by circumstances in which providers cannot meet face-to-face, cannot easily deliver necessary resources, and may themselves be frightened, dysregulated, and without critical relationship supports. Health care professionals are leaving the field or retiring in large numbers, further straining access to care and further amplifying health inequities. And, as a result of the racial justice movement, we see with a new clarity just how profoundly the families and communities with whom we work have suffered from intergenerational and centuries-long violations of basic human rights. These changes will have ripple effects for years, if not decades, to come, and our practices will undoubtedly be changed or modified as we adapt to the many realities before us. It is in this spirit that we have tried to keep these reckonings and conversations alive throughout this book, informing our discussions of how to best support families in their desire to raise healthy, whole children, and clinicians in their efforts to listen and speak with open hearts and minds.

Acknowledgments

Relationships matter, and this book evolved out of myriad relationships: with the families to whom we dedicate this volume and with the many colleagues, students, funders, and organizations who joined us on our journey. Beginning in 2002, an interdisciplinary group of researchers and clinicians from the Yale Child Study Center, the School of Nursing, and the Department of Pediatrics joined together with primary care providers at the Fair Haven Community Health Center (FHCHC) to create a home visiting program that would meet the needs of highly stressed parents living with socioeconomic risk and other forms of adversity. Linda Mayes, Director of the Yale Child Study Center, led the group and provided the initial inspiration and seed funding necessary to found the *Minding the Baby* (MTB) home visitation program. Her support and encouragement have been unwavering since. Jean Adnopoz, Kate Mitcheom, Laurel Shader, Karen Klein, and John Leventhal were essential to this effort; the late (and extraordinary) Katrina Clark, then Executive Director of FHCHC, believed in the MTB mission from the start and in every way ensured that MTB would be welcomed and would flourish at FHCHC.

Lois S. Sadler, Arietta Slade, Janice Currier-Ezepchick, Denise L. Webb, and Cheryl Dedios-Kenn made up the original MTB team. As time passed, Sarah Fitzpatrick, Rosie Price, Dana Hoffmann, Bennie Finch, Tanika Eaves, and Heather Bonitz-Moore brought their many clinical gifts and wisdom to the team as home visitors. Nancy Close supervised the clinical teams for many years, sharing her warmth, optimism, insight, and exquisite understanding of babies and young children with all of us. Together this core group worked over many years to shape the clinical model that is described in this volume. Crista Marchesseault came on to help administer the program and guide training and implementation in 2010, and within 5 years she had established the MTB National Office. Her remarkable resourcefulness, great spirit, and deep intelligence had an enormous impact on all of us. Andrea Miller worked tirelessly for over a decade to track and follow families and monitor data collection and research protocols. Patricia Miller likewise monitored data collection and research protocols. We were blessed with an extraordinary research team: Maggie Holland brought her remarkable talents as a statistician and methodologist to our research program, as did Tony Ma, Kris Fennie, and Sangchoon Jeon. Along the way, a number of doctoral students and psychiatric residents joined the project and became active research collaborators and colleagues. These include Jessica Gorkin Albertson, Lisa Braun, Eileen Condon, Serena Flaherty, Brianna Jackson, Amalia Londoño Tobón, Monica Roosa Ordway, Hanna Stevens, and Madeleine Terry. Undergraduate and master's students Holly Robinson, Lisa Strouss, and Deborah Caselton Trahan helped as well. We also thank Emily Bly, Libby Graf, Melissa Ilardi, Olga Poznansky, and Jasmine Ueng-McHale for their help coding parent interviews and mother–child interaction data. We are especially grateful to Betty Carlson for coding all of our Strange Situations and consulting with us at critical points over the years. JoAnn Robinson also provided helpful consultation along the way. And none of our work would have been possible without the ongoing support of the clinicians and supervisors at our partners in Connecticut: FHCHC, the Hill Health Center, Yale New Haven Hospital, Family Centers, and the Family and Children's Agency. Special thanks to Chris Prokop, Beth Moller, Leslie Sexer, and Mary Kate Locke for their tremendous help guiding expansions in Connecticut.

As the program developed, we began to collaborate with colleagues outside of Connecticut, first in Florida and later in the United Kingdom, Denmark, and Brazil. We are most grateful for all of their support: Barbara White and her colleagues at the Young Parents Project at Florida State University; Chris Cuthbert, Gwynne Rayns, Lucy Morton, Chrissie Rickman, Gary Mountain, and their colleagues at the National Society for the Prevention of Cruelty to Children; and Lislaine Aparecida Fracolli and her colleagues at the University of São Paulo. In 2016 we began a large-scale implementation in Denmark. In addition to the many gifted home visitors who delivered the program, a number of colleagues have helped bring the project to scale: Bjarke Nielsen, Simon Østergaard Møller, Anne Blom Corlin, Jeppe Budde, Conny Sig Overgaard, Merethe Vinter, Birgitte Cortz Ammitzbøll, Inge Kjærgaard, Stinne Nygaard, Helle Skovgaard, Susanne Nilsson, Gitte Berit Jørgensen, Dan Jelling-Petersen, and Brit Holmstrup. We are also grateful to Pasco Fearon, who led the clinical trial of MTB in the United Kingdom, and Maiken Pontopiddan, who led the clinical trial in Denmark.

There are also so many friends and colleagues who helped in a variety of ways over the years, reading drafts, offering moral support, and just being there: Larry Aber, Vicky Bijur, the "BI Crew," Jessie Borelli, Jude Cassidy, Nancy Crown, John Grienenberger, Wendy Haft, Mary Hepworth, Denise Hien, Jeremy Holmes, Jill Lepore, Alicia Lieberman, Alison Locker, Ruth Paris, Chris Pendry, Emma Pendry-Aber, Patty and Tom Rosbrow, Alison Steier, Victoria Stob, and Joe Woolston. Jon Allen offered wise counsel and warm enthusiasm and read numerous drafts of several chapters. And the "B5 Group"—Ann Stacks, Kristyn Wong, Ruth Paris, Michelle Sleed, Sanna Isosävi, and Marjo Flykt—inspired us to think deeply about the assessment of parental reflective functioning.

We are, of course, most grateful to those who provided financial support for our endeavors. For over 15 years, the FAR Fund and its Executive Director, Shirlee Taylor, have been unwavering in their support for the clinical program, clinical trials, as well as statewide and international expansions of MTB. Their generosity made it possible for MTB to grow and flourish in so many ways, and for that we are thankful beyond measure. We are also hugely indebted to the Irving Harris Foundation for providing the seed funding necessary to get MTB off the ground and flourish over the course of the next decade. Other critical funding was provided by the W. K. Kellogg Foundation, the Grossman Family Foundation, Metodecentret, the National Center for the Prevention of Cruelty to Children, the Stavros Niarchos Foundation, the Generativity Trust, the Child Welfare Fund, the Patrick and Catherine Weldon Donaghue Foundation, the Annie E. Casey Foundation, the Pritzker Early Childhood Foundation, the Seedlings Foundation, the Schneider Family Foundation, and the Edlow Family Foundation. MTB was also supported by a number of federal grants: National Institutes of Health/National Institute of Nursing Research (NIH/NINR; No. P30NR08999), National Institutes of Health/National Institute of Child Health and Human Development (NIH/NICHD; Nos. R21HD048591 and RO1HD057947), National Institutes of Health/Clinical and Translational Science Award (NIH/CTSA; No. UL1RR024139), NINR (Nos. F31NR011263-05, 5T32NR008346-06, and F31NR016385), and National Center for Advancing Translational Sciences (NCATS; No. TL1 TR001864).

These acknowledgments would be incomplete without a giant thank you to Anna Kilbride, who served as our assistant throughout the 3 years that it took to write this book. We were so very lucky to have her. Not only was she a discerning, creative, and tireless researcher who chased down innumerable references with unflagging good humor and speed, but she was a marvelous editor and—as a burgeoning psychologist-to-be—understood the material inside and out. And she could make a perfect slide when presented with nothing more than an iPhone picture of a drawing on a napkin.

Seymour Weingarten, Editor-in-Chief of The Guilford Press, gave his blessing to this project from the start, and our editor, C. Deborah Laughton, saw us through the process with unflagging optimism and support. She was always there with a helpful suggestion, a word of encouragement, a deep read, a good laugh, and a willingness to think and talk things through. Even through the dark days of the pandemic, she never doubted that the book would come to fruition and championed us all along the way. Jessica Blume, Carolyn Graham, Elaine Kehoe, Andrea Lansing, Katherine Sommer, and Jeannie Tang were wonderfully responsive and made the move to contract and production easy and seamless.

Finally, we thank our families—especially Sam Felder, Rick Sadler, Anissa and Gabby Simpson, and Denise Duclos—for their patience, good humor, and love. Life just wouldn't be as rich and fun and safe without them. Relationships matter.

Contents

Glossary of Acronyms and Abbreviations

AAI (Adult Attachment Interview)

ACEs (Adverse Childhood Experiences)

AMBIANCE (Atypical Maternal Behavior Instrument for Assessment and Classification)

APrON (Alberta Pregnancy Outcomes and Nutrition)

BCEs (Benevolent Childhood Experiences)

CF-PRF (Child-Focused Parental Reflective Functioning)

CMS (Certainty about Mental States)

COS (Circle of Security) Intervention

COS-PP (Circle of Security Perinatal Protocol)

CPP (Child–Parent Psychotherapy)

EF (Executive Functioning)

EMBP (Emotional, Mental, and Behavioral Problems)

FaPI (Father Pregnancy Interview)

HPA (Hypothalamic–Pituitary–Adrenal) Axis

IC (Interest and Curiosity in Child's Mental States)

IMH-HV (Infant Mental Health Home Visiting)

IPP (Infant–Parent Psychotherapy)

MTB-HV (*Minding the Baby* Home Visiting)

PCEs (Positive Childhood Experiences)

PDI (Parent Development Interview)

PDI-R (Parent Development Interview—Revised)

PEM (Parental Embodied Mentalization)

PI (Pregnancy Interview)

PM (Prementalizing)

PRF (Parental Reflective Functioning)

PRFQ (Parental Reflective Functioning Questionnaire)

RCT (Randomized Clinical Trial)

RF (Reflective Functioning)

RF-T (Trauma Reflective Functioning)

RFR (Relational Foundations of Reflection)

RPS (Reflective Parenting Scale)

SF-PRF (Self-Focused Parental Reflective Functioning)

SSP (Strange Situation Procedure)

WMCI (Working Model of the Child Interview)

Chapter

1

Minding the Baby™ and Reflective Parenting

AN INTRODUCTION

Expectant and new parents[1] are full of hope. They hope to be good parents, to love, provide, teach, and protect and, in so many ways, ensure their child's safety and security. They hope to meet the challenges of parenthood without faltering too much or too often. They hope for a happy child, a healthy child, a successful child, a child with more emotional or material opportunities than they themselves had. They hope for a deep, meaningful, and abiding connection that will enrich their lives. They hope for everything. And they are full of courage.

The more vulnerable they are, however, the more their hope and courage are challenged. For parents who suffered grave assaults and adversity as children (Felitti et al., 1998; Lieberman et al., 2015; van der Kolk, 2014), who grew up in families struggling with addiction and mental illness, or who have had to grapple, often for years on end, with a range of chronic, toxic stressors (Shonkoff et al., 2012)—such as severe poverty, both overt and systemic racism (Bailey et al., 2017; Ghosh Ippen, 2019; Kendi, 2019; Shonkoff et al., 2021; Trent et al., 2019), cultural oppression, and health, social, economic, and educational disparities—building safe and loving relationships can be difficult. Day in and day out, hope and courage fight

---

[1]In line with current practice, throughout this book we use the gender-neutral terms *parent* and *caregiver* when referring to the person or people primarily responsible for the child's care. This is meant to recognize the diversity of individuals responsible for the child's emotional and physical health and safety.

against despair and hopelessness, or against anger and fear that disrupt and destroy.

Practitioners working with young families do their best to maintain parents' hope and courage and support them in being "good-enough" parents. This wonderful term, coined by pediatrician and psychoanalyst D. W. Winnicott (1965), was meant as an antidote to the notion of a "perfect" parent, in which there is, essentially, no room for failure or difference. All parents (and humans!) are imperfect. No one gets it right all the time; in fact, there is no *right*, and even if there were, there is plenty of evidence to suggest that children of all ages learn much from moments of discord and repair (Sander, 1962; Tronick & Gold, 2020; Winnicott, 1965). What matters is that a parent is reflective *enough*, safe *enough*, supportive *enough*, emotionally available *enough*, and able—most of the time—to provide for the child's emotional safety and security, safeguard the child's health and well-being, and create a loving environment in which the child can flourish.

Reflective Parenting

The term *reflective parenting* has been around for the last two decades (Cooper & Redfern, 2015; Gold, 2011; Grienenberger et al., 2015; Pally, 2017; Slade, 2002, 2005, 2007), and refers—broadly speaking—to a parent's capacity to reflect upon or mentalize the child's experience. What this means, quite simply, is that they are able to envision or imagine the child's thoughts, feelings, desires, and intentions (Fonagy et al., 1995). Here is a common example:

> A mother is trying to do some last-minute shopping on her way home from picking her toddler up at day care. Tired, hungry, and wanting to be home, he starts to tantrum almost as soon as they arrive at the store. A reflective parent would fairly quickly realize why her child is fussing: He does not want to go shopping, and he wants to go home. He has a mind of his own, and he and his mother are clearly of different minds. She sets about meeting his mind in order to make this brief but necessary stop bearable for both of them. She gives him a drink, something to eat, calms him with her voice, and tries to distract him because she understands what he is feeling and knows that addressing it will lessen his distress. He will feel heard, and he will calm down. A less reflective parent would be more concerned, by contrast, with controlling the child's behavior and much less so with understanding the feelings triggering his meltdown: "Sit down and be quiet. This is what we have to do." This kind of interaction is an invitation to escalating distress, and they would likely both be very upset by the time they leave the store. And neither would feel heard or understood.

Sally Provence, one of the founders of both the Yale Child Study Center and the national infant mental health organization ZERO TO THREE, advised parents: "Don't just *do* something. Stand there and pay attention. Your child is trying to tell you something." A reflective parent asks, in action and with language, enough of the time, *"What is that something, and how can I address/ameliorate/regulate/understand it? Let me try to imagine what you are feeling so I can figure out what you need to help you feel better."* The stance of curiosity, of wondering about the child's experience, allows the parent(s) to implicitly or explicitly ask the child: *"Who are you, what happened, what do you feel, what do you need, and how can I help?"* It also allows parents to ask the same of themselves: *"Who am I, what happened to me, what do I feel, and what do I need?"*

The capacity to be curious about the child's internal experience, to understand the child's behavior in light of mental states, to appreciate the complexity, dynamics, and developmental aspects of mental states, and to understand their basic nature is what is known as *parental reflective functioning* (PRF; Slade, 2005). As we describe in Chapter 4, researchers have, over the past two decades, consistently linked this parental capacity with a number of positive outcomes, notably the security of the child's attachment (cf. Slade et al., 2005) and the quality of the parent–child interaction (cf. Grienenberger et al., 2005). This accumulating evidence spurred a number of clinicians to focus their intervention work on developing and enhancing PRF to promote *reflective parenting*. The *Minding the Baby* (MTB) home visiting program (MTB-HV; Sadler et al., 2006, 2013; Slade, 2002, 2007; Slade et al., 2005, 2017a, 2017b, 2019) was the first of these. Our aim in this book is to introduce an MTB-informed clinical approach to working with parents, which in this volume we refer to as MTB-P. This reflective parenting approach derives from our two decades' experience developing and implementing the *Minding the Baby* home visiting program.

The *Minding the Baby* Home Visiting Program

Background

MTB-HV was developed in 2002, when a group of community health and mental health providers—working out of the Yale School of Nursing, the Yale Child Study Center, and two federally qualified health centers (FQHCs)—came together to address the pressing needs of young parents-to-be living in underserved and poorly resourced neighborhoods in New Haven, Connecticut. These parents, typically teenagers, fell beyond the reach of traditional services at local health centers; often unable to attend school or keep office appointments for pre- and postnatal care, they needed much more intensive, comprehensive services than those available.

MTB-HV grew out of an effort to provide these broad and deep levels of support, bringing together health and mental health care, relationship support, developmental guidance, and concrete services in a single intervention.

Linda Mayes, now the Chair of the Yale Child Study Center, brought together Lois Sadler, a pediatric nurse practitioner, and Arietta Slade, a clinical psychologist, to found and develop MTB-HV. The program was rigorously tested in two federally funded randomized controlled trials (RCTs; Sadler et al., 2013; Slade et al., 2019) at sites in New Haven, Connecticut. In 2014, MTB-HV was designated as an *evidence-based* model by the U.S. Department of Health and Human Services. This designation made MTB-HV services one of only 20 models eligible for federal funding through the Maternal, Infant, and Early Childhood Home Visiting (MIECHV) Program. MTB-HV was later replicated at other sites in Connecticut, Florida, the United Kingdom, where a three-site replication was conducted from 2011 to 2016 (Longhi et al., 2019), and Denmark, where a nine-site replication began in 2017. An adaptation of the MTB-HV model has also been implemented in São Paulo, Brazil. In the following sections, we briefly describe the MTB-HV model and the evidence for its efficacy.

The Intervention Model

MTB-HV was developed with the aim of enhancing young parents' capacities to *see* and *hear* their children, capacities that we saw as essential to a range of positive attachment, health, and mental health outcomes and that were so often challenged by the ubiquitous structural and interpersonal stressors in their lives. We recruited young pregnant women in their second trimesters of pregnancy and continued visiting them, along with their babies and other family members, on a weekly basis until the children turned 1 year old, at which point we visited every other week. The intervention was delivered by an interdisciplinary team made up of a nurse and a licensed clinical social worker, who alternated visits across the whole of the intervention. They worked collaboratively, layering their work with families to provide coherent and organized care. Both home visitors focused on parental reflectiveness, parent–infant attachment, developmental guidance, parenting support, and maternal life course outcomes. The nurse also addressed physical health and wellness, nutrition, reproductive health care, and physical safety. The social worker provided therapeutic services and a range of concrete supports, linking families with resources for housing, food, diapers, transportation, and education. MTB-HV was intensive; the target dose was approximately 90 home visits across the 27 months from pregnancy to the child's second birthday, delivered in equal parts by the nurse and social worker. From the start, the program was interdisciplinary, as we quickly discovered that pregnant women, new mothers, and their infants, as well as other family members, needed *both* health and mental health services to address their vulnerabilities and support their strengths. Socioeconomic risk, extreme health disparities, and long histories of trauma, adversity, and toxic stress exposure (see Chapter 6) led to a range of health concerns, as well as numerous challenges in the realm of attachment, affect regulation, and mental health. The notion that physical and emotional health are profoundly intertwined is fundamental to the program model and to all of our clinical approaches (Marchesseault et al., 2019, 2020; Slade et al., 2018; Webb et al., 2019).

Population

MTB-HV was optimized to serve families with high economic and social needs who are underresourced and underserved, with a history of developmental trauma and adverse childhood experiences. The mothers who participated in our two clinical trials were between the ages of 14 and 25 and having their first babies. Only mothers who were abusing drugs prenatally, had a debilitating medical condition, or were actively psychotic were excluded from enrolling. In our RCTs, the majority of participants (65%) were Latina, 18% were African American, and a very small proportion identified as non-Hispanic White or other ethnoracial categories. The mean age was 20, and the mean level of education was 11.5 years, with 15% of the sample having dropped out of school before high school graduation. All but a very small number of families were receiving public assistance. Those who were employed had low-wage hourly jobs with shifting schedules and no benefits; housing instability was common. A large proportion of the parents seen in MTB-HV had experienced a range of early adverse experiences, including sexual and physical abuse, neglect, homelessness, family mental illness, and addiction and had come to the attention of child protective services while they themselves were children. At the same time, there were also parents who possessed impressive survival skills and many inherent strengths; home visitors identified and enhanced these strengths.

Results

A total of 237 New Haven families were recruited through prenatal providers at two local FQHCs into two separate RCTs beginning in 2002. Of these, 133 received MTB-HV, and 104 were enrolled in the control group. Participants in the control group received "treatment as usual" at the FQHC, along with intermittent newsletters mailed from MTB staff. In the research, health, mental health, developmental, and relationship assessments were collected at baseline (pregnancy) and at 4, 12, and 24 months postpartum. The goal was to improve intervention group outcomes in all of these areas, relative to outcomes in control group families. Comparisons with control families revealed impacts on a number of public health variables: significantly lower rates of obesity and higher rates of normal weight in toddlers in the MTB condition (Ordway et al., 2018), significantly higher rates of on-time pediatric immunization and lower rates of rapid subsequent childbearing, as well as a trend toward lower rates of child protection referrals in families receiving MTB (Sadler et al., 2013). Attachment outcomes included significantly higher levels of secure attachment and lower levels of disorganized attachment in infants in the MTB condition, as well as significantly enhanced reflectiveness in parents receiving MTB (Sadler et al., 2013; Slade et al., 2019). Finally, parent–child interactions were less disrupted in teen mothers receiving MTB (Sadler et al., 2013). It has been well established that positive mother–child interactions, maternal reflectiveness, and secure infant attachment contribute to socioemotional development, a key ingredient in school success as well as future wellness (Jones et al., 2015; Sroufe et al., 2005).

At 1- to 3-year follow-up, a subsample of preschoolers in the MTB condition had significantly lower rates of maternally reported externalizing (acting-out) behaviors when compared with those in the control group (Ordway et al., 2014). In a longer term follow-up study of data from families in the MTB condition with 4- to 9-year-old children, parents who received MTB had significantly lower levels of impaired mentalizing and hostile/coercive parenting than mothers in the control group, and their children had fewer externalizing and total problem behaviors than their control group peers (Londoño Tobón et al., 2022). Behavior problems in general and externalizing problems specifically directly predict suspension and expulsion in preschool- and elementary-age children, which in turn are linked to both academic failure and later psychopathology (Gilliam et al., 2016). Londoño Tobón and her colleagues (2023) also reported long-term impacts of MTB-HV on biomarkers of stress and inflammation. Condon and her colleagues (2022) found that MTB mitigated the impact of mothers' own history of childhood maltreatment on their capacity to parent reflectively.

Despite the many positive outcomes associated with participation in the MTB-HV intervention, its cost and complexity proved a considerable impediment to its wider dissemination. Today, in 2023, the only current implementations of MTB-HV are at multiple community agencies in Denmark. However, based on our experiences developing, testing, and disseminating MTB-HV, we began over a decade ago to provide training and consultation in reflective parenting to a wide range of practitioners working with parents and young children. These trainings allowed us to distill the core principles of MTB-HV into a broader reflective parenting model, MTB-P, the focus of this book. MTB-P is not an intervention, per se, but rather a clinical approach designed to support practitioners working with vulnerable infants, toddlers, preschoolers, and their parents. These vulnerabilities can be manifested in poor health, disrupted attachments, disrupted development, social isolation, and lack of access to critical resources. MTB-P practitioners include a range of professionals: infant mental health specialists, mental health practitioners (social workers, family therapists, psychologists, psychiatrists), health care providers (nurses, nurse midwives, primary care providers), as well as teachers and early interventionists (such as occupational therapists). The tenets of MTB-P can be used in a variety of settings and, indeed, have direct relevance to a broad array of providers, including those delivering programs such as Child–Parent Psychotherapy (CPP; Lieberman et al., 2015, 2020), the Circle of Security (COS; Hoffman et al., 2017; Powell et al., 2013), the Nurse–Family Partnership (NFP; Donelan-McCall & Olds, 2018), and a range of attachment-based infant mental health programs (see Steele & Steele, 2018; Zeanah, 2019).

MTB-P: Core Principles

Begin with the Relational Foundations of Reflection

When we began our work, we focused our efforts on helping parents become more aware of their own and their children's internal experience. But we quickly learned that mentalizing, per se, was very difficult for many of the parents we were seeing. Often they were in states of fear and threat, and often they were dysregulated. They were slow to trust and slow to engage. They were in survival mode, the parts of their brains that registered danger were on high alert, with little potential for connection or reflection. Many lived in states of fight, flight, and freezing (McEwen, 2000). The capacity to mentalize, or reflect, is built on the foundations of safety, regulation, and trusting relationships, whereas threat, dysregulation, and isolation are the antitheses of mentalization (Allen, 2013). Distrust and fear made it almost impossible to create the "we" space (Fonagy et al., 2021; Gallotti & Frith, 2013) from which reflection emerges. It also made it difficult for parents to experience the pleasures and rewards of attachment and intimacy.

These observations led us to a critical insight: We could not even begin to think about parents' becoming reflective until (or unless) we could lessen their sense of threat, help them become regulated, and slowly come to trust us and what we had to offer. As we describe fully in Part II, we came to think of these as the *relational foundations of reflection* and to understand that direct attention to these relational foundations is essential to the development of reflective capacities and reflective parents. We conceptualized these relationships as a pyramid, with reflection at the top of the pyramid. At the base of the pyramid are safety and regulation, which together support the development of a trusting relationship (see Figure 1.1). As such, we saw our clinical goals as, first, establishing a parent's sense of safety and, second, helping the parent to become more regulated and less defensive. These steps would pave the way to the development of a therapeutic relationship, with trust at its core (Allen, 2022; Fonagy & Allison, 2014). From this base, mentalizing and reflecting, knowing oneself and the other, could begin.

As is evident throughout this book, the relational foundations of reflection (RFR) model has guided our thinking in a myriad of ways. When clinical work is going well, and we are able to provide safety, support the pleasures of parenting, and help to regulate fear, shame, and despair, multiple "we" spaces are created: between clinician and parent, parent and other family members, and—finally, and, of course, most important—parent and child. These are the "playspaces" (Winnicott, 1971) for reflection. However, if parents are threatened, dysregulated, or unwilling or unable to connect, reflection will be impossible. Removing and regulating threat and establishing trust and connection are thus our first steps.

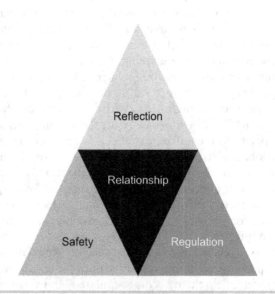

FIGURE 1.1 The relational foundations of reflection.

Maintain a Reflective Stance

The clinician's ability to establish safety and regulation and to build a relationship is dependent upon their *own capacity* to mentalize, to wonder, and to be curious and to thus create a mentalizing *environment* for the parent and child. To paraphrase Sally Provence, "Don't just do something. Stand there and pay attention. The parent (or child) is trying to tell you something." Maintaining a mentalizing stance begins with the clinician's own sense of safety, capacity to regulate, and willingness to connect, to be open to another person, whoever they are. Working with complex, traumatized, and disenfranchised families can challenge our sense of safety and regulation, as well as our capacity to mentalize. But this is where the change process starts, with the clinician, and their capacity to create safety and regulation and to connect with the parent. It is from this environment that the parent's and ultimately the child's curiosity, openness, and understanding flow. MTB-P is not about "getting" a parent to reflect; rather, the work begins with the clinician's capacity to create a safe space for the parents. As we emphasize throughout Part II, the clinician's capacity to mentalize is the key mechanism of change in promoting *parental* mentalizing (Suchman et al., 2012, 2016, 2018).

Develop Strategies to Support PRF

When we developed MTB-HV, we were focused on helping parents become more "reflective." Over time, however, we realized that rather than being a starting point, mentalizing in even the most basic ways was, in fact, an *outcome* of the intervention process. Parents came to mentalize slowly, over time, as the relational foundations of reflection were established and reestablished again and again. This allowed clinicians to shift their focus to safety, regulation, and the relationship and to feel less frustrated that parents weren't "*being* reflective." The process of becoming more reflective is rarely straightforward; rather, it is often a bumpy road, with fits and starts, as parents begin to feel freer and more comfortable moving into this uncharted and often frightening territory. For traumatized individuals, exploring one's inner life can simply be terrifying. Many parents move only from being highly defended to finding a basic language for thoughts and feelings. In Chapters 10 and 11, we describe the stepwise techniques we developed to move the parent into or toward a reflective mode: engage the relationship, observe/listen, mirror, wonder, hypothesize, and (when necessary) repair. These make it possible for parents to explore their thoughts and feelings in a gradual, nonthreatening way. Moving too quickly can disrupt the process and send parents back into survival mode, often manifest in fight, flight, or freezing.

Cultivate Cultural Awareness and Responsiveness

Another core principle of MTB-P is the importance of cultural responsiveness (Ghosh Ippen, 2019; Hart, 2017) or "cultural humility" (Tervalon & Murray-Garcia, 1998), "an openness on the part of . . . treatment providers to reflect on their own beliefs and decisions" (Suchman et al., 2020, p. 109). Professionals working with young families are so often working across racial, cultural, ethnic, class, and gender lines: a White nurse working with an African American mother, a Colombian psychiatrist treating a Puerto Rican father, a Native American male psychologist working with a White mother, a gay male social worker seeing a trans woman, and so forth (see Ghosh Ippen & Lewis, 2011). Working in these intersections requires great awareness, care, and compassion. Sometimes cultural responsiveness is taken to mean that we should—as clinicians—be familiar with the key aspects of another culture. But we can never be "competent" in another culture (Hart, 2017). We learn by being responsive, curious, open, and ready to learn from families who are so often willing to help us make sense of what we do not understand. This is a mentalizing stance. At its best, it is antiracist (Kendi, 2019), anti-"us/them," and antiphobic and conveys a willingness to approach difference with curiosity, humility, and a readiness to learn (Hart, 2017). But without safety, regulation, and a deep willingness to connect, mentalizing is impaired, and the barriers to such openness are great. Without openness, curiosity, and genuine interest, clinicians risk being yet another of the "mundane, extreme environmental stressors" (Peters & Massey, 1983) that disempower and harm racially marginalized individuals.

The Inspirations for MTB

If I have seen further, it is by standing
upon the shoulders of giants.
—ISAAC NEWTON

In the sections that follow, we describe the programs and perspectives that inspired us and provided the frameworks and ways of thinking that profoundly shaped MTB-HV and the MTB-P approach.

The Nurse–Family Partnership

The NFP was developed over 40 years ago by David Olds, a developmental psychologist, and Harriet Kitzman, a nurse researcher; today it is the most widely tested and disseminated home visiting program in the world, with NFP implementations in 41 states in the United States and 7 countries other than the United States (England, Australia, Canada, Scotland, Northern Ireland, Norway, and Bulgaria; see *www.nursefamilypartnership.org*). The NFP model is delivered in the home by public health nurses over a 27-month period beginning in pregnancy, with visits occurring weekly or biweekly, depending on the phase of the program, until the child is 2. Services are offered to economically disadvantaged first-time mothers. The program is most helpful to those families experiencing multiple challenges, such as intellectual disabilities, mental health issues, and being a teenage mother (Olds et al., 2007).

The program was tested in three large RCTs during the 1980s and 1990s; many of the mothers and children who were part of the original studies have also been followed in a series of longitudinal follow-up studies (e.g., Olds, 2002, 2006; Olds et al., 2002). The program has been linked to a range of short- and long-term outcomes in the domains of (1) sensitive, competent care of the child, (2) child abuse, neglect, and injuries, (3) prenatal health behaviors and pregnancy outcomes, (4) parental life course, and (5) child/adolescent development outcomes (see Donelan-McCall & Olds, 2018).

The outcomes of NFP make several things clear: (1) The support of skilled nurses during the transition to parenthood makes a significant difference to both parent and child; (2) the *relationship* that develops with the nurse over 27 months is at the center of the parent's ability to change and grow; and (3) intervening before the baby is born is critical to short- and long-term success. These principles informed every aspect of our work.

Nursing Support

The transition to parenthood is a period of dramatic change and growth for both parents. With a first child, there is so much to learn; most everything is new, and little is clear. The availability of nurses in the home, on a frequent and regular basis, can—to put it simply—be a godsend. Indeed, in a number of Western European countries, postnatal nurse home visiting is standard care for all mothers (regardless of income level) after each birth (Kamerman & Kahn, 1993). As Olds described it, nurses

> are charged with improving the outcomes of pregnancy by helping women improve their prenatal health-related behaviors (i.e., reducing use of cigarettes, alcohol, illegal drugs, identifying and obtaining treatment for emerging obstetric complications); with improving children's postnatal health by helping parents provide more responsible and competent care of the child early in life; and with improving parents' economic self-sufficiency by helping parents develop a vision for the future, plan subsequent pregnancies, complete their educations, and find work. (Olds et al., 2007, p. 377)

Nurses guide the woman through the latter stages of pregnancy, prepare her for childbirth, support her feeding and caring for her child, provide developmental guidance and health information, and serve as a link to the family's medical home. They also help the mother address the changes in her body, attend to her own health and wellness, and focus on her own development and plans for the future. Finally, and critically, they support the emerging mother–child and father–child relationship in myriad ways. All of these supports and information are a balm against the isolating, overwhelming, and frightening aspects of new parenthood. And they are *especially* important for families who have limited access to even the most basic health care.

Despite these many positive impacts, nurses in NFP were often challenged by the task of *"addressing maternal mental illness and intimate partner violence in the home"* [emphasis added] (Olds et al., 2007, p. 381). Efforts to address this issue led to various solutions: Some NFP programs provide mental health consultation to nurses (Boris et al., 2006), whereas others make available short-term, focused, in-home cognitive-behavioral therapy (CBT; Ammerman et al., 2006). As described earlier, the complexity of the families we were seeing in MTB-HV led us to include mental health support in our basic service delivery model. As we saw it, just as families would benefit from stable and consistent nursing support, so would they benefit from stable and consistent infant and adult mental health support.

As we describe more fully throughout this book, and explicitly in Chapter 11, the inclusion of nurses in the MTB-HV model led us to the concept of *reflective nursing*. This term describes an approach to health care delivery that is grounded in the establishment of safety, regulation, relationship, and reflection. Now central to the MTB-P approach, it is an antidote to health care delivery based on "systems checks," offering instead an opportunity to use the nurse–parent relationship to strengthen the parent–child relationship and bring about deep change in parents' relationship to their children's health, their own health, and their sense of themselves as effective and competent people in the world. Reflective nursing also provides a chance to *slow down* health care and address the many questions that come up during the transition to parenthood. It also scaffolds the "anticipatory guidance" that helps parents understand and manage developmental changes and health- and safety-related needs in the child and paves the way toward a more relationship-based, trauma-informed, and reflective form of nursing practice.

Building a Relationship

Today, relationship-based practice is essential to many forms of parent–infant intervention. In 1977, when NFP was founded, the idea of a practitioner building a long-term, stable relationship that would provide a corrective emotional experience for vulnerable young mothers and their families and a model for the parent–child relationship was revolutionary. Olds found inspiration in attachment theory, to which he was exposed when he worked with Mary Ainsworth while an undergraduate student. Though Ainsworth's work was still relatively unknown in the United States at that point, it had a profound impact on Olds's career:

> The home visitors seek to develop an empathic and trusting relationship with the mother and other family members, because experience in such a relationship is expected to help women eventually trust others and to promote more sensitive, empathic care for their children. To the extent that the nurse's relationship with parents (primarily the mother) is characterized by deep appreciation for the mother's needs, and helps her gain control over a host of challenges that are of concern to her, the nurse will have demonstrated the essence of an effective attachment relationship. (Donelan-McCall & Olds, 2018, p. 81)

As is evident throughout this book, the clinician–parent relationship is at the heart of both MTB-HV and MTB-P.

Beginning Prenatally

Olds, Kitzman, and their colleagues made the wise decision to begin working with families *before* the baby was born, with the aim of *preventing* later difficulties and *promoting* a range of health outcomes. This contrasts with programs that *intervene* once the child, the parent, or both are in trouble. For similar reasons, we decided to enroll MTB-HV families in the second trimester of pregnancy. The brain changes that set the stage for parenthood (Hoekzema et al., 2017, 2020; Kim et al., 2016; Martínez-García et al., 2021; Pawluski et al., 2022; Toepfer et al., 2017), as well as the parent–child relationship itself, begin well before birth. Especially with a first baby, this is also a time in life when pregnant women and their partners have many questions, as well as fears, about labor and delivery. Thus the more time spent making room for the baby—emotionally, physically, and relationally—the better (Lieberman et al., 2020).

Infant–Parent Psychotherapy

At around the same time that Olds and Kitzman were developing NFP, the child psychoanalyst Selma Fraiberg and her colleagues (notably Alicia Lieberman and Jeree Pawl) were developing the model that became known as infant–parent psychotherapy (IPP; Fraiberg, 1980; Lieberman et al.,

1991; Lieberman & Pawl, 1993). With the publication of the classic *Clinical Studies in Infant Mental Health* (Fraiberg, 1980), the infant mental health movement was born. Interestingly, despite the fact that their goals and methods had much in common and that the two models greatly complement one another, it seems that the developers of NFP and IPP were largely unaware of each other's efforts. This likely had to do with the fact that NFP was a research program informed by developmental and attachment theory and IPP was a clinical model informed by psychoanalytic theory and practice. In the 1970s, they were worlds apart.

IPP was developed when Fraiberg and her colleagues were approached by local child protection workers asking for help with dire cases of child neglect and abuse, specifically with mothers who were about to have their children removed. Thus IPP was a clinical intervention born in the trenches, a last-ditch effort by a small group of psychoanalytically oriented child clinicians to avoid family separation in highly distressed families. Their approach was entirely novel at the time: They worked *dyadically* with mothers (and, when possible, fathers) and babies. They also worked in the home. Their approach was explicitly psychoanalytic in that they believed that the roots of disturbed caregiving were to be found in the mother's and father's childhood experiences with their own parents. But even within the framework of psychoanalytic practice, IPP marked an enormous leap forward. In that era there was as yet little emphasis placed on the importance of the relationship in promoting change. The notion of a "relational psychoanalysis" was a decade away (Mitchell, 1988). For Fraiberg and her colleagues, as for Olds and Kitzman, the parent–clinician relationship was a primary agent of change.

Although so much of Fraiberg's work was revolutionary, we focus here on several key aspects: (1) the importance of *dyadic* relationship-based work, (2) the description of the force and power of "ghosts in the nursery," and (3) the importance of bringing to light the unbearable memories and affects distorting the mother's capacity to "hear her baby's cries" (Fraiberg et al., 1975). These were the first iterations of what we think of today as trauma-informed infant mental health practice.

Dyadic Work

From the start, Fraiberg and her colleagues specifically worked with parent and child (no matter how young) *together.* They did so because they quickly learned that working with mothers alone was unproductive because, in the atmosphere of social service concern and potential removal, parents felt shamed and persecuted and quickly shut down. But having the baby in the room was—to quote Fraiberg—like "having God on your side" (1980, p. 53). Together, the clinician and mother observed the baby, with the clinician taking the mother's lead rather than dispensing child care advice that was potentially threatening to mothers, who easily felt inadequate and criticized. Out of this work the now-common techniques of "speaking for the baby" and "speaking for the mother" were born, with clinicians providing developmental guidance by giving voice to the baby's needs and abilities, as well as the mother's. So much that was inaccessible when mothers were seen alone came alive with the baby included in the sessions. The baby became the conduit to the mother's inner world, and thus to transformation.

Fraiberg and her colleagues built the relationship with mothers with great care, offering kindness and understanding at every turn, remaining exquisitely attuned to the disruptions that followed any perceived threat or empathic failure and working tirelessly to repair the relationship whenever there were ruptures (which were, of course, frequent). They were greatly aided in this work by psychoanalytic notions of transference, countertransference, and resistance, which provided a means of understanding the powerful affects that regularly invaded the clinician–parent relationship. All these ideas are central to MTB-P.

Ghosts in the Nursery

The following oft-cited passage is arguably the most significant in the entire infant mental health literature:

> In every nursery there are ghosts. They are the visitors from the unremembered past of the parents; the uninvited guests at the christening. Under all favorable circumstances, the unfriendly and unbidden spirits are banished from the nursery and return to their subterranean dwelling place. The baby makes his own imperative claim upon parental love and, in strict analogy with the fairy tales, the bonds of love protect the child and his parents against the intruders, the malevolent ghosts. . . . [In some families,] intruders from the past have taken up residence in the nursery, claiming tradition and rights of ownership. They have been present at the christening for two or more generations. While no one has issued an invitation, the ghosts take up residence and conduct the rehearsals of the family tragedy from a tattered script. (Fraiberg et al., 1975, pp. 387–388)

Thus was born an application of psychoanalytic theory that was meaningful and organizing for generations of infant mental health practitioners and that brought vividly to life the tremendous power of past, unresolved experiences in shaping the parent–child relationship from its very earliest days. Unearthing these ghosts is key to loosening their hold on the present.

Freeing Affects Locked in the Past

One of Fraiberg and her colleagues' critical discoveries was that identifying these ghosts is *not enough*. Most of the parents Fraiberg worked with were able to describe the horrific events of their childhoods; what they did not have access to, however, were the feelings that accompanied them. Rather than remembering their own unbearable feelings, they instead identified with the aggressor. Thus, for example, a mother could remember being beaten, but told the story with cold laughter, often poking her own baby a bit too harshly as she did so. The clinicians used the baby's reactions to illuminate other feelings the mother might have experienced as a child: fear, confusion, and hurt. This allowed the mother to identify with the lonely, frightened child and to slowly relinquish her identification with an aggressive, scary parent. As these feelings were expressed, the child and their actual needs and feelings became clearer to the mother, allowing her to respond with much greater sensitivity and understanding.

Fraiberg's work in this area was groundbreaking in another way: She was the first to identify a parent's trauma as playing a central role in disrupted parent–child relationships. Needless to say, this emphasis on trauma was to have a profound impact on contemporary infant mental health practice. In particular, it was *instrumental* to the development of Child–Parent Psychotherapy (CPP) by Alicia Lieberman and her colleagues (Lieberman et al., 2015; Lieberman & Van Horn, 2008), which we discuss next. It also became a central focus of both MTB-HV and MTB-P.

Child–Parent Psychotherapy

Lieberman and her colleagues (Lieberman et al., 2015; Lieberman & Van Horn, 2005, 2008) used the IPP model as the basis for CPP, which is a "relationship-based, trauma-responsive, multitheoretical intervention through which joint sessions between the parent and the young child center on spontaneous interactions and play as vehicles to promote protective caregiving and secure attachment, target maladaptive mutual attributions between parent and child, and help the parent understand and respond in developmentally supportive ways to the child's signals of need" (Lieberman & Van Horn, 2005, 2008, as cited by Toth et al., 2018). CPP extends the age range of IPP up through age 5 and focuses specifically on addressing the impact of the child's exposure to relational or attachment trauma. CPP also broadens the psychoanalytic foundations of IPP to include the perspectives of attachment, developmental psychopathology, and neuroscience.

Families are typically referred to CPP as the result of recent traumatic events (e.g., maltreatment, witnessing domestic violence); in many cases, children are beginning to show signs of posttraumatic stress disorder (PTSD; Scheeringa & Zeanah, 2001). The parent and child are seen dyadically, in home or office settings, for a period of 6–12 months; this time frame can be modified to meet clinical need. Although CPP is aimed at promoting and, in some cases, restoring a reciprocal, loving, and safe parent–child relationship, it is its specific trauma focus that distinguishes CPP from the other interventions described here. Interestingly, though the focus of CPP has only recently expanded to include the prenatal period (Lieberman et al., 2020), Lieberman applied IPP to the prenatal period in two papers more than 40 years ago (Lieberman, 1983; Lieberman & Blos, 1980).

Today, the CPP model has been rigorously tested in at least 5 RCTs (see Toth et al., 2018, for a review). CPP is consistently linked with a range of positive outcomes (relative to control conditions): attachment security (Lieberman et al., 1991; Cicchetti et al., 2006; Stronach et al., 2013; Toth et al., 2006), intellectual functioning (Cicchetti et al., 2000), more positive representations (Toth et al., 2002), decreased behavioral problems (Lieberman et al., 2005b, 2006), and stability of cortisol levels (Cicchetti et al., 2011b). CPP also led to secure attachment in maltreated infants regardless of variation in *5-HTTLPR* and *DRD4* genes (Cicchetti et al., 2011a). Training in the CPP model has grown exponentially over the past 20 years; to date, there are well over 2,000 CPP practitioners working in the United States, and many more in Europe, Scandinavia, and Israel.

The elements of CPP that have had a profound impact on our work with MTB-HV and MTB-P include (1) the direct and specific emphasis on trauma, seen within the framework of attachment, developmental psychopathology, and neuroscience; (2) "angels in the nursery," the sister concept to "ghosts in the nursery" (Lieberman et al., 2005a), and the related emphasis on the importance of "benevolent childhood experiences" (BCEs; Narayan et al., 2017, 2018, 2019, 2021); and (3) the importance of cultural awareness in infant mental health practice.

Attachment-Based, Trauma-Informed Practice

When Fraiberg and her colleagues developed IPP, there was little, if any, explicit focus on trauma in the fields of psychoanalysis, adult or child mental health, pediatrics, or child and adult development (which is, in part, why Fraiberg's work was so revolutionary). This was to change dramatically over the ensuing years, thanks to Lieberman's pioneering work on child trauma (Lieberman, 2004; Lieberman & Van Horn, 2008), and Judith Herman (1992a, 1992b) and Bessel van der Kolk's (2014) work with adults.

In her work with traumatized parents and their young children, Lieberman—who had also been a graduate student of Mary Ainsworth's—saw firsthand how dramatically even the smallest children were affected by

exposure to violence and trauma, particularly when their primary attachment relationships were disrupted (Lieberman & Van Horn, 2008). Their
sense of safety, their relationships, and their ability to think and explore the
world around them were profoundly disrupted. As she and her colleagues
put it: "Witnessing violence and being the victim of violence shatter the
child's confidence that his well-being matters and that adults will take care
of him" (Lieberman et al., 2015, p. 1). Thus trauma that occurs within
the child's primary attachment relationships is particularly devastating.
This led Lieberman and many others to reframe clinicians' understanding
of the behavioral and mental health problems of small children (Zeanah,
2019; Zeanah et al., 2016). From the perspective of CPP, so many of the
symptoms that bring very young children to clinical attention are best
understood through a trauma lens. Often, they are "big" traumas, such
as domestic violence or maltreatment, but sometimes they are less tangible
and overt traumas, such as neglect and isolation or prolonged exposure to
parental mental illness or substance use.

Trauma invariably affects the security of the child's attachment
(Ainsworth et al., 1978), namely, the crucial sense that their caregivers will
keep them safe and provide them with a basic sense of trust in themselves,
the world around them, and the people in it. Insecure attachment reflects
varying levels of chronic fearful arousal in the child (Slade, 2014), which
results from caregivers' inability to provide safety and regulation, or—in
the worst case—when they are frightening to the child (Lyons-Ruth et al.,
1999b; Main & Hesse, 1990). In CPP, every effort is made to give voice to
the traumas the child has experienced and to the unspeakable feelings that
stem from what the child has seen and heard. Thus the ghosts in the *child's*
nursery are as relevant as those of the parent. It is in this way that the parent comes to understand the child more fully and deeply and becomes able
to mirror and empathize with the child's feelings rather than defend against
and deny them. The experience of being seen by the parent in a new way
can be transforming and organizing for the child.

Angels in the Nursery and Benevolent Childhood Experiences

In 2005, Lieberman and her colleagues (Lieberman et al., 2005a) published
a paper as radical in its own way as Fraiberg's original description of ghosts
in the nursery: "Angels in the Nursery: The Intergenerational Transmission
of Benevolent Parental Influences." In this paper, the authors draw attention to the critical importance of recovering or discovering memories of
benevolent and loving interactions with caregivers; these memories, they
argue, play a crucial role in buffering and attenuating the impact of trauma
exposure. This makes their recovery essential to transformation and therapeutic progress. Angel memories are messages of "intrinsic goodness and

unconditional love" (Lieberman et al., 2005a, p. 506). As such, they argue that

> the uncovering of angels as growth-promoting forces in the lives of traumatized parents is as important to therapeutic work as the containing, taming, and exorcizing of ghosts . . . the recovery and integration into consciousness of early experiences of safety, intimacy, joy, and other pleasurable experiences can promote a more nuanced appreciation of early relationships with primary caregivers and encourage a greater sense of self-worth and emotional investment in developmentally appropriate goals. (Lieberman et al., 2005a, p. 507)

The parent's ability to remember these crucial experiences, often stored at a bodily level, provides essential counterpoints to frightening, disorganizing memories of pain and abandonment. Focusing exclusively on negative experiences—as often occurs in trauma treatments and even relationship-based infant–parent work—potentially deprives the parent of sources of hope, reorganization, and resilience. The reawakening of positive memories can serve as powerful therapeutic agents, promoting the parent's identification with the *protector*, rather than the aggressor. Although there are parents for whom there are few, if any, angels in the nursery, the openness to listening for them and responding to them is crucial to the therapeutic enterprise. As we describe in Chapter 6, the clinical power of "angel memories" led Lieberman and her colleagues, notably Angela Narayan, to describe the ways such memories could offset or buffer the impact of traumatic memories in predicting both maternal symptomatology and child trauma exposure (Narayan et al., 2017, 2018).

Cultural Responsiveness

The first families to receive IPP were living in the economically and socially deprived suburbs of Detroit, Michigan. Soon thereafter, Lieberman began working with families from communities surrounding the new home of the IPP program, San Francisco General Hospital. Here she began seeing families who hailed from an array of diverse countries, home to a myriad of cultures and subcultures: Central and South America, Mexico, the Caribbean, and a range of African American communities in the United States. Almost without exception, families were grappling with considerable economic hardship, as well as the ongoing and toxic effects of racism; often they were also forced to live without access to basic resources (shelter, food, health care, transportation, etc.). Immigration, migration, poverty, and racism provided points of commonality among many of the families served. The exposure to such diversity, combined with her own experiences as a Latina immigrant, powerfully informed Lieberman's understanding of the impact of culture on families *and the practitioners who treat them.* Despite the homogeneity of exposure to poverty and other forms of socio-economic risk faced by families who come to clinical attention, there are enormous differences within and among populations. Heterogeneity not only among cultural groups but also *within* them is the norm, and it plays a powerful role in informing a parent's belief about parenting and childrearing practices (Ghosh Ippen, 2019; Lieberman et al., 2015).

For the developers of CPP (and MTB-P), the role of the clinician necessarily includes an awareness of and curiosity about such cultural heterogeneity. This kind of openness makes it possible for clinicians to learn from families what factors and belief systems are informing and often guiding their choices. When cultural practices are harmful (for instance, in the case of corporal punishment), clinicians must work sensitively to help parents consider the ramifications of their choices and align themselves with other, more benign practices.

The Circle of Security Intervention

The Circle of Security intervention (COS) was developed over 20 years ago by Glen Cooper, Kent Hoffman, and Bert Powell. When the three of them began this work—in partnership with Robert Marvin—they were working as psychoanalytically oriented psychotherapists consulting to local Head Start programs. Fortuitously, their Head Start work led them to attend a training workshop on attachment assessment led by Jude Cassidy, an accomplished and well-known attachment researcher. Interestingly, she, too, had been a student of Mary Ainsworth. Struck by the relevance of attachment theory and research to clinical intervention, the COS developers worked closely with Cassidy to immerse themselves in attachment study. The result was COS, an intervention that translates attachment essentials to parents in an accessible and meaningful way. The original COS intervention was administered to parent groups over a 20-week period; outcome studies have linked this form of the intervention with significant increases in attachment security and significant decreases in disorganized attachment from pre- to postintervention in independent samples (Hoffman et al., 2006; Huber et al., 2015). Since then, the program has been adapted in a number of ways to promote broader implementation in a range of settings (Woodhouse et al., 2018). Many of these adaptations have been empirically tested. For example, when implemented as part of a jail diversion program, the COS Perinatal Protocol (COS-PP) showed rates of attachment security and disorganization among infants that were comparable to low-risk, middle-class samples and better than typical high-risk samples (Cassidy et al., 2010). A short home visiting protocol (COS-HV4) significantly improved attachment outcomes for highly irritable infants relative to control infants receiving a brief home-based psychoeducational intervention (Cassidy et al., 2011). The program has been implemented extensively in the United States and around the world. At the core of each adaptation is the effort to help parents recognize their children's attachment needs and understand their own defenses against them. In the more clinical applications of the model, clinicians use attachment assessments of various kinds to address and modify both the child's and parent's attachment organization.

The COS model and its application of the basic principles of attachment theory have had an enormous impact on infant and young child mental health practice. This has to do, in large part, with their successful translation of the essentials of attachment theory into highly accessible materials that have proven enormously useful for parents, clinicians, teachers, and community intervenors alike. Those include (1) the attachment "Circle," (2) the notion of shark music, and (3) the deceptively simple formula for secure base parenting: "Always be bigger, stronger, wiser, and kind. Whenever possible: follow the child's need. Whenever necessary: take charge" (Powell et al., 2013).

The Attachment "Circle"

From its inception, a core element of all COS interventions has been the use of a graphic that illustrates in a straightforward, compelling, and clear way the parental supports that are necessary to meet the child's basic attachment needs: providing a haven of safety and a secure base for exploration. The process is conceptualized as a circle (see Figure 1.2), with two adult-sized hands drawn on the left-hand side of the circle. The top hand is labeled "secure base," and to its right is a picture of a child moving away from the parent, labeled "support my exploration." The bottom hand is labeled "safe haven," and to its right is a picture of the child moving toward the parent, with the label "welcome my coming to you."

This graphic, which is first introduced to parents as a way of "teaching" them about the attachment system, brilliantly captures what children most need from their parents if they are to feel safe and free to explore the world, able to maintain the crucial "attachment–exploration balance" (Ainsworth et al., 1978) so essential to attachment security. The graphic is then used to help clinicians determine and parents understand their own challenges, when—for instance—they avoid the child's bids for closeness or insist on proximity at the expense of exploration. Finally, it is used as the basis for reflection upon the impediments to being able to provide safety, security, or both.

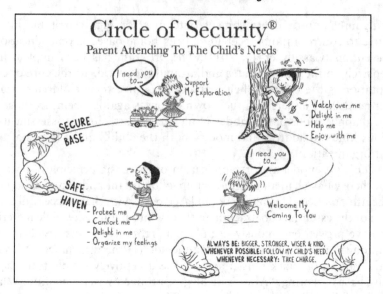

FIGURE 1.2 Circle of Security™ visual map. Copyright © 2018 Glen Cooper, Kent Hoffman, and Bert Powell; Circle of Security International. Reprinted by permission.

Shark Music

Another deceptively simple but enormously effective concept introduced by the COS developers was "shark music" (Hoffman et al., 2006). Clinicians use the contrast between a soothing piece of classical music and the dramatic, intensifying theme from the movie *Jaws,* which for most listeners connotes approaching danger, to make the simple point that the emotions surrounding an event can dramatically affect one's experience of it. Thus, for instance, a child's approach may signal great danger for the mother, eliciting and provoking a range of hard-won defensive maneuvers that can affect the child's sense of safety. This begins the process of the parents identifying and reflecting both upon what they do when they feel endangered and why they do so. Usually this involves reflection upon their own childhood attachment experiences as well.

Providing a Safe, Secure Base

In what again turned out to be a simple, clear map for parents and practitioners, the COS developers offered a concise mantra for secure-base parenting: "*Always:* be BIGGER, STRONGER, WISER, and KIND. *Whenever possible:* follow my child's need. *Whenever necessary:* take charge." The first, be bigger, stronger, wiser, and kind, is inspired by Bowlby's (1969/1982) conviction that—in order to promote both security and safety—an attachment figure, namely, the parent, must be "stronger and wiser," someone the child can trust, feel safe with, and learn from. The addition of "bigger" speaks to the child's need not only for protection but also for someone who can see the *bigger* picture and—in the colloquial sense of the term—be a "big"—that is, good, humane, decent—person. And, finally, "kind," a much-needed addition that speaks to the child's need for kindness, warmth, and affection.

The second and third elements of the COS "mantra" are interrelated. Following the child's need is essential to acknowledging their autonomy, separateness, and personhood. Doing otherwise risks "compliance" and the development of a "false self" (Winnicott, 1965) or, more perniciously, an "alien self," as in the case of more disrupted attachments (Fonagy et al., 2002). At the same time, it is crucial, as someone bigger, stronger, wiser, and kind, for the parent to take charge when necessary: when the child is hurt, distressed, in danger, or needs help becoming regulated and organized.

This framework serves as a touchpoint for parents to remind themselves of what is essential to meeting their child's attachment needs and for clinicians to identify areas that require more work and specific intervention.

What MTB-P Is and Is Not

As we describe throughout this book, the MTB-P model provides a framework for training and supporting clinicians working with parents and young children in a range of interventions in a range of settings. As we describe in Part I, MTB-P is based in attachment, mentalization, and trauma theories; as such, we take as a given that transforming developmental trajectories depends upon a parent's ability to *understand* the child's (as well as their own) experience. Most behavioral programs are focused on changing parent or child behaviors, not on understanding their root causes and thus transforming underlying representations and emotional experience. We believe that true and deep change follows from understanding "What *happened* and how did that feel?" in a moment with the child, in a parent's childhood, in an interaction with a romantic partner, rather than, "What's wrong with you/the baby and what should they/you do?" This is why, as we noted above, MTB-P is not about the clinician or parent "doing" something. To once again paraphrase Sally Provence's sage advice to parents, MTB-P reminds clinicians of the following: "Don't just do something. Stand there and pay attention. The child/parent is trying to tell you something!"

MTB-P is not a curriculum with specified content, structure, and protocols. Rather, MTB-P provides a set of principles and practices that can be applied in a flexible way to the clinical situation at hand. Programs that are curriculum-based often pay scant attention to *how* to implement a given approach or to the transferability of interventions to particular families and settings. This can leech the humanity out of human service, with clinicians pressured to "do" rather than to be present and attentive to what a parent needs in a given moment. There are many settings in which curricula (or treatment plans) cannot easily be implemented because of the exigencies that parents and children bring to the table. In these situations, practitioners are often left with few tools for managing complexity and chaos. This is particularly the case when practitioners are not equipped with the basic skills intrinsic to building a relationship, responding to the person in front of them, getting to know them and their stories. If they have only the methods of a particular curriculum or evidence-based approach, the work will suffer. Thus we believe that it is particularly important to provide deep and wide support and training to beginning clinicians, both in their own disciplines and in the work of building and sustaining relationships, supporting attachment, mentalization, and reflective parenting. To these ends, MTB-P applies a range of approaches in a flexible way, meeting parents "where they are," *wherever* that is. MTB-P is also not time-limited. Time limitations can leave practitioners without the resources to extend and tailor the work to the situation at hand. We believe that in order to truly help a family, it is necessary to take time, slow down, and understand the often complex and layered situations that bring them to clinical attention.

Finally, unlike MTB-HV, the MTB-P approach is not specifically interdisciplinary. Nevertheless, we have come to understand that close collaboration with other professionals is critical to providing families with the kinds and levels of care they require. The isolation and "silos" that are so common within and between health, social service, mental health, and educational systems are truly and deeply detrimental to families, who need us to see the breadth and depth of their needs and respond to them. MTB-P practitioners have learned again and again, for example, that issues that surface as mental health concerns (e.g., depression, passivity, lethargy) can be powerfully linked to physical health concerns (e.g., severe anemia, malnutrition) or that issues of compliance with health directives (e.g., the failure to use birth control when a mother wants to delay further pregnancies) can have deep psychological roots (e.g., the mother is powerfully attached to a partner who wishes her to have another baby). Likewise, the absence of supports in a young mother's own family of origin can lead to truancy, the result of which is typically the end of her schooling, with lifelong economic and social consequences. Thus, helping young families in a meaningful way depends upon "keeping in mind" a larger view of the systems and providers affecting the parent's everyday life and collaborating actively to make sure that—to the extent that it is possible—systems are cooperating to keep the family safe, healthy, and engaged members of society. Collaborative, interdisciplinary practice also provides a secure base for each member of the clinical team.

Outline of the Book

The book's structure reflects our emphasis on building reflection from the ground up. Part I provides a general introduction to the MTB-P approach and the theoretical, scientific, and clinical foundations upon which it was based. Part II provides specific guidelines for establishing safety and regulation in clinicians and families and for promoting and sustaining the relationships that are essential to reflection—the clinician–parent, clinician–child, and clinician–parent–child relationships. In Part III, we begin by outlining a range of strategies for enhancing reflective parenting once the foundations of reflection are in place. We then turn to a discussion of reflective nursing, the impact of parental mental health disturbances on MTB-P and other early intervention approaches, and the clinical applications of the Pregnancy Interview (Slade, 2003) and Parent Development Interview (Slade et al., 2004a). Part IV examines the application of MTB-P principles through three case studies. Throughout Parts I–III, we close each chapter with a brief summary of its key points. We also outline what we see as the clinical applications of the ideas presented in each chapter. In this way, we try to bring theory, science, and other abstract principles to life for the working practitioner.

Part

I

Theoretical and Scientific Bases for *Minding the Baby* Parenting

Chapter

2

The Foundations
of Attachment Theory and Research

As we described in Chapter 1, we began MTB with the aim of supporting young, highly stressed, and underserved parents through the transition to parenthood, beginning in pregnancy and continuing through the infant's first 2 years of life. From the start, we saw the establishment of a resilient, reciprocal, loving parent–child relationship as key to both parent and child development. Attachment theory and research, which emerged from the foundational work of John Bowlby and Mary Ainsworth, provided us with a key conceptual framework for our efforts. Here we review this work, with an eye to making its key points meaningful and accessible to clinicians working with young children and their caregivers. Given that attachment study began nearly 80 years ago with the publication of Bowlby's classic paper on juvenile thieves (1944), we recognize that it is impossible to do justice to many of the subtleties of subsequent advances in the field in a brief review (see Cassidy & Shaver, 2016). Nevertheless, we hope that the reader will come away from this and the next chapter with a grasp of the principles that make attachment such a meaningful and helpful construct for clinicians. And one that—despite its limitations—offers a rich and deep view of how living beings become the human beings that they are.

John Bowlby and Mary Ainsworth: The Pioneers

John Bowlby, a psychiatrist and psychoanalyst, founded attachment theory after observing that the delinquent adolescents with whom he was working all had histories of early trauma and loss (Bowlby, 1944), or—in today's parlance—complex or attachment trauma (Allen, 2013; Courtois, 2004; van der Kolk, 2014). The evident link between disruptions in early relationships and long-term psychopathology led him to eventually propose that all human beings are born with a predisposition to become attached to those who care for them (Bowlby, 1969/1982, 1973, 1980, 1988; Cassidy, 2016; Holmes, 2014; Slade & Holmes, 2013) and that disruptions in these early relationships cause long-term psychological distress. It is in a child's *very nature* to seek proximity to a "stronger and wiser" attachment figure (in most cultures, a mother or maternal figure) when they feel threatened, in need of comfort and nurture, or wish to explore in safety. They signal their need for proximity in whatever way they are able (raising their arms, crawling, crying). Bowlby saw such behaviors as evidence of an inborn biological mechanism, namely, the "attachment behavioral system," which functions to promote and sustain the child's primary attachments. Bowlby further proposed that the child's predisposition to seek safety and care is evolutionarily privileged because it ensures *their literal and emotional survival*. With this formulation, Bowlby also identified an evolutionary *motive* behind the often mysterious ways children will *adapt* their behavior in order to maintain critical attachment relationships, even when such adaptations come at great cost to their functioning.

Bowlby's emphasis on survival as a prime motive in the development of attachment gave particular importance to *fear and threat detection* (Porges, 2011; Slade, 2014). Without the capacity to detect threat, we would not survive. The perception of threat activates the child's attachment system, a dynamic mechanism that propels the child to seek safety when threatened and caregivers to provide it. The child's fear signals the parent to provide safety. When safety is achieved, the attachment system is *deactivated*. Thus the attachment system is, in effect, a fear regulation system, and the emphasis on survival crucially focuses us—as clinicians, in particular—on the central role of *fear, threat,* and *threat detection* in shaping the child's most significant relationships. As Bowlby put it: "examination shows . . . that, so far from being irrational or foolhardy, to rely initially on the naturally occurring clues to danger and safety is to rely on a system that has been both sensible and efficient over millions of years. For, it must be remembered, we have but one life" (Bowlby, 1973, p. 139). Ideally, the infant will have only the most benign and passing threats to contend with, threats that will be readily addressed, fears that will be readily regulated within the context of their relationships.

It may seem peculiar to put survival at the center of a theory of human relationships, but of course Bowlby meant much more than *literal* survival. He also meant emotional survival, which above all depends upon relationships. Bowlby did not often use such words as *love* and *pleasure* and *delight* in his work, and yet there is no question that he viewed the human need for close relationships as another of the motives for attachment and goals of the attachment behavioral system (Richard Bowlby, personal communication, 2008). He was profoundly influenced by Harlow (1958), who opened his famous paper, "The Nature of Love," with the words, "Love is a wondrous state, deep, tender, and rewarding" (p. 673). And though Harlow suggested that psychologists had largely failed in the mission to understand "love and affection" (p. 673), these were, for Bowlby, essential aspects of secure and meaningful attachments. Just as there is no survival without the capacity to detect threat, so there is no real emotional survival without the rewards of relationships. Mary Ainsworth, Bowlby's partner in the development of attachment theory and research, was more explicit; in the closing chapters of *Infancy in Uganda* (1967), she noted that: "We are here concerned with nothing less than the nature of love and its origins in the attachment of a baby to his mother" (p. 429).

What Bowlby and Ainsworth termed "insecure" attachments result not from a lack of love but from the degree to which the child is *anxious* about the caregiver's availability as a safe and secure base. For children who are insecurely attached, the attachment relationship is to some degree a source of relational threat rather than a source of safety and pleasure, of reward and joy. Relational threat results when a parent pushes a child away (overtly or covertly), inhibits the child's autonomy out of their own anxiety, or frightens the child, such that the relationship itself threatens the child's sense of safety. The child is left with no choice but to achieve safety in whatever way is possible, even if it compromises their freedom, flexibility, and emotional health. To put it simply, "better safe than dead."[1] As reflected in Figure 1.1 in Chapter 1, and as we discuss more fully in Chapter 7, disruptions in safety seeking and regulation powerfully weaken the foundations upon which secure attachments develop. The child does what they must to guarantee the parent's care, despite the reality that these defensive adaptations shape the child's core sense of the universe and the people in it, typically not for the better.

Clearly, parents play a critical role in the development of attachment, and in fact Bowlby described an evolutionarily privileged system recipro-cal to the attachment–behavioral system in parents, which he termed the "caregiving system" (Bowlby, 1969/1982; George & Solomon, 1996, 1999, 2008; Solomon & George, 1996). By this he meant that, just as children are programmed to seek protection and care from their primary caregivers, so are parents programmed to provide it. We can see this at so many levels, from the hormonal to the behavioral to the psychological, beginning from the moment pregnancy is affirmed (Feldman, 2015). The child's survival

---

[1] We thank Nancy Crown for putting this so clearly.

depends upon the parent's capacity to provide care. What we see in disrupted relationships is that the parent's orientation to caregiving has been, in some way or other, disabled.

The work of Mary Ainsworth, an American-Canadian clinical psychologist, was foundational to the enormous body of research testing and expanding upon Bowlby's fundamental ideas. In particular, her work identified the various ways children adapt to preserve even the most fraught attachment relationships. After working with Bowlby in London, Ainsworth began her own study of attachment while living in Uganda (Ainsworth, 1967); there she followed a group of postpartum women in a small rural village and tracked the natural development of infant–mother attachment over the course of the first year of life. Seeking to replicate her observations when she returned to the United States, she recruited a second group of 26 mothers and babies and began observations in the home shortly after the babies were born. This was known as the Baltimore study. When the babies turned 1 year old, she observed them in a brief separation procedure she had developed called the Strange Situation Procedure (SSP; Ainsworth et al., 1978; Ainsworth & Wittig, 1965). The brilliance of this simple procedure, which has been used in thousands of studies over the last 50 years (see Cassidy & Shaver, 2016; Slade & Holmes, 2013), is that it serves to mildly stress the child, activating the attachment system. When an infant is left first with a stranger, and then alone, the biological system that propels them to seek safety when danger looms is set in motion. Just as the baby bird in Martin Waddell's (1992) wonderful children's book *Owl Babies* cries "Where's my MOMMY?" upon awakening to find her missing, the child in the SSP is singularly focused on reuniting with their caregiver.[2]

Ainsworth discovered that, although many of the children cried or became distressed upon separation, what differentiated them was their response when the parent returned. Some greeted the mothers readily and sought their comfort. They settled quickly and happily returned to play. Ainsworth classified these children as "secure." Others avoided their mothers and hid their distress, even if they had been crying mightily in their mother's absence. She described these children as "avoidant." And some, despite being obviously upset, resisted their mothers' help and seemed unable to find solace or settle down. Ainsworth originally used the term "ambivalent" to describe these children, but ultimately settled on the term "resistant" because these children both sought and resisted care.

The differences Ainsworth observed in reunion behavior were lawfully related to differences in caregiver responsiveness during the first year: Those mothers who had responded to their infants over the first year by

---

[2]The SSP, though originally tested with mothers, can be reliably used with any primary caregiver.

picking them up when they cried and holding them close when they needed comfort were more likely to have secure children. Those whose mothers avoided close bodily contact and rejected their bids for comfort were more likely to be avoidant. And those children whose mothers had been preoccupied and inconsistently available were more likely to be resistant. Thus the child's response upon reunion revealed what the child had come to expect from the parent at times of stress or distress. The child's actions upon reunion revealed the *history of their efforts* to find safety and to manage (hopefully slight) fear and threat. The child's expectations derived from actual relational experiences, and specifically from the caregiver's capacity to be sensitive to their cues.

Attachment Classification: A Poetic Frame

Sharon Olds's poem "Bathing the Newborn" (1984) describes a mother giving her infant son one of his first baths. At its center is a moment when she senses her child's fear as she guides him into the water; she regulates his trepidation by reassuring him, crooning her comfort, and easing him into the pleasures of the water. At a moment of threat, of potential "trouble," the mother meets his fear and calms it: "I love that time/when you croon and croon to them, you can see/the calm slowly entering them, you can/ sense it in your clasping hand,/the little spine relaxing against/the muscle of your forearm, you feel the fear/*leaving their bodies*" [emphasis added]. The poem offers a lesson in "security" and what it means, and as such exemplifies many of the key themes that we return to again and again throughout this book.

Secure Attachment

As the infant is lowered into the bath in Olds's poem, he senses threat in his nakedness, in the approaching water, in the sensation of it against his skin he stiffens. He communicates his apprehension through his eyes, his limbs, his movements. And we can imagine that his tiny heart beats ever so slightly faster. He is momentarily distressed. The mother senses his unnamed fear in her fingers and in her *bones*; she croons to him and holds his body safely in the crook of her arm. With words, with her arms, she holds him "exactly right," providing the "holding" (Winnicott, 1965) that allows him to explore. She tells him he is wonderful and that the world is wonderful. And within the safety of her arms, he can begin to feel this, to trust her and her view of the world. In this moment of comfort and safety, the fear *leaves* him, the calm *enters* him, and he can abandon himself to the pleasures of the bath and precious intimacy with his mother.

The mother *loves* to remember the times when she transforms her newborn's fear into pleasure through her soothing, so that he can explore from the safety of her arms. She has transformed his trepidation into calm, his apprehensiveness into exploration. She feels she is good for him. There is deep satisfaction in knowing him and seeing just what he needs (Benedek, 1959). The mother's pleasure in the child is palpable, as are the rewards that flow from caring for him in a way that feels so right. She is a little frightened, too, but that is framed by her awe and wonder. She all but *bathes* him in her happiness.

When the child's attachment system is activated, and he seeks safety from someone "stronger and wiser," he learns that he is not alone and that he needn't be afraid. In this moment, his distress has—in Bowlby's terms—activated his mother's reciprocal caregiving system, namely, the proclivity to protect and care for one's young (Bowlby, 1969/1982). She moves *toward* his fear with the aim of calming him and providing him the security to explore (Ainsworth et al., 1978). This ensures that his fear is transformed—*through her care*—into curious and pleasurable exploration. This is, as we discuss later, the essence of a "reflective," "sensitive," or "mentalizing" parent who can contain the child's distress, meet it, and in so doing soothe him and delight in him. To use Winnicott's (1965) wonderful words, she—as a "good-enough" mother—"facilitates" the child's "going on being" so that he can discover the world. She diminishes the threats and regulates the fear that would otherwise disrupt his sense of himself and his own agency.

When exchanges like this are repeated again and again, the child gradually comes to feel secure in knowing that they can trust in the world around them. This does not imply that the parent is *always* there. That is the beauty of the notion of a "good enough" parent (Winnicott, 1965); moments of discord are normal and in fact critical to building flexible and resilient relationships (Tronick & Gold, 2020). Within a secure relationship, there is room for the gamut of emotions, as well as the opportunity to ameliorate loss with pleasure, rupture with repair, and fear with safety. Threat, discomfort, and distress (including physical discomfort and distress) are a part of everyday life; their regulation and management begin with the parent's capacity to recognize them and frame them in trust and safety. From these moments, the child begins the journey through life and its many hardships with the deep, embodied knowledge that they can find safety, comfort, and pleasure in others. Pain need not be private but can be communicated in a way that brings relief, if only from the comfort of sharing it. The more the child and parent can experience the inevitable disruptions of daily life within the context of the pleasures of intimacy and connection, the more the stresses and pains of life can be managed and overcome.

But what of the parent who struggles to remain present and loving in moments of distress, in the face of the infant's varied needs for closeness and exploration? For generations of attachment theorists and researchers, building upon the foundational work of John Bowlby and Mary Ainsworth, the answer is relatively straightforward: The child would have a greater chance of being "insecure." What does this mean and what does it look like?

Insecure Attachment

Insecurity means just that—"*I'm not sure you'll be there for me.*" As attachment researchers have demonstrated consistently for over 50 years, insecurity or anxiety typically manifests itself in one of three fundamental ways: the two categories described by Ainsworth, namely, avoidance or resistance, and a third, described by Mary Main and Judith Solomon (1986, 1990): disorganized attachment. We explain these three terms next.

THE AVOIDANT PATTERN

Let us return to Olds's poem and imagine a different baby and mother and the moments that, over time, might lead to an insecure–avoidant attachment. This time, the mother feels her baby's slight fear but—likely because it is somehow *threatening* to her—tries to shut it out. Her arm tenses slightly against his body, she slips him into the water more quickly, and she does not croon. The activation of the child's attachment system triggers *her* anxiety, but instead of feeling and holding it, she in subtle ways avoids and even disavows his fear. He enters the playground of the tub with his stress levels slightly elevated, with the following threat registered: "*My fear pushes my mother away.*" As he enters the water, she withdraws her arm; now, perhaps, she smiles brightly, says a few words, and splashes him with water. Another observation is registered: "*She seems happier when I am exploring; keeping my distance is the way to stay connected with her.*" These are the essentials of an avoidant stance; the child maintains a connection to others via exploration and *down-regulates* distress; genuine pleasure often seems missing. That is, a kind of limited closeness is achieved through distance and engagement in the outside world. What is crucial is that the child's fear of losing the mother is managed via avoidance and minimizing negative affect (Cassidy, 1994), or what Main (1981) termed "avoidance in the service of proximity."

THE RESISTANT PATTERN

Let us imagine a third mother and baby and an exchange that might, were it to characterize the dyad's exchanges, lead to a resistant attachment. The baby's transient fear of the water startles the mother. She feels anxious and grips him more tightly. She may even pull him back from the water and lay him against her chest. Anxiety in her face and in her voice, she croons,

"*You OK? You OK?*" Suddenly his utterly normal, minor perception of threat has been amplified by the mother's. In his infantile way, he observes, "*Exploration scares my mother; maybe I should be scared, too. Better stay close to her, even though this feels overwhelming.*" He fusses, "*I neeeed you.*" The pleasures of intimacy are infused with anxiety. An insecure–resistant child achieves proximity by limiting exploration, and negative emotion is up-regulated or maximized to preserve closeness (Cassidy, 1994; Cassidy & Berlin, 1994).

Mary Ainsworth was the first to describe the avoidant and resistant patterns of attachment (Ainsworth et al., 1978). Later, Mary Main, originally a student of Ainsworth's, was to describe these insecure patterns as "organized" (Main, 2000), meaning that they are coherent, stable, and well-established strategies for regulating attachment-related affects. The difference between these strategies is the amplification of one set of developmental needs over another. The avoidant child feels safer exploring and keeping bids for closeness at a minimum, whereas the resistant child feels safer maintaining proximity and distress and diminishing natural interest in the larger world. Thus the attachment and exploratory systems are—in effect—shaped by the child's goal of preserving life-sustaining relationships. As such, the avoidant and resistant patterns are *adaptations* that preserve whatever kind of literal and emotional proximity to the parent is possible. They differentially privilege positive and negative affect, such that the avoidant child learns to damp down distress and keep up a happy face; the resistant child amplifies distress at the expense of joy and pleasure.

THE DISORGANIZED PATTERN

Some 20 years after Ainsworth's initial discovery of the avoidant and resistant patterns of insecure attachment (Ainsworth & Wittig, 1965), Mary Main and Judith Solomon (Main & Solomon, 1986, 1990) discovered a third insecure pattern of attachment that they labeled *disorganized attachment*. They called this a "dis"organized pattern because it reflects a collapse of behavioral strategies for gaining proximity in moments of distress. That is, rather than consistently avoiding or seeking contact when distressed, the child falls apart, stilling, freezing, or behaving in erratic or contradictory ways. Far more pernicious than either of the other two insecure categories, disorganized attachment—which is most common in highly stressed populations and has been consistently linked with child maltreatment (Cicchetti et al., 2006)—is associated with a range of problematic outcomes across childhood and early adulthood (Carlson, 1998; Lyons-Ruth & Jacobvitz, 2016). And it seems that—regardless of the cultural context—attachment disorganization indicates a breakdown in the attachment system and thus should be both a cause for concern and a focus of prevention.

The disorganized pattern emerges most often when the caregiver is the source of fear. Let us return to the dyad in the Olds poem and imagine two different scenarios, one in which the mother is actively frightening, one in which she withdraws in his moment of distress. In the first, when the baby tenses as he is lowered into the water, his mother becomes enraged (likely because she was startled and frightened). "*What is the **matter** with you??*" She lowers him roughly into the water, her voice and body harsh. His body stiffens even more and he lets out a little yelp. The mother seethes. He searches her face, his mouth in a wavering smile, hoping to placate her, fear in his eyes. He cannot lose his focus on her, as she has become dangerous; he must keep her in his sights. Needless to say, he can enjoy little about the warmth of the water or the ways it supports his limbs as he floats. In a second iteration, the mother, frightened by the baby's anxiety, "disappears," as it were, and withdraws or dissociates while she is bathing the child. This, too, is frightening to the child, but in a different way. He is alone, left to manage his fear and the inherent danger of the water on his own.

When the awareness of danger, most perniciously from the caregiver herself, persists even at low levels, the fear system is chronically elevated and dysregulated and begins to infiltrate the child's experience, his sense of the other, his sense of his own body, and his sense of his autonomy and freedom to explore. The child feels helpless, angry, and more frightened. Here, the capacity to defend and adapt, to *organize* a response, is shattered in the face of unmanageable threat. The experience of danger effectively wipes out the potential for regulation, the result being an attachment relationship dominated by fear, in which neither the pleasures of autonomy nor closeness are genuinely possible.

The Clinical Relevance of Attachment Classifications

Ainsworth's research gave rise to thousands of studies, nearly all of which link a range of positive developmental, academic, social, and health outcomes to secure attachment, whereas more negative outcomes are typically associated with insecure and *particularly* disorganized attachment (Cassidy & Shaver, 1999, 2008, 2016; Slade & Holmes, 2013). On balance, the findings of thousands of studies suggest that, although a secure attachment does not ensure an easy life course, it certainly makes life easier (van IJzendoorn, 1995; Verhage et al., 2016, 2018). They also suggest that, although an organized–insecure attachment *may* forecast trouble later down the line, it also may not (Verhage et al., 2018). As we discuss later in this chapter and in Chapter 3, in some cultural contexts avoidant and resistant organizations are entirely adaptive and culturally congruent. A disorganized attachment, however, is nearly always associated with maladaptation and compromised development (Carlson, 1998; Lyons-Ruth & Jacobvitz, 2016). It is for this reason that a major emphasis of MTB-HV was to increase the likelihood of child attachment security and to decrease the likelihood of attachment disorganization, which is associated with relational threat and fear and most clearly predicts a range of negative outcomes.

In the preceding section, we used Sharon Olds's poem to bring to light the differences between various insecure strategies and the relational environments from which they emerge. Although these vignettes vastly oversimplify enormously complex processes, they demonstrate the ways in which the infant will adapt to preserve life-sustaining attachments and regulate threats to these attachments. These adaptations, though potentially costly, are ultimately *rational* within the context of their history in relationships—this is what the young child has had to do to survive. These vignettes also illustrate an essential aspect of attachment theory and research, which is the conceptualization of these adaptations along the following dimensions: overregulation (avoidance), underregulation (resistance), and the collapse of regulatory strategies (disorganization).

We represent these distinctions graphically using the "arousal curve," to which we return again and again throughout this volume. T. Berry Brazelton first used this graphic nearly 40 years ago to describe variations in infants' states of consciousness (Brazelton, 1984). As he conceptualized it, the left-hand side of the curve represents "too little" arousal and the right-hand side, "too much." At the curve's apogee is the state of being alert and awake, with arousal modulated and contained. In this state, infants

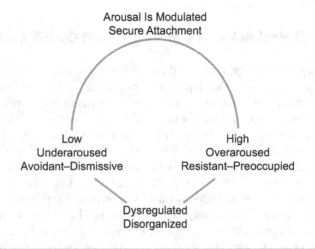

FIGURE 2.1 Attachment and arousal.

have remarkable capacities for engaging and attending, and their "best" performance can be readily elicited. When shut down or overstimulated, however, they cannot be fully available.

We find the metaphors of "too little" and "too much" arousal to be extremely helpful in understanding the avoidant, resistant, and disorganized patterns of attachment. As represented in Figure 2.1, the left-hand side of the curve represents the avoidant organization, namely, strategies or defenses that suppress affect (too little affect, diminished arousal). The right-hand side represents the resistant organization, namely, the relative failure to contain and organize strong affects (too much affect or arousal). At the apogee of the curve is the secure organization, where affects are modulated and organized and threat is minimal. Below the curve is the disorganized pattern, where threat prevails, causing the collapse of affect and self-regulatory strategies. The beauty of using the arousal curve as a way of understanding attachment organization is that it makes evident that there are *degrees* to which an individual relies on any particular strategy or defense. It also allows room for movement between poles, such that, for instance, an avoidant individual might become flooded in certain situations, or a resistant individual might become overwhelmed and shut down. The closer one comes to the end of the curve, the more entrenched and potentially problematic the strategy. From any but a research perspective, a categorical approach to attachment seems too narrow; using a more continuous approach allows room for movement and complexity.

Ainsworth originally used the term *anxious* rather than *insecure* attachment. She abandoned the term *anxious*, however, likely because within the psychoanalytic literature the term primarily connotes a response to intolerable internal experience rather than to a fear of loss and abandonment. But in many ways *anxious* is the right word. Insecure children are, in fact, *anxious about whether they can get what they need*. The *fear system is continuously elevated in all three insecure adaptations, though to different degrees* (Hesse & Main, 1999; Slade, 2014). The insecure child "must continuously attend to the safety versus threat implicit in current conditions" (Hesse & Main, 1999, p. 494). The insecure–avoidant child regulates the fear of losing the parent via emotion-depleted exploration, and the insecure–resistant child regulates the fear of losing the parent via elevated (and often ineffective) bids for closeness. Although these adaptations may ensure a degree of safety, multiple studies of insecurely attached children have demonstrated that they do not eliminate stress (Gunnar et al., 1996; Luijk et al., 2010a, 2010b; Sroufe & Waters, 1977), and genuine positive affect is largely missing. Insecure adaptations ensure that the attachment system is perpetually activated, with threat a chronic presence in children's psychological lives and their internal representations of attachment (Cassidy, 2021). As threat increases, the degree of defensiveness and insecurity increases, with the most threat being associated with disorganized attachment.

Mary Main[3]: A Move to the Level of Representation

The Adult Attachment Interview

Before 1985, attachment research had focused almost exclusively on young children. This was to change dramatically with Mary Main's work on adult attachment. A student and mentee of Mary Ainsworth's, Main had begun her career at the University of California, Berkeley, studying infant–mother attachment. As the participants in her longitudinal study grew older, she began to wonder about their parents. What were their attachment stories? How did these affect their children and the children's sense of security? These questions led her to develop, along with Carol George and Nancy Kaplan, the Adult Attachment Interview (AAI; George et al., 1984/1988/1996). This 16-item interview invites adults to remember and reflect upon their childhood relationships with their own parents. They are asked, again and again, what happened in critical moments of distress and need and how they felt about it. As such, the AAI is, in many ways, analogous to the SSP, as it asks the adult to describe in words the very same experiences that are evoked behaviorally in the SSP.

What Main and her colleagues (1985) discovered was that the *process of remembering and describing childhood experiences of seeking care from primary attachment figures* activates the attachment system in much the same way that separation from the parent does during the SSP. In other words, it is possible to see, in an adult's response to being asked to describe early attachment experiences of distress, loss, and separation, the same patterns of defense *in language and representation* that are revealed behaviorally in the SSP. Some adults have little difficulty recalling childhood attachment experiences or describing them in coherent and emotionally authentic ways. Even when childhood experiences have been difficult, complexity and mixed feelings can be managed nondefensively. For other adults, however, dipping into childhood memories of needing and seeking care triggers intense feelings and well-worn, characteristic defenses against them.

Based on verbal responses to the AAI, Main and her colleagues identified three distinct patterns of attachment, each of which reflects distinct *representations* of attachment. She conceived of these as analogous to patterns of infant attachment: the secure or autonomous pattern (analogous to

---

[3]We mourn the passing of our brilliant colleague on January 6, 2023. Her work, which so inspired generations of researchers and clinicians, profoundly transformed attachment study and dramatically expanded its reach.

the secure infant pattern of attachment), the dismissing pattern (analogous to the infant avoidant classification), and the preoccupied pattern (analogous to the infant resistant classification). These patterns were not only derived from an analysis of the *content* of the narrative(s) (i.e., what *happened* to the parent) but were also based on *how* the story was told (Main et al., 1985; Schafer, 1958). Like the secure child, autonomous adults have free access to positive *as well as negative* childhood memories and value attachment, and they can describe their experiences coherently, fluently, and with emotional authenticity. Insecure representations, by contrast, reflect distinct patterns of defense against attachment-related affects and memories.

Dismissing adults, like their avoidant infant counterparts, minimize negative affect and keep any strong (including positive) emotion and attachment at bay. Their interviews tend to be short, their memories sparse, and descriptions of childhood experiences barren, idealized, and contradictory. A different sort of incoherence is manifest in the interviews of adults whose narratives are described as preoccupied. These interviews are long, full of negative affect and oscillations, with vague, inchoate, and baldly contradictory narratives. In a sense, preoccupied individuals defend against loss by clinging to negative affect. Both types of insecure adult attachment narratives, like their infantile behavioral counterparts, are considered "organized" in the sense that they rely on a strategy that—for the most part—*works* to regulate the adult's relationships and emotional life (Main, 2000). Main later described a third insecure adult representation of attachment—the unresolved pattern (Main & Hesse, 1990). This state of mind in relation to attachment is most apparent in adults who have suffered loss or trauma (and is thus also associated with fear). Analogous to the disorganized pattern of infant attachment, it lacks the coherence and organization of the dismissing and preoccupied organizations. Basic discourse features such as language fluency and meaning, narrative monitoring, and sense of time and space are missing. Like the speaker, the listener feels disoriented, confused, and unable to find a footing in the story.

The insecure adult utilizes a range of defensive strategies that, although emotionally costly, are protective. In dismissing and preoccupied individuals, these defenses are typically well organized and effective, such that the dismissing adult or avoidant child down-regulates and suppresses need and distress to protect themselves against unfulfilled longing, whereas the preoccupied adult or resistant child up-regulates or maximizes need and distress so as to protect themselves from the fear that autonomy leads to loss (Cassidy, 1994). In unresolved adults and disorganized children, such defenses are disorganized and chaotic, manifest in dissociation and disorientation. In this, they are ineffective and leave the individual frightened, alone, and overwhelmed.

Both Bowlby and Main understood attachment representations to be manifestations of an individual's "internal working model of attachment," namely, representational models that are built up over the course of relational experiences (Bowlby, 1969/1982, 1973, 1980; Bretherton, 1985; Main et al., 1985). A child who has multiple experiences of feeling loved and cared for develops an internal working model of themselves as good and lovable, of caregivers (and others) as safe and trustworthy, and of intimacy as joyful and safe. And one who is treated harshly develops a representation of themselves as unworthy and others as untrustworthy. That is, experiences of threat (of abandonment, of harm) in the relationship lead to the development of distinct representational models of attachment. As Main put it, mental representations of attachment provide "a set of conscious and/or unconscious rules for the organization of information relevant to attachment and for obtaining or limiting access to that information" (Main et al., 1985, p. 67). Clearly, then, a parent's representation of attachment in and of itself profoundly influences the way they respond (both behaviorally and internally) to attachment-related affects in themselves and in the child.

The Intergenerational Transmission of Attachment

Main and her colleagues' description of categories of adult attachment analogous to those in children was groundbreaking. But even more groundbreaking was the discovery that mothers' attachment classification predicted children's attachment classification more than 75% of the time. Thus parents whose state of mind in relation to attachment on the AAI was secure were more likely to have secure infants, dismissing parents were more likely to have insecure–avoidant infants, and preoccupied parents were more likely to have insecure–resistant infants (Main et al., 1985). Later, Main and Erik Hesse documented a link between unresolved adult attachment status and infant attachment disorganization (Main & Hesse, 1990). Main's findings were subsequently replicated in numerous studies spanning three decades (e.g., Benoit & Parker, 1994; Fonagy et al., 1991a; Slade et al., 2005; Ward & Carlson, 1995; Waters et al., 2000), with two major meta-analytic studies (van IJzendoorn, 1995; Verhage et al., 2016) confirming, across 95 studies, that intergenerational transmission of attachment is the rule rather than the exception, *for mothers as well as fathers* (Verhage et al., 2016). This link is strongest when the parent is autonomous, in which case the child is highly likely to be secure. Main's method of measuring adult attachment also made possible three generational studies of attachment. These longitudinal studies make clear that not only do attachment patterns remain fairly stable across childhood and adolescence (see Grossman et al., 2006), but their impact persists into the next, third generation, when the children themselves become parents (Benoit & Parker, 1994; Hautamäki et al., 2010). Wordsworth (1807) said it simply: "The Child is father of the Man . . . ," to which attachment researchers would now add, ". . . who is parent of the child, who is parent of the wo/man."

Main's finding of a link between parent and child attachment provided evidence for what dynamically oriented clinicians (Winnicott and Fraiberg being prime examples) had been saying for decades: The internal world of the child is shaped by the internal world of the parent. Her work also raised a critical question: How is a parent's state of mind in relation to attachment *transmitted* from parent to child? What are the *mechanisms* for the intergenerational transmission of attachment? How does the parent's orientation to attachment shape the child's? As we show in Chapters 3 and 4, the search for answers to these questions led in a number of directions, with researchers identifying a range of pathways to secure and insecure attachment. We argue that these all unite around parents' capacity to make sense of the child *and* remain present in moments of distress, the child's as well as their own.

Attachment Processes and MTB-P

The core premises of attachment theory and the core findings of attachment research influenced our work in several distinct ways. First, as we mentioned earlier, we focused on the establishment of secure attachments, seeing these as critical to a range of later developments. Second, we kept our eyes on relational threat and tried in a variety of ways to address situations in which babies and toddlers might feel frightened. Third, we used the idea of "too little" and "too much" to guide our clinical efforts. As Talia (Talia et al., 2014) and others (Dozier, 1990; Holmes & Slade, 2018) have noted, secure adults in therapy tend to express distress openly, ask for help, and show gratitude. Dismissing patients tend to minimize any disclosure, convey self-sufficiency, and downplay their distress. Preoccupied patients tended to obstruct the therapist's attempts to intervene, fail to enlist the therapists' own points of view, and convey their experience in vague or confusing ways. It is particularly fascinating that preoccupied patients not only seek contact but also *resist* it (Talia et al., 2014). This is, of course, completely in line with Ainsworth's observation of ambivalence in resistant infants' behavior (Ainsworth et al., 1978) and very much clarifies why working with preoccupied adults can be so challenging. Studies of attachment and psychotherapy also underscore how important it is for clinicians to attend to the ways a parent's language invites understanding or in some ways obscures communication or pushes others away. These dynamics will have a significant impact on the parent's capacity to come to trust in and rely upon the clinician. A dismissing, shut-down parent requires an approach that gently encourages them to tolerate more and more affect, whereas a preoccupied, overwhelmed parent requires an approach that helps them manage and contain negative affect (Dozier, 1990; Holmes & Slade, 2018; Talia et al., 2014). We also used the idea of "too little" and "too much" to understand clinicians' own responses to families.

Critiques of Attachment Theory and Research

There have been many critiques of attachment theory and research over the past 80 years. Space does not allow us to describe these in full, but in the next section we turn briefly to the question of attachment's biological bases. We then turn to the question of whether attachment theory and research have adequately considered the question of culture and, in particular, the ways attachment security and insecurity are expressed in different cultural contexts.

Biological Bases of Attachment

One of the earliest critiques of attachment theory was that it failed to take biological differences into account. The first version of this criticism was the suggestion that attachment classifications were, in fact, measures of infantile temperament, not of the parent–child relationship (e.g., Campos et al., 1983; Kagan, 1995). Thus avoidance was simply a measure of a "slow to warm up" temperament, resistance a manifestation of the temperamental trait of negative emotionality, and so forth. In this view, measures of individual differences in attachment reflected temperamental differences and not relationship quality. Thus, individual differences in attachment were reflections of features intrinsic to the *baby*, not the relationship.

Attachment theorists, notably Sroufe (1985), countered that, from the moment of birth, relationships shape biology, generally, and temperament, specifically; thus measures of the temperament are always, to a certain extent, measures of relationship. And although babies naturally differ in their emotional reactivity and sensitivity to stimuli, these qualities do not determine attachment quality. To this point, van den Boom (1994) demonstrated—with an intervention focused on sensitive responsiveness—that even mothers with the most temperamentally disrupted babies could learn to calm and soothe them and build secure attachment relationships. In related work, Belsky and Rovine (1987) proposed that while temperament does not determine the quality of attachment, it may influence the way insecurity is expressed (i.e., slow-to-warm-up babies are more likely to be avoidant, and highly reactive babies are more likely to be resistant).

Contemporary support for this position comes from Verhage and her colleagues' (2016) finding that dismissing mothers do not necessarily have avoidant children or preoccupied mothers resistant children, but simply that an insecure parent is more likely to have an insecure child. Thus, while attachment quality is a measure of relationship quality and not the child's level of emotional reactivity, variations in emotionally reactivity may well determine the way the child responds to the parent's unavailability.

As the years went on, and methodologies became more sophisticated, the temperament argument became much more nuanced, with multiple investigators looking for underlying genetic causes for differences in attachment and testing the hypothesis that particular genes might be associated with particular manifestations of attachment. Nevertheless, despite tremendous advances in the study of genetics and epigenetics, there is today no clear evidence of such associations; almost without exception, environmental influences remain the most reliably and significantly predictive of a child's attachment classification (Bakermans-Kranenburg & van IJzendoorn, 2016; Fearon et al., 2006b; Oliveira & Fearon, 2019; Plomin, 2013; Verhage et al., 2016).

What has gained more traction, however, is the notion that children may be *differentially susceptible* to environmental influence (Belsky, 1997; Belsky et al., 2007; Belsky & Pluess, 2009; Vaughn & Bost, 2016). Rather than determining a child's orientation to attachment, genes may well affect *how* a child responds to a given environment. Some children thrive despite adversity, and others collapse in its face. Described as the "orchid hypothesis," this is a more sophisticated way of thinking about the baby's contribution to the attachment process and to the ways an individual's genetic makeup may convey a sensitivity to *both* negative and positive environments. From this perspective, more delicate "orchid children" suffer greatly in difficult environments but do particularly well in positive ones. In this way, environmental impacts are experienced differently depending upon levels of genetic vulnerability. Although this epigenetic approach shows considerable promise, the science is very much in its infancy, and we are still learning *how* biological and hereditary factors matter (Bakermans-Kranenburg & van IJzendoorn, 2016; Bokhorst et al., 2003; Oliveira & Fearon, 2019). Bowlby (1969/1982) himself presented one of the first arguments for gene × environment interactions: "Just as area is a product of length multiplied by width so every biological character . . . is a product of the interaction of genetic endowment with environment" (p. 38). Given the overwhelming evidence that the parent–child relationship has a substantive and meaningful impact on the child's sense of themselves in the world and the fact that clinicians cannot (at least at this point) modify genetic or biological factors, we are left to focus on the relationship and the ways we can enhance and support it.

Cultural Differences in Attachment

Another of the most common criticisms of attachment research is that the theory and the research upon which it is based are culturally biased. This raises a number of complex issues that we try to untangle here and again in Chapter 3. Let's begin with several of the theory's core assumptions. Bowlby (1969/1982) and Ainsworth (1967) believed that infants, almost without exception, form a preferential bond with one or more of their trusted caregivers. This is (or these are) the person(s) to whom the child will turn when threatened and from whom the child will learn about the ways of people and of the world. This is where the child first learns about love and about conflict. As we discussed earlier, there are powerful evolutionary reasons for the development of attachment bonds: They protect the child from danger and ensure their humanity. Evidence for the notion that infants will become attached to their caregivers in infancy has been demonstrated again and again in hundreds of empirical, ethnographic, and naturalistic studies across a range of populations around the world (including Ainsworth's original Uganda study; Mesman et al., 2016). Indeed, it seems hard to argue with the basic idea that infants are born with a universal need for love and safety with another. *Every child in every culture* needs to feel beloved *by* and safe *with* one or more caregivers. Their survival and the survival of the species depends upon it.

Ainsworth also believed that, although the search for the secure base is universal, the way security is sought and achieved varies across cultures. "I think that environmental influences play no significant role in the infant's basic need for an attachment figure who can be trusted. But culture-related differences in ecologies and expectations will certainly affect how some specific aspects of that organization are expressed" (Ainsworth & Marvin, 1995, p. 8). That this is the case has been demonstrated time and again by researchers working in a range of cultures and settings. On the one hand—unless they are being raised in a context in which their survival is threatened—the majority of children across studies are classified as secure using standard measures of attachment assessment or ethnographic observations. Thus it appears unlikely that secure attachment is "just a North American invention or a Western ideal, but instead is a widespread and preferred phenomenon" (Mesman et al., 2016, p. 866). At the same time, cross-cultural studies have also consistently demonstrated that what Ainsworth described as "insecure" strategies of avoidance and resistance may be normative in certain contexts (Mesman et al., 2016) and are not necessarily associated with poor outcomes (Verhage et al., 2016, 2018). Thus, as we discuss more fully in Chapter 3, avoidance, or minimizing displays of emotion, might well be a good and even lifesaving adaptation in certain cultural or racially dangerous contexts (e.g., for a Black person living in a largely White community; Dunbar et al., 2022; Stern et al., 2022c).

Klaus and Karin Grossmann (Grossmann et al., 1985) made this point in one of the earliest studies of cross-cultural variation in patterns of attachment, noting that in a North German sample, organized avoidance was common and culturally congruent (see also Grossman et al., 2005). Likewise, Miyake and colleagues (Miyake et al., 1985) noted that resistance was far more common and thus normative in Japanese samples. They also reported quite different distributions of attachment patterns across the United States, Germany, Japan, Sweden, and Israel. Thus, insecure–*organized* attachment organizations—namely, avoidance and resistance—may be typical and normative in a variety of contexts and cultures, and, as such, not associated with poor outcomes. At the same time, these adaptations may in some instances have originated in response to historical trauma (e.g., slavery, war, and genocide). Disorganized attachment, however, is almost always associated with fear and threat, as well as a range of negative outcomes.

Despite the fact that there has been no shortage of cross-cultural attachment research, critics have consistently and correctly argued that such studies make up only a fraction of the larger opus of attachment research (see Mesman et al., 2016) and that, as such, the concepts of security and insecurity are still based in Western European, largely White notions of what "good" relationships look like. And, as vividly described in a recent issue of *Attachment and Human Development*, edited by Jessica Stern, Oscar Barbarin, and Jude Cassidy (2022a), attachment researchers have tended to either ignore or pathologize populations living *with* racism, cultural oppression, and historical trauma or *without* access to basic resources such as food, shelter, or the opportunity to work and lead a productive life. These criticisms require our attention and concern, particularly as clinicians are often working with marginalized populations whose ways of coping and adapting they may not fully understand.

We believe that redressing these failures begins with a closer look at the meaning and *function* of an individual's attachment organization and, specifically, at the meaning and function of avoidance and resistance. Although we label both as indications of insecurity, it is often the case that patterns of avoidance and resistance are congruent with patterns within the individual's culture or subculture, and thus normative. For example, we can all think of fully functioning individuals who tend to be emotionally reserved. We can also think of fully functioning individuals who are more emotional and reactive. By contrast, we can also think of individuals whose avoidance and resistance seems driven by ongoing relational threat. In these instances, such defenses are likely to be clinically relevant and likely to be associated with poorer outcomes. With insecure–disorganized and unresolved patterns of attachment, the picture is clearer, as the presence of disorganization, disorientation, and dissociation almost always indicates pervasive relational threat and the consequent collapse of any strategies for regulating and organizing attachment-related affects. The sequelae include a range of negative social, emotional, behavioral, cognitive, and neurobiological outcomes (Lyons-Ruth & Jacobvitz, 2016).

As such, we must approach the families we see with humility and an open mind. In particular, it is critical to think about avoidance and resistance in a more nuanced way. We have represented this in Figure 2.2 using the arousal curve, shading the upper third of the curve to indicate that there are many circumstances in which avoidance or resistance has emerged not in response to relational or interpersonal threat but instead is congruent with the expectations of a particular culture or subculture and will not necessarily be associated with poor outcomes.

It is so important to think about patterns of seeking and receiving care dynamically and to use the notion of attachment patterns in ways that are rich and clinically meaningful. Clinicians need to be concerned about those children and parents who fall outside the shaded area, who are shut down, inaccessible, ready to fight, easily dysregulated, or dissociated and disorganized. Do their defenses and ways of managing affect seem rigid and entrenched, overwhelmed, or absent altogether? Observing these differences clinically tells us about the degree to which fear has infused the attachment system, such that the child distorts their need for trust and closeness in order to maintain whatever relationship with the caregiver is possible. As we noted previously, Hesse and Main (1999) make the key point that the insecure child "must continuously attend to the safety versus threat implicit in current conditions" (p. 494). These are the children and adults we are concerned about and for whom a range of attachment-based interventions have been developed (Steele & Steele, 2018).

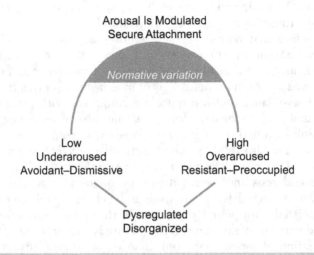

FIGURE 2.2 Normative variations in attachment.

Summary

Bowlby described the baby as born seeking safety in relationships, both literal safety and the safety of love and connection. Children need to feel loved to survive emotionally; they need (to return to the words of President Obama in the frontmatter) to feel important and beloved by *someone*, to feel that they light up someone's (or many someones'!) world. We have learned over the past eight decades that it doesn't have to be just the mother or the father and that often (indeed optimally) the child is attached to several primary caregivers. We have also learned that culture dramatically shapes the way the baby comes to feel that they *belong*. But the feeling of being precious, of being cherished by another human being is central to one's humanity. Equally important, the child is most likely to flourish when their pivotal and essential relationships are largely free from fear. The intrusion of fear into the child's earliest relational experiences is at the heart of what attachment theorists call insecurity. It is at the heart of feeling alone, alienated, angry, and unsafe. Families in pain come to us not because of a shortage of love but because love is battling fear, anger, and other demons. It has become fraught.

We now summarize the basic premises that guided our clinical aims and approaches. Beginning in earliest infancy, children have the capacity to detect threat and danger. When threatened, they are evolutionarily programmed to seek proximity and care from the stronger and wiser caregivers meant to protect and care for them. Moments of "trouble," when the child is distressed, are critical moments in the child's developing sense of self and of others. Ideally, they find safety from danger and pleasure in connection with those closest to them. They learn that although ruptures are inevitable, repair is, as well. When threats go unmodulated, the child adapts in whatever way is necessary to maintain the relationship with the caregiver. The defensive maneuvers of shutting down ("too little") or maximizing negative affect ("too much") reflect the effort to manage threat and danger and to preserve whatever pleasure in intimacy is possible. These adaptations invariably involve disruptions in affect regulation and manifest themselves in forms of flight, fight, and freezing; as such, they are often quite costly to the child. They also greatly diminish the pleasures that flow from safety in closeness.

It is important for clinicians to remember that the insecure categories of child and adult attachment, as well as the behavioral and narrative markers described previously, are shorthand for the individual's dynamic efforts to regulate threat and fear and preserve whatever intimacy and closeness is possible in their primary relationships. *And it is these dynamics rather than the categories themselves that deserve our clinical attention.* A child's or parent's adaptations—to push away and/or cling (some individuals fluctuate between the two), to collapse, to flee, fight, or freeze—are the focus of our clinical work. *Our goal is to identify the threats that propel an infant, child, or adult to defend themselves, remedy their intensity, help the individual develops ways to manage them more flexibly, and to find pleasure in genuine, unfettered closeness.*

QUESTIONS FOR CLINICIANS

Clinical situations provide multiple opportunities to observe dynamic attachment processes as they unfold between child and parent or child and a trusted caregiver (a family member, teacher, etc.). Here we list some of the phenomena clinicians can look for in assessing the child's orientation to attachment. We address ways to approach these therapeutically in Part III.

▶ Moments of separation, reunion, or interpersonal conflict reveal a great deal about what happens—within the child, and between the child and their caregiver—when the child's attachment system is activated.

  ▷ How does the child respond when they are mildly threatened?
  ▷ Are they able to seek care freely from the caregiver?
  ▷ Do you see evidence of avoidance or dampening down negative affect ("too little")?
  ▷ Do you see evidence of the child's being overwhelmed with distress ("too much")?
  ▷ What do you notice about the parent's behavior at these moments?
  ▷ Is the parent comforting or protective?
  ▷ Is the parent frightening or frightened?

▶ What do you observe in moments of pleasure between parent and child? Does it build? Does it feel authentic? Is it reciprocated and shared?

▶ What happens in the dyad when the child seeks closeness? When the child explores away from the parent? When the child forges new relationships?

▶ What does the parent tell you about their experience with their own parents?

▶ What do you notice about the way the parent describes interactions and family relationships? What can they talk about? What is missing? Can you follow the parent's story? Are you filling in the blanks? Are you lost and overwhelmed?

▶ When a parent talks to you, do you feel they want to help you understand, or that they are pushing you away, or "resisting" your input, fighting what you have to offer (see Talia et al., 2014)?

Chapter

3

Pathways to Secure Attachment
CAREGIVER SENSITIVITY

In Chapter 2, we outlined the reasons behind our focus on helping parents and children develop secure attachments and diminishing the likelihood of fearful or disorganized attachment. Security, the feeling of being safe and loved and valued, of *unconditionally mattering* to another (Stern et al., 2022b), is not a guarantee of ease in life, but it does make life easier. In this and subsequent chapters, we examine the relational pathways to security. What features of the caregiver–child relationship contribute to the child's feelings of safety and *belonging* in the world? Understanding this was key to our clinical approach. What elements of the relationship were most essential for us to support? What were the foundations we needed to build? Where did we need to intervene and guide parents in their interactions with the child? Needless to say, and as we make clear in the chapters that follow, the answers to the question of how caregivers nurture feelings of safety and belonging in their children are complex and layered, depending on a variety of contexts and perspectives. Yet in many ways the answer is very simple: The child needs—within the framework of their culture—to feel safe, heard, known, and *important* to somebody (and optimally multiple somebodies!).

One of the ways parents communicate emotional presence and safety to their children is through their behavior. The abundant research on caregiver behavior can be described in three waves. The first focused on caregiver sensitivity, which Ainsworth identified as essential to the infant's sense of safety and trust. The second wave focused on efforts to define insensitive or anomalous caregiver behavior, which Main and Lyons-Ruth saw as prime contributors to the development of disorganized attachment. The third and present wave returns to the question of culture and the necessity of broadening the notion of caregiver sensitivity to include a range of cultural variations. Although this has been a subject of discussion among cross-cultural researchers for decades, today—when, in the wake of the social justice movement, the relative failure of attachment researchers to understand the strengths and struggles of minoritized parents has become all too clear (Murry et al., 2022; Stern et al., 2022a)—the need is clearly urgent.

Caregiver Behavior

Caregiver Sensitivity

In her earliest studies of mother–infant attachment in Uganda, Mary Ainsworth (1967) observed that parents' sensitive responsiveness to infant cues played an enormous role in the development of what she was later to call secure attachment in the infant. Upon her return to the United States, she sought to examine the link between sensitive maternal behavior and infant attachment empirically. She observed a group of mothers and babies at home for a year. During that time, she observed how *receptive* mothers were to their infants' signals, how much they *cooperated* with their children in meeting the children's needs, and the degree to which they *remained psychologically and physically available* and *accepted* their children's needs. She described these as the core components of "maternal sensitivity" (Ainsworth et al., 1978). When the babies were 1 year old, she observed them in the SSP (Ainsworth et al., 1978; Ainsworth & Wittig, 1965), the brief separation procedure we described in Chapter 2. Mothers who were more sensitively responsive during the first year were more likely to have infants who, at 12 months, sought them out readily when distressed or in need of comfort. Mothers who did not pick the baby up when distressed, who were uncomfortable with close bodily contact, who were intermittently available, or who failed to respond to infant cues were more likely to have avoidant or resistant babies in the SSP (Ainsworth et al., 1978).

Sharon Olds's poem "Bathing the Newborn" (1984), which we described in Chapter 2, captures some of what Ainsworth meant by caregiver sensitivity. The mother conveys her presence to the baby in a variety of ways: she coos, she holds him "just right," she tells him he is wonderful, and she watches closely for signs that he is distressed. She leans in, adjusts her body, her hands, her grip, and her voice to let him know that he is OK and watches as he calms and begins to feel the water against his "silky limbs." She attends to every inch of his "wonderful body." She feels his spine relaxing, the fear *leaving* him. Attuned to his pleasure and his distress, she sees what he needs, what he wants, what brings him relief, and what pleases him, and she responds accordingly. She has him in mind. Perhaps most important, she does not fade away, criticize, challenge, or shut down when she senses her infant's apprehension. She continues to hold him and his distress with compassion and love.

Ainsworth's original hypothesis that caregiver sensitivity was essential to the development of secure attachment has been tested in hundreds of studies over the past 40 years. Most of these studies assess sensitivity using measures based on Ainsworth's original scale, which rates the parent's capacity to recognize the child's cues, interpret them correctly, and respond to them in a timely and appropriate way. Meta-analytic studies confirm that—almost without exception—such measures consistently predict the child's attachment classification (De Wolff & van IJzendoorn, 1997; Verhage et al., 2016). But caregiver sensitivity is hardly a certain predictor of secure attachment, as it predicts only 6% of the variance in attachment security across samples and only 2% of the variance in low socioeconomic status (SES) samples (De Wolff & van IJzendoorn, 1997).

Caregiver sensitivity has also been identified as a primary mechanism for the intergenerational transmission of attachment in two large meta-analytic studies (van IJzendoorn, 1995; Verhage et al., 2016). Parents classified as securely attached on the AAI are more likely to respond sensitively and contingently, and their children are more likely to be secure. Parents classified as insecurely attached are less likely to respond sensitively, and their children are less likely to be secure. Here, too, however, caregiver sensitivity accounted for only a small proportion of the variance in explaining the link between a parent's attachment classification and that of their child. Thus, as van IJzendoorn (1995) put it succinctly, there is a "gap" in understanding how attachment is transmitted from one generation to the next and the multiple contexts that lead a child to feel that they "unconditionally matter" (Stern et al., 2022b). We return to this issue again in upcoming chapters.

It is important to note that attachment researchers were hardly the only researchers and clinicians to emphasize the importance of caregiver sensitivity. The work of Daniel Stern (1977, 1985), T. Berry Brazelton (1984), Beatrice Beebe (Beebe et al., 2010), Ed Tronick (2007), and Colwyn Trevarthen (1979) (to name only a few) makes crystal clear the subtlety and power of early dyadic interactions: the ways both parent and child contribute to the interaction and its quality, the ways the child's sense of themselves and of their emotions is shaped by parental attunement, reciprocity and mutual regulation, and how the absence of attunement leaves the child alone in a profound way. The child's sense of themselves of their internal world, and of their body emerges over the course of thousands and thousands of interactions with their closest others. When things are going well, this is a wonderful process, but when they are not, early interactions become the source of building darkness and pain.

Insensitive or Anomalous Parental Behavior

Beginning about 30 years ago, researchers began to focus more directly on caregiver *insensitivity*, specifically on identifying what parental behaviors might preclude or *interfere with* the development of secure attachment. This effort began with Main and Hesse's (1990) observation that disorganized attachment results when the parent—who is meant to protect the child in moments of danger—becomes a "source of alarm" (p. 163). When the child's attachment system is activated, when they would naturally seek comfort and proximity from a stronger and wiser caregiver, the parent *threatens* them, either by actively frightening them or withdrawing. The critical insight that some parents threaten the child in moments when the attachment system is activated highlighted the importance of the parent's capacity to respond sensitively *when the child is distressed.* (i.e., when they are in the throes of negative affect and *most* need their parents). Even the most insecure dyads can at times find pleasure in each other, and even the most anxious parents can at times respond sensitively to the child, but insecure and particularly disorganized dyads really differ in the regulation of stress and distress in the interaction. Specifically, parents behave in "anomalous" (Lyons-Ruth et al., 1999b) ways that run *counter* to their evolutionarily privileged role of providing safety and comfort in times of distress (Lyons-Ruth et al., 1999b; Main & Hesse, 1990). These responses invariably leave the child feeling afraid and alone (Allen, 2013).

In the first descriptions of these phenomena, Main and Hesse (Main & Hesse, 1990; Hesse & Main, 2000) noted that some mothers appeared menacing, threatening, aggressive, and overtly frightening to their children. In interaction, they might hiss, growl, bare their teeth, and in some cases raise their lips on one side (a common primate threat gesture). These actions were not playful and appeared and disappeared without cause. Another group of mothers responded to their babies as if frightened by them, showing a "fear face" at the baby's approach, shrinking from the child, and responding behaviorally as if they were helpless and overcome by the child. Some spoke in a haunted way and would at times freeze, still, or appear to dissociate. Main and Hesse (1990) reasoned that—because both frightened and frightening behaviors signal so clearly that the parent cannot be relied on for protection—they would be deeply frightening to the child. The link between such parental behaviors and disorganized attachment has since been confirmed in a number of studies and meta-analyses (Madigan et al., 2006; Schuengel et al., 1999), making evident the link between threatening parental behavior and disorganized attachment and, in particular, the dilemma of seeking protection from a caregiver who is also the "source of alarm" (Main & Hesse, 1990).

Several years later, Karlen Lyons-Ruth and her colleagues (Lyons-Ruth et al., 1999b) took a closer look at anomalous parental behavior. Building on Main and Hesse's (1990) observations, she and her colleagues developed the Atypical Maternal Behavior Instrument for Assessment and Classification (AMBIANCE; Bronfman et al., 1992–2008), which identifies five dimensions of atypical parental behavior in response to the child: affective errors (in which the parent gives contradictory, nonresponsive, or inappropriate cues); disoriented, frightened, or confused behavior; verbal or physical negative intrusive behavior; role confusion (role reversal or sexualization of the child); and withdrawal (verbal or physical distance from the child). Lyons-Ruth and her colleagues found that mothers who displayed more atypical or anomalous caregiving behaviors upon reunion were more likely to have disorganized infants than mothers who displayed few such behaviors (Lyons-Ruth et al., 1999b). Grienenberger and his colleagues (2005) later replicated this finding. Note that the AMBIANCE system, like Main and Hesse's system for assessing frightening maternal behavior (FR), links a parent's threatening behavior to disorganized attachment. Note that both systems also distinguish between two primary modes of parental behavior: intrusion and withdrawal, or, to use the distinction we introduced in Chapter 2, "too much" and "too little." Lyons-Ruth described this as the hostile–helpless relational diathesis (Lyons-Ruth et al., 1999a). Later, as we describe in Chapter 5, she used these same dimensions to describe adults' representations of their parents on the AAI.

In a 2006 meta-analysis of the relationship between anomalous parental behavior and disorganized attachment, Madigan and her colleagues found Main and Hesse's FR system and Lyons-Ruth's AMBIANCE measure equally predictive of disorganized attachment. Given the prevalence of disorganized attachment in clinical samples (Bakermans-Kranenburg & van IJzendoorn, 2009), the value of both instruments in informing clinical observation and intervention cannot be overemphasized. The AMBIANCE system, in particular, provides clinicians (and researchers) with a great deal of specificity in identifying the anomalous parental behaviors that provoke fear in the child and lead to disruption and disorganization of the attachment system. As we describe in subsequent chapters, the more clinicians can become aware of the many sorts of subtle parental behaviors that can frighten the child, the more they can address the issues that lead to behavioral and relational disruptions.

Beebe and her colleagues (2010) later provided yet another level of specificity regarding the link between anomalous parental behavior and disorganized attachment. Microanalysis of face-to-face interactions between future disorganized 4-month-old infants and their mothers revealed that mothers became less contingent and were less likely to respond in synchronous, attuned ways *when their infants were distressed*. That is, when infants displayed high levels of negative affect, their mothers emotionally withdrew in a variety of ways that compromised "interactive agency and emotional coherence" (Beebe et al., 2010, p. 7). The child was left alone and unknown in moments of distress, and vital opportunities for repair (Tronick & Gold, 2020) were missed. These findings, along with those of Main and Hesse and of Lyons-Ruth and her colleagues, bring home the clinical significance of observing *precisely what happens* between parent and child when the child is distressed, and particularly whether the parent frightens or is frightening to the child in that moment.

Ecological Constraints on Caregiver Sensitivity and the Intergenerational Transmission of Attachment

The discovery that caregiver sensitivity predicts both infant security and intergenerational transmission led researchers to ask: (1) What are the contexts that make it more difficult for a parent to be sensitive? and, relatedly, (2) what are the contexts that weaken the intergenerational transmission of secure attachment, namely, the likelihood that a parent's attachment security will be transmitted to the child? The ecological constraints hypothesis (Sagi et al., 1997) suggests that, as ecological stresses increase, caregiver sensitivity decreases, and the effect of a parent's attachment organization on the child's weakens (Verhage et al., 2018). Ecological stresses are often framed in terms of societally imposed risks such as family separation, parental risks such as a history of abuse or psychopathology, or sociodemographic risks such as chronic poverty, adolescent parenthood, marital status, and the like. Importantly, these risks are often conflated, both in research and in real life. In so many instances and across cultures and subcultures, parents with high levels of early trauma and PTSD are also those who are living below the poverty line, who become parents at an early age, who have limited access to a range of educational and social resources, and so forth. They also tend to be members of ethnically, racially, or culturally oppressed groups.

Verhage and her colleagues (2018) conducted a meta-analysis of the findings of 58 studies to examine the impact of both parent and child risk on attachment transmission. They defined parental risks as adolescent parenthood, maternal psychopathology, parental substance abuse, parental abuse or childhood trauma, child abuse (i.e., the parent's parents were maltreating), and demographic risk/poverty. Child risks included a non-biological relationship to the parent, preterm and/or low birth weight, and the health of the child. They found that the likelihood of a parent's attachment organization predicting the child's diminishes as both parent and child risks increase, specifically that "attachment transmission was weaker in samples of known risks (e.g., teenage mothers, parents with psychopathology, socioeconomically stressed families, and preterm-born children)" (Verhage et al., 2018, p. 2024). These findings drive home the point that stress makes parenting very hard indeed—whether it is the internal stress of PTSD, depression, or another form of mental illness, the challenges of having a child who is ill or disabled, being young, living in a violent relationship or community, or struggling with a chronic lack of economic and social resources.

Socioeconomic Risk

A range of studies make clear that "socioeconomic risk" poses especially great challenges to both parental sensitivity and the intergenerational transmission of secure attachment. "Socioeconomic risk" is typically defined as including a variety of factors, such as income level, minoritized status,[1] and a range of other sociodemographic risks, such as a history of substance abuse, single parenthood, being an adolescent mother, or having less than a high school education. Thus it is not only poverty but also its structural and social determinants that constitute socioeconomic risk. Again and again, studies make clear that, although other factors (i.e., parental psychopathology and child maltreatment) have an impact on the child's attachment security in a number of ways, socioeconomic risk consistently *equals* these risks in their effects.

As an example, in a major review of studies using the AAI, Bakermans-Kranenburg and van IJzendoorn (2009) found that parental psychopathology and socioeconomic risk are equally predictive of adult insecurity on the AAI. Individuals drawn from clinical populations were more likely to be insecure and unresolved (73%) than participants in normative samples (42%). When the impact of risks such as poverty and adolescent parenthood on AAI status was examined, 70% of the adults were insecure, with approximately half dismissing and half unresolved. *Thus socioeconomic*

---

[1] This is a term used by Black scholars in place of "ethnic minority status." It is meant to connote the fact that Blacks (as well as Latinx, Asians, Native Americans and immigrants fleeing their countries of origin), rather than being inherently "less than," have been *treated* as "less than" by European Americans and other groups in positions of power.

risk was nearly as likely to be predictive of adult insecurity as parental psychopathology. In another major meta-analysis, Cyr and her colleagues (2010) found that, just as child maltreatment robustly predicted infant disorganization, so did socioeconomic risk. Although maltreated children had lower levels of attachment security and higher levels of attachment disorganization than both low-risk children and non-maltreated high-risk children, when socioeconomic risks accumulated to the *point that parents had five or more risk indicators,* their children were as much at risk for disorganized attachment as the maltreated children. *In other words, high levels of socioeconomic risk are just as likely to lead to disorganized attachment as frank maltreatment.*

Socioeconomic Risk, Race, and Attachment

In numerous studies, minoritized status is often included in composite measures of socioeconomic risk, thus conflating poverty and race or ethnicity. Black and Latinx populations are often described as "high risk," which conflates race with experiences of living below the poverty line, having less than a high school education, and experiencing underemployment and housing and food insecurity. Parents considered "high risk" are often adolescent and/or single parents who may have been diagnosed with a substance use disorder or mental illness. The conflation of socioeconomic factors and race in this way affirms historically racist narratives regarding diverse members of a given society. Researchers began trying to tease these variables apart nearly 20 years ago, albeit using language we would find offensive today. Racist tropes aside, what research in this area has consistently made clear is that *when income is held constant,* minoritized parents are as likely to be sensitively responsive and have secure children as White parents.

The first study specifically designed to study the impact of race on attachment was published in 2004 by Bakermans-Kranenburg and colleagues. Initial analyses revealed that African American children were less likely to be securely attached and their mothers less likely to be sensitively responsive than their White peers. However, when they eliminated the variance associated with income, maternal age, and levels of sensitivity, they found no differences between the two groups in levels of security. These findings suggest that the primary route to infant security is caregiver sensitivity and that, regardless of their ethnicity, when mothers are sensitive, their children will be secure. The authors concluded that "our findings provide support for the *no group difference* hypothesis," (p. 429) namely, that African American and White children are equally likely to be secure when their parents are sensitive. In a similar study carried out two decades later, Dexter and his colleagues (2013) also found that parenting behaviors, and particularly sensitive, responsive parenting, led to child security regardless of race.

The no-group-difference hypothesis received further confirmation in a review of 27 cross-cultural studies of attachment (Mesman et al., 2012). The authors reported that U.S. studies found lower levels of caregiver sensitivity in African American as compared both with Latinx and European American parents, with European American mothers having the highest levels of sensitivity. In addition, ethnic minority families typically had lower SES backgrounds than European American parents. *Thus, when researchers controlled for SES, the differences in sensitivity between ethnic minority parents and their European American counterparts disappeared or became much smaller.* That is, ethnic minority mothers were just as likely to be sensitive as those in the dominant cultural group when the effects of poverty were statistically controlled. Caregiver sensitivity is associated with secure attachment no matter the caregivers' cultural group, race, or ethnicity.

Attachment researchers have consistently been reassured when their findings prove the no-group-difference hypothesis, namely, that a Black or Latinx parent is as likely to have a secure child as a White parent, because it is sensitivity, and not race, that predicts security. When parents are less stressed, their race has no bearing on their capacity to be sensitive. This is a very important thing to prove, again and again. The problem with this hypothesis, however, is that it overlooks the fact that cumulative socioeconomic risks are very high in many minoritized families (McLoyd, 1990). The no-group-differences hypothesis also overlooks the fact of the particular and pernicious impact of prejudice, bias, racial discrimination, and systemic racism on both parents and children (Murry et al., 2022). Racism, a particularly devastating form of toxic stress (Shonkoff et al., 2021), is an everyday reality for BIPOC[2] families, regardless of their socioeconomic status. So, yes, in the absence of stress, most parents would be responsive, and their children would do well. But the environments in which many minoritized families are raising their children are extremely, relentlessly stressful, through no fault of their own. It is harder to be sensitive and to derive pleasure from caregiving when you lack the basic resources to survive and when you are under constant, chronic threat, particularly the hateful threat of racism. In that sense, there *is*, in fact, an enormous group difference. To return to our fear hypothesis, the daily threats inherent in dire poverty and cultural and racial oppression all too often put parents in survival mode when they most need and want to be connected to those most precious to them. All things being equal, parents and children would do fine. But all things are not equal.

---

[2]Black, Indigenous, people of color.

Until late in 2021, these issues had received little attention in the attachment literature. This oversight is but another example of the racial bias built into psychology research (Buchanan et al., 2021; Roberts et al., 2020), and that has led to the widespread failure—at multiple levels—to confront and confirm the realities of racism. The killing of George Floyd, along with a number of other Black men and women, forced attachment researchers to reckon with this profound oversight directly. In 2022, the journal *Attachment and Human Development* published a remarkable series of papers in a special issue devoted to attachment perspectives on race, prejudice, and antiracism (Kendi, 2019), with a particular focus on Black Americans. Edited by Jessica Stern, Oscar Barbarin, and Jude Cassidy (2022a), these collected papers reflect a unique and much-needed effort to bring together scholars in both attachment and Black youth and family development to look closely at the bias inherent in attachment research before 2021 and at the ways the field can work toward "antiracist perspectives in attachment theory, research, and practice" (Stern et al., 2022b) going forward.

The first issue noted by many of the contributors is a consistent bias in measurement, such that researchers have failed to identify the positive ways that many African American parents have been able to adapt to the ever-present reality of racism in order to "raise secure and stable children" (Murry et al., 2022, p. 322). The writings of African American slave mothers tell us that they desperately missed the children from whom they were routinely and savagely separated and describe the many ways they found to sustain these attachments despite the threat of violence and death (Harriet Jacobs's [1861] *Incidents in the Life of a Slave Girl* and Tiya Miles's [2021] *All That She Carried*). Nevertheless, little (if any) attention has been paid to the many ways that caregiving patterns in Black parents have evolved to protect children from the effects of racism. Racial/ethnic socialization (Murry et al., 2022) and other forms of secure-base provision (Woodhouse et al., 2020) are ways that parents help children thrive in an environment of evolutionary adaptedness where threat is real and ever present.

For example, as described by Dunbar and her colleagues (2022), Black parents prepare their children for bias by supporting them in their distress, while at the same time gently suppressing its expression. This is an essential part of helping children self-regulate when they are under constant threat. Thus behaviors that might appear to be insensitive, namely, emotion suppression, are actually critical forms of "secure-base provision" (Woodhouse et al., 2020) and lead to positive outcomes in the child. The message is clear: "*I know this hurts so much, but for you to be safe it's best to dampen down your distress and not challenge the aggressor.*" Teaching the child to be mildly avoidant in some circumstances but not necessarily others (Lozada et al., 2022) is both loving and protective. Stern and her colleagues (Stern et al., 2022c, p. 314) likewise suggest that, particularly within the context of neighborhood racism, attachment avoidance "may serve as an adaptive strategy for Black adolescents in guarding against the multiple social, emotional, and physical stressors of racism; in this context, we might consider whether a certain degree of avoidance in social interactions represents a 'hidden talent' within a harsh environment (Ellis et al., 2022)." These findings hark back to the point we made in Chapter 2 about culturally "normative" patterns of avoidance and resistance.

Coard (2022) makes the related point that many White researchers pathologize the fact that African American children are often cared for by an extended kin network that includes grandparents, aunts, and other close family members or friends. The extended family has been the source of strength, resilience, and survival for African American children who—historically facing the terrible family disruptions that were part and parcel of slavery—developed the capacity to flexibly bond with immediate family, extended family, and multiple caregivers. Today, given that those African American families who are living in poverty lack the resources to pay for organized child care, the ability to turn to one's kin for care is particularly important. Thus research that focuses solely on the parent–child dyad overlooks the "social context of caregiving" (Coard, 2022) and the ways that multiple caregivers can serve as a secure base for the African American child.

Related to concerns about bias in measurement is the criticism that Ainsworth's original measure of caregiver sensitivity fails to reflect the positive adaptations parents make to help their children thrive in the face of adversity (Coard, 2022; Dunbar et al., 2022; Stern et al., 2022b). As we noted previously, caregiver sensitivity—as Ainsworth conceived of it—accounts for only 6% of the variance in child security across studies and only 2% in studies of low-SES families (De Wolff & van IJzendoorn, 1997). Thus, even from the standpoint of empirical evidence, this gold standard is quite weak. Recently, Susan Woodhouse, Jude Cassidy, and their colleagues introduced a new measure of caregiver responsiveness that assesses "secure-base provision" in parents (SBP; Woodhouse et al., 2020). They found—in a low-SES sample, in which 66% of the mothers were BIPOC (and the majority of these were Black)—that caregiver sensitivity did not predict attachment security. However, and importantly, SBP did, with an effect size *eight times larger* than has been found in large meta-analytic studies of attachment and caregiver sensitivity in low-SES families. These findings raise the clear possibility that Ainsworth's measure fails to include an assessment of the multiple ways parents can provide what their children need to feel safe and loved, even when facing economic and social adversity.

Woodhouse and her colleagues defined SBP as *providing* a secure base for the child's needs for closeness *and* exploration, while at the same time *avoiding* frightening them. The SBP scale was inspired by Cassidy and her colleagues' earlier observation (2005):

> the infants of the low-SES mothers they studied appeared to tolerate a high level of maternal insensitivity and develop a secure attachment to their mothers, as long as two conditions were met: First, certain negative caregiving behaviors must not be present (e.g., frightening or extremely hostile behaviors), particularly during distress when the attachment system is activated. Second, mothers must show behaviorally that they are sufficiently responsive to infant signals related to both aspects of the attachment–exploration balance by ultimately meeting both attachment and exploration needs" (Woodhouse et al., 2020, p. e251)

Thus, apparent insensitivity mattered less than the mother's capacity to support the child's evolutionarily privileged needs for closeness and autonomy and refrain from frightening the child. As such, the SBP scale brings together many aspects of what we have thus far highlighted as key to attachment security: the capacity to support both closeness and exploration, to respond to distress and avoid frightening the child, and to join in the child's delight and pleasure. Woodhouse's SBP measure essentially assesses whether the caregiver is able to assist the child in their evolutionarily privileged efforts to seek closeness, delight, and safety on the one hand and to explore the world on the other. As such, it brings together many aspects of what we have thus far highlighted as key to attachment security: the capacity to support both closeness and exploration, to join in the child's delight and pleasure, to respond to distress and avoid frightening the child. The measure also takes into account the crucial role of fear in disrupting the development of secure attachment.

A final point made by many authors in this special issue is that attachment researchers have generally failed to appreciate the profound impact of discrimination, racial inequity, and systemic racism on African American parents, children, and families (Murry et al., 2022). Up until 2021, many attachment researchers used the "family stress model" (Conger & Elder, 1994) to describe the accumulating stresses on at-risk families. Murry et al. (2022), Coard (2022), and others argue that the concept of stress is simply inadequate to describing the profound impact of relentless and pervasive "bias, racial discrimination and systemic racism on all areas of American family life, particularly parenting, parent–child bonds, and other familial relationships in African American families" (Coard, 2022, p. 373). In light of the contempt, derision, and sheer hatred with which a majority of African American parents have to contend every day, the fact that many have developed myriad and flexible ways to protect, support, and love their children is particularly impressive. As such, it is crucial to identify the strength-based cultural practices that lead to security in the face of threats that have to do only with racist ideologies and historical narratives, and not with a person's essential worth and value. Moving the field toward antiracism will require not only major shifts in perspective but shifts in measurement as well (Stern et al., 2022b).

We return to these issues again in Chapter 6, in which the data make clear that Black and Latinx families face levels of adversity and stress that are qualitatively and quantitatively different from those facing even the most challenged White families. As we consider again and again in the chapters to come, just as these findings have a myriad of implications for social and policy change, they also inevitably shape how we think about our clinical work.

Summary

Identifying the pathways to security was essential to our clinical approach. The first wave of attachment research, along with the work of Stern, Brazelton, Tronick, Beebe, and others, made clear the importance of interactions that give children a sense of their own agency, a sense that they matter and that they are heard. Across cultures, a sensitive parent allows the child a meaningful "place" within the interaction; children are heard, seen, and—to again use Winnicott's term—"held." Today, spurred on in part by the social justice movement, attachment researchers are working to broaden the definition and measurement of sensitive caregiving to be more inclusive and reflective of the multiple ways that caregivers, even in the face of tremendous strain and stress, can support children's needs for closeness and autonomy.

The emphasis on identifying and remedying anomalous parental behavior, behavior that runs contrary to the parent's evolutionary goal of protecting the child, also deeply informed our work by focusing us on the negative consequences of a caregiver—wittingly or unwittingly—scaring the child. As we discuss throughout the rest of this book, this can happen in a variety of ways and for a variety of reasons but is most pernicious when the child is distressed. Its negative consequences for the child's sense of wholeness and safety cannot be overemphasized. Equally critical is the parent's ability to stay present for the child's distress so that they may learn to regulate and tolerate negative emotions such as anger, fear, and sadness.

So much depends upon the parent's own sense of safety and self-worth. The more these are challenged and the parent's or the child's survival is threatened, the more fear floods the attachment–behavioral system, the more difficult it is for caregivers to experience the rewards of parenthood, and the more at risk is the child's sense of the world's essential goodness (Winnicott, 1965). It is much easier to provide security, reflection, and unfettered love, to be "good enough" (Winnicott, 1965), when you yourself are not traumatized, threatened, and afraid.

▲▲▲▲▲▲▲▲   QUESTIONS FOR CLINICIANS   ▲▲▲▲▲▲▲▲

One of the clear paths to a child's sense of safety and belonging is parental behavior. Clinical situations provide multiple opportunities to observe how caregivers respond to the child's needs for closeness and safety on the one hand and for exploring and discovering the world on the other. Here we list some of the phenomena clinicians can look for when observing caregivers and children in interaction. We address ways to approach these therapeutically in Part III.

▶ Is the parent receptive to infant signals? Do they appear attuned to the child's cues?

▶ Does the caregiver follow the child's lead and allow the child agency in the interaction?

▶ Does the caregiver remain emotionally available to the child, both in times of pleasure and distress?

▶ Does the caregiver seem accepting of the child's needs?

▶ Is the caregiver comfortable with close bodily contact?

▶ When the child is distressed or in danger, does the caregiver move to comfort and protect the child?

▶ Alternatively, does the caregiver "abandon" the child in these moments by becoming frightening (menacing, threatening, shaming)? We can think of this as an example of the parent's intense affect overwhelming the child's self-experience (i.e., "too much" on the arousal curve).

▶ Or does the caregiver "abandon" the child in these moments by becoming frightened, confused, or dissociated? We can think of this as an example of the parent retreating from affective experience, leaving the child to organize their own distress (i.e., "too little" on the arousal curve).

▶ Is affective communication *disrupted* in moments of distress? Do you see signs of mixed signals from the caregiver? For example, the child appears to be smiling, but upon closer observation, it becomes obvious that there is fear or distress in their eyes. Or the mother is laughing while poking the child, who is clearly uncomfortable (though likely smiling weakly).

▶ Does the caregiver support the child's needs for exploration of the larger world? Do they invite the child to try new things, to widen the circle of discovery?

▶ Do you observe moments of mutual delight between parent and child?

▶ In highly stressed parents, do you see evidence of their helping the child adapt positively to the larger and potentially hostile environment?

▶ Do you see evidence of extended caregiving support networks that can provide additional sources of protection, comfort, and discovery for the child?

Chapter

4

Pathways to Secure Attachment

PARENTAL MENTALIZING

In this chapter and the next, we turn to another relational pathway to attachment security: parental mentalizing. The study of mentalizing processes—which was pioneered by Peter Fonagy, Miriam Steele, Howard Steele, and Mary Target (Fonagy et al., 1991b, 1995, 2002; Fonagy & Target, 1996, 1997; Steele & Steele, 2008)—grew out of an effort to understand the very same questions that had dominated attachment research for decades: What are the relational antecedents of a child's capacity to be open, trusting, and engaged in the world? What are the relational factors that establish the foundation for secure attachment in the child and the orientation to people and to learning that the term *security* implies? Fonagy and his colleagues' work began with the identification of the critical role of a parent's reflective functioning (RF)—the ability to consciously reflect upon or reason about mental states—in creating the context for secure attachment (Fonagy et al., 1991b, 1995). They soon came to see RF as but one manifestation of a more general *underlying* capacity, that of *mentalizing* (Fonagy & Target, 1997, 1998); namely, the capacity to envision the contents of one's own or another's mind, to keep minds in mind.[1] Later, Dana Shai (Shai & Belsky, 2011, 2017) identified mentalizing

---

[1] In this chapter, we focus primarily on parental RF, as measured by the Parent Development Interview (PDI), the Pregnancy Interview (PI), and the Parental Reflective Functioning Questionnaire (PRFQ). We also focus on mentalization-in-action, as exemplified by the work of Shai and her colleagues (Shai & Belsky, 2011, 2017; Shai et al., 2017) and Ensink and her colleagues (Ensink et al., 2017b). Meins and her colleagues' measure of mind-mindedness (Meins et al., 2001) and Oppenheim and Koren-Karie's

processes in parental behavior, which she termed *parental embodied mentalization* (PEM). Thus what began as a study of parental language evolved into a much broader consideration of mentalizing as it is manifest across a range of contexts. As we describe in this chapter, research has consistently linked parental mentalizing with attachment security, as well as a range of other positive outcomes. This oriented us to the importance of supporting parental mentalizing, beginning as early in the caregiver–child relationship as possible, and led us to develop clinical approaches aimed specifically at enhancing these capacities. We describe each of these developments in this chapter, but first we begin by defining mentalizing.

Mentalizing: A Definition

As human beings,[2] one of the most natural things we do is try to understand one another. It is essential to our survival. This is what makes it possible for us to get along, to connect with others, and—in so doing—to discover our own humanity. To quote Marvin Gaye's 1971 song "What's Going On?," we want to know: "What's going on? Talk to me, so we can see, what's going on. . . . " Making sense of others underlies our ability to love, and build the relationships that anchor our lives. It also allows us to make sense of ourselves, how we feel, and who we are. Peter Fonagy—in collaboration with numerous colleagues, most prominently Mary Target, Miriam and Howard Steele, Jon Allen, Anthony Bateman, and Patrick Luyten (Allen, 2012, 2013; Bateman & Fonagy, 2004; Fonagy et al., 1991a, 1991b, 1995, 2002; Fonagy & Target, 1996, 1997; Luyten & Fonagy, 2015; Steele & Steele, 2008)—described this critical interpersonal capacity as *mentalizing,* or the capacity to envision or imagine our own or another's "mental states," namely, thoughts, feelings, desires, beliefs, and intentions. It is an awareness of one's own and others' internal, mental, subjective life. Whether conveyed behaviorally or through conscious reflection, the capacity to process (observe, respond to, reflect upon) what is going on in our own or another's mind gives rise to a *mentalizing stance.* "I am interested in what is in my mind and yours. I want to know you, I see you, I am curious about you, I am open to you" can all be communicated in a tilt of the

---

measure of parental insightfulness (Insightfulness Assessment [IA]; Koren-Karie et al., 2002; Oppenheim & Koren-Karie, 2013) also measure parental mentalizing capacities. See Zeegers et al. (2017) for a full review. A number of researchers have also studied parental representations of the child, using the Working Model of the Child Interview (WMCI; Zeanah et al., 1986). See Vreeswijk et al. (2012) for a review.

[2]Several primate species also show evidence of rudimentary mentalizing capacities (Hrdy, 2009).

head, an opening of the chest, and a softening of the eyes, or in words or conscious reflection.

To return to Sally Provence's words: "Don't just *do* something. Stand there and pay attention. Your child is trying to tell you something." A "good-enough" parent asks, in *one way or another,* enough of the time: "*What is that something, and how can I address/ameliorate/regulate/ understand it? Let me try to imagine what you are feeling so I can figure out what you need to help you feel better.*" The stance of curiosity, of wondering about the child's experience allows the parent(s) to implicitly or explicitly ask the child: "*Who are you, what happened, what do you feel, what do you need, and how can I help?*" This stance also allows parents to ask the same of themselves: "*Who am I, what happened to me, what do I feel, and what do I need?*" The parents respond with warmth, comfort, and support *because they can see, feel, and understand what the child is feeling and thinking, what the child needs.* They are able to *mentalize.*

Pasco Fearon and his colleagues (Fearon et al., 2006a) offer this wonderful description of a mentalizing stance:

> The heart of good mentalizing is not so much the capacity to always accurately read one's own or another's inner states, but rather a way of approaching relationships that reflects an expectation that one's own thinking and feeling may be enlightened, enriched and changed by learning about the mental states of other people . . . mentalizing is more like an attitude than a skill, an attitude that is inquiring and respectful of other people's mental states, aware of the limits of one's knowledge of others, and reflects a view that understanding the feelings of others is important for maintaining healthy and mutually rewarding relationships. (p. 214)

This quote makes so clear the pleasures of a mentalizing relationship. Imagine a world in which we all treated each other in this way!

A Note about the Term *Mentalizing*

Unfortunately, *mentalization* is an "ungainly" (Holmes, 2010) term. It sounds mechanistic and would seem to favor thinking (i.e., mentation) over feeling (Allen, 2013). However, the term actually refers to both "thinking about feeling and feeling about thinking" (Mary Target, personal communication, December 11, 2003), as it relies on a number of both prefrontal and more emotional centers of the brain (Luyten & Fonagy, 2015). The ungainliness of the term *mentalizing* is, in part, why many clinicians prefer to use the terms *reflection* or *reflective capacities*; certainly, these are more user-friendly and intuitively obvious to both professionals and parents. Indeed, we describe MTB-P as a "reflective parenting" approach, and we use these terms frequently throughout the book. But it is important to recognize that, although they are conflated throughout the literature (and, regrettably, likely at points in this book), mentalization and reflection are not synonymous. As we mentioned earlier and describe more fully in this chapter, reflection typically refers to a more conscious process that relies upon a certain amount of cortical processing (Luyten & Fonagy, 2015). Mentalizing, by contrast, refers to the more general underlying psychological capacity that makes both reflection and behavioral sensitivity possible. One can reflect on what to eat for dinner or to plant in the garden,[3] whereas *mentalizing* is a term that is reserved for making sense of states of *mind*. By describing MTB as *reflective* and as aimed at promoting *reflective* parenting, we have chosen the more familiar, benign term that aligns nicely with the focus on reflective practice and reflective supervision in infant mental health work (Fenichel, 1992; Gilkerson, 2004; Heffron & Murch, 2010). Nevertheless, we recognize that the term *reflection* is inherently less specific and descriptive than *mentalizing*. As such, it does not really capture the range of psychological processes that are key to positive child and parent outcomes, and that can become atrophied and distorted in the face of trauma and other severe relational disruptions (Fonagy et al., 1995).

Mentalizing and Distress

Mentalizing is most difficult in times of distress. Fear, anger, and significant stress trigger the primitive "emotional brain" (LeDoux, 1996), namely, the amygdala and other parts of the limbic system. Strong emotion disables the parts of the brain that are essential to mentalizing; the more upset we are, the harder it is to reflect (Mayes, 2006), to think and feel straight. And yet these are the moments when we most need to do so. Allen (2013) describes this as the "mentalizing Catch-22," namely, that "you most need to mentalize when you are least capable of doing it" (p. 241). This has special relevance to parenting, when stress and distress—both the caregiver's and the child's—are inevitable and frequent.

> Imagine a father who is trying to simultaneously get his toddler son and restless dog out for a walk. The baby was awake several times in the night, and everyone is exhausted. At the precise moment they're about to set out, the mailman arrives, and the dog barks frantically and pulls at the leash. The toddler bursts into tears. He clings to his dad and starts to wail. Naturally, the father's stress level rises, and it takes all his self-control not to yell at his son to stop crying and yank at the dog's collar with force. But he is able to keep the

---

[3] We thank Jon Allen for his very helpful comments on how to think about and use these terms.

child's fear and exhaustion, as well as the dog's territorial instincts, in mind. This gives him a handle on a stressful situation.

This is a very benign, everyday example. Imagine a situation in which the stakes are much higher. The more stress builds, the harder it is to keep the big picture in mind, to stay physically calm and emotionally regulated. And the harder it is to keep the other—in this case, the child—in mind.

Mentalizing and Pleasure

In Chapter 2, we noted that secure relationships not only guarantee safety but bring pleasure and reward in closeness as well. The same can be said of mentalizing. It is very pleasurable to understand another and to *be* understood, and so often it makes us closer to one another. Imagine a toddler taking her first steps. She is absolutely thrilled. The parent, waiting with outstretched arms, feels the same thrill and delight. *"You really wanted to get up and WALK! You DID it! Wow!! YAY!!!!!"* Singular pleasure becomes mutual, shared joy, deepened for them both. Or imagine that mother who figures out that her baby is crying because he thinks Mom is about to leave. *"Oh, no, baby, I just went in the other room to get something. Let's have a hug."* The child soon relaxes and smiles, again ready for play. He is rewarded by feeling known; Mom "got" what was wrong. And Mom is rewarded not only with a big smile but with the knowledge that she made a difference, she helped. She feels like a good mother. In this way, mentalizing is essential not only to distress and stress regulation but also to the establishment, maintenance, and deepening of pleasure in connection and closeness. As such, as we discuss in subsequent sections of this chapter and throughout this book, it might well be considered a resilience (Berthelot et al., 2015) or protective factor in the intergenerational transmission of attachment and trauma.

The Relational Roots of Mentalizing Capacities

"Mutual understanding" (Hrdy, 2009) grows out of relationships and from the humans who teach us how to care and be with others. The capacity to mentalize is "prewired" for its survival value; the vast majority of infants are born with a readiness to attend to the minds of others, scanning eyes and mouths and bodies from the first days of life (Porges, 2011). The full development of mentalization takes years, however, and depends upon a range of cognitive and other neural capacities, as well as safe and loving relationships. In a secure or "good enough" attachment relationship, the parent is—from the very start—engaged with and responsive to the child's internal experience, actively trying to make sense of what the child might be thinking and feeling, to organize, regulate, name, and contingently respond to the child's cues. The parent's observations of the moment-to-moment changes in the child's mental states—namely, what is going on in the child's mind—and their representation of these, first in gesture and action and later in words and play, are at the heart of sensitive caregiving and are crucial to the child's ultimately developing mentalizing capacities of their own. The parent who can, in action and in words, make sense of a broad range of the child's experiences is most likely to have a child who feels safe and secure coming to know themselves and to know others. By contrast, the child whose parent amplifies some experiences and denies others (and all parents do this to some extent) will have a less textured view of their mental life and a potential sense of threat and danger in relation to certain affects and experiences. Gergely, Fonagy, and their colleagues have described these iterative processes as "marking," such that the parent mirrors and expands upon the child's emotion expressions, re-presenting the child *to themselves* as having feelings, desires, and intentions (Gergely & Watson, 1996; Fonagy et al., 2002). As Winnicott (1971) put it: "The mother gazes at the baby in her arms, and the baby gazes at his mother's face and finds himself therein" (p. 89).

An atmosphere of calm, interpersonal sharing and the sense of being known and heard allows the child to trust the myriad kinds of information and knowledge the parent provides (Fonagy & Allison, 2014); together, parent and child can make sense of the world together, collaborating in a "we" mode, or relational mentalizing (Fonagy et al., 2021; Gallotti & Frith, 2013). The child comes to trust the parent's view of him or her, to trust and incorporate the parent's view that there can be safety and pleasure in the broader world. In insecure attachments, the child's cues are ignored or distorted; as such, they cannot be seen and do not become fully known, and the child's experience is refracted through the parent's projections and misattributions. As a result, the child's mentalizing potential can be distorted or—in extreme instances—atrophy altogether.

Parental Reflective Functioning

The First Studies: RF on the AAI

The empirical study of mentalizing processes began when Peter Fonagy, Miriam Steele, and Howard Steele set out to replicate Main's finding that attachment could be transmitted across generations, from parent to child. They began their study in pregnancy and administered AAIs to mothers and fathers before their babies were born. They found—as had Main and her colleagues (1985)—that securely attached parents were more likely to have securely attached children, as measured by the SSP when their children were 1 year old (Fonagy et al., 1991a). Importantly, their work did not end there. As psychoanalytic clinicians, they wondered what internal psychological processes might *underlie* the hallmarks of secure adult attachment on the AAI. In other words, what *within* the parent makes it possible for an adult to describe their experiences in a coherent, emotionally vital way? Studying the transcripts closely, Fonagy, Steele, and Steele discovered that adults differed in the capacity to think about their *own parents'* psychological lives, motivations, intentions, and desires. Whereas some parents had a rich and dimensional sense of their own and their parents' inner lives, others defaulted to banal explanations, to projection, or to dismissing affective experience altogether (Fonagy et al., 1991b, 1995; Steele & Steele, 2008). They also differed in their capacity to wonder about *their own* experiences as children and to make sense of themselves in terms of their own thoughts and feelings, or mental states. Fonagy et al. (1998) termed this the capacity for "reflective functioning" (RF), namely, the capacity to reflect upon or reason about mental states and to understand behavior in light of mental states.

The RF Scale for the AAI

On the basis of their observations, Fonagy, the Steeles, and Target developed a scale to measure the level of RF, which they applied to the AAIs of parents who had participated in their research. Individual questions and the overall interview receive a score from low to high RF, from the denial or distortion of mental states (thoughts, feelings, and intentions) to high and fluid, complex, and sophisticated reflection about mental states (Fonagy et al., 1998).

Reflective Functioning Scale (RFS)

Prementalizing

–1 Bizarre, hostile, or negative RF

1 Disavowed or absent mental states

The Foundations of Reflective Functioning

3 Identifying thoughts and feelings

Reflective Functioning

5 Average RF; reflecting on the nature and impact of thoughts and feelings

7 Complex or sophisticated RF

9 Exceptional RF

The lower scale points (–1 through 2) are meant to capture various forms of *prementalizing,* namely, the inability to describe one's own or another's mental states. Here references to one's own or others' internal states are either missing altogether or are inaccurate, malevolent, or bizarre. At the lowest end of the scale (–1) are frankly bizarre or extremely hostile attributions or projections. *Disavowal* (1) refers to the absence of language for mental states, the denial of mental states, or lesser forms of intrusive mentalizing. We describe prementalizing processes more fully in Chapter 5.

The next level, *identifying thoughts and feelings* (3), marks the emergence of a rudimentary capacity to recognize mental states and refers to the individual's capacity to name internal experiences ("I want," "I know," "I feel sad/joyful/angry/confused," etc.). Importantly, the capacity to identify thoughts and feelings, although a critical building block in the development of the capacity to mentalize, *is not indicative of RF.* One cannot mentalize without having the capacity to identify internal experience, but one can identify internal experience without having the capacity to mentalize. Clinically, we often see parents begin to name their own or the child's thoughts and feelings as treatment proceeds; it is yet another step to actually mentalize.

Level 5 marks the transition to true RF, namely, the capacity to recognize the *nature* and *impact* of mental states on the self or other. For example, a mother realizes that she cannot be sure what her child is thinking or feeling but is prepared to guess. Or a father realizes that his son has thrown his toys across the room because he is angry that his dad has to go to work. Or a mother realizes that her own sadness is having an impact on her child, who is seeming lethargic and unhappy. In all these instances, the parent is not only recognizing the presence of thoughts or feelings but also reasoning about them and understanding their dynamic and interpersonal properties. Higher levels (6 and above) refer to increasingly complex types of reflection, in particular the capacity to describe mixed or extremely painful emotion and the awareness of interaction and interplay between one's own mental states and those of others. Trevarthen (1979) referred to this as "intersubjectivity," the recognition that subjective, internal states can be shared (Stern, 1985) and mutually influence each other (Tronick, 2007).

Fonagy and his colleagues first used the scale to examine whether differences in RF predicted differences in adult or child attachment. They hypothesized that a parent's reflective capacities would predict both their own attachment security as well as their child's. Indeed, they found that parents with high levels of RF on the AAI were more likely to be classified as secure on the AAI; they were also more likely to have a secure child (Fonagy et al., 1995). Importantly, RF was more predictive of overall AAI classification than was the coherence scale of the AAI. These findings led them to suggest that what Main had described as the hallmarks of adult security—coherence, emotional authenticity, affect tolerance—were, in fact, manifestations of the capacity to reflect upon, tolerate, and integrate complex thoughts and emotions. They also proposed that this particular ability is also what allows a parent to be sensitive and to respond in ways that ensure the child's security and that it is thus at the heart of the inter-generational transmission of attachment (Fonagy et al., 1995).

PRF on the Parent Development Interview

Fonagy and his colleagues' scale was designed for use with the AAI; thus a high score referred to the adults' capacity to reflect upon their child-hood experiences with their parents. A group of us—Arietta Slade, John Grienenberger, Elizabeth Bernbach, Dahlia Wohlgemuth Levy, and Alison Locker—reasoned that evaluating the parent's capacity to reflect upon the *mind of the child* would be more relevant to child and parenting outcomes than their capacity to reflect upon their own childhood experiences. That is, we made a distinction between more general reflective capacities (as measured by the AAI) and *parental* RF (PRF), namely, the parent's capac-ity to mentalize about the child and about themselves as a parent (Slade, 2005). We measured PRF using the Parent Development Interview (PDI; Aber et al., 1985[4]; Slade et al., 2004a), which we scored using an adapta-tion (Slade et al., 2004b) of Fonagy and his colleagues' RF scale (Fonagy et al., 1998). The PDI is a semistructured interview that focuses on the parent or caregiver's[5] view of the child, of their relationship, and of themselves as a parent. Parents are asked to reflect upon the child's feelings, as well as their own emotional experience of parenting, and to consider how their own childhood experiences influence their parenting. This interview appears in Appendix I in this book.

Our goal in shifting to an assessment of PRF (Luyten et al., 2020; Slade, 2005) was to focus specifically on the parent's capacity to reflect upon the live, complex, and emotionally intense relationship with their child, and particularly the strong emotions intrinsic to parenthood, rather than upon past experiences that were likely to be somewhat less activating. Thus PRF refers specifically to parents' *conscious* reflections on the child's mental states, or thoughts, feelings, desires, and intentions. It also refers to parents' capacity to make sense of and nondefensively envision both their

---

[4]The PDI was developed by J. Lawrence Aber, Arietta Slade, Brenda Berger, Ivan Bresgi, and Merryle Kaplan (Aber et al., 1985). It was revised in 2004 (Slade et al., 2004a). This is the version used in all of the research described here.

[5]The interview can be given to any of the child's caregivers. It has also been used with teachers and other child care providers (Stacks et al., 2013)

own and their child's mental states (Fonagy et al., 1995; Slade, 2005; Luyten et al., 2017b). This is distinct from (though, as shown below, closely related to) caregiver sensitivity, which refers to what parents *do* as opposed to what they *consciously think and say* about their experience of the relationship. In the following sections, we describe research that assesses PRF using the PDI (Slade et al., 2004a), the Pregnancy Interview (PI; Slade, 2003), and the Parental Reflective Functioning Questionnaire (PRFQ; Luyten et al., 2009; Luyten et al., 2017a). We discuss the clinical applications of the PDI and PI in Chapter 13. As will be obvious throughout the rest of this book, however, as useful as interviews and questionnaires can be, listening for and enhancing PRF in clinical material is a consistent focus of MTB-P. And it is at the heart of reflective practice.

In our first study with a low-risk sample of 40 mothers and babies, we used the PDI to measure PRF at 10 months (Slade et al., 2005). It was significantly associated with both maternal attachment (measured prenatally using the AAI) and child attachment (measured using the SSP at 14 months). In addition, PRF was linked to attachment categories in theoretically meaningful ways. Free/autonomous mothers had significantly higher PRF scores than dismissing, preoccupied, and unresolved mothers, and both dismissing and preoccupied mothers had higher PRF scores than unresolved mothers. Thus maternal adult attachment security and high PRF were strongly associated, whereas insecure and, particularly, preoccupied and unresolved attachment were associated with lower PRF. In addition, mothers of secure infants had significantly higher PRF scores than those of either resistant or disorganized children. Finally, PRF mediated the relationship between adult and child attachment, meaning that the mother's RF was, in effect, the vehicle whereby the parent's security (or insecurity) was transmitted to the child. Though this was a small study, our results supported Fonagy's suggestion (Fonagy et al., 1995) that PRF might help explain some more of what van IJzendoorn (1995) described as "transmission gap" between adult and child security.

In a second study carried out with the same sample, Grienenberger and his colleagues (2005) examined the relationship between disrupted dyadic affective communication using the AMBIANCE measure developed by Lyons-Ruth and her colleagues (Bronfman et al., 1992–2008) and PRF. Recall from Chapter 3 that high levels of disrupted affective communication (manifest in a range of anomalous maternal behaviors) were associated with infant disorganization in Lyons-Ruth's original study (Lyons-Ruth et al., 1999b). Grienenberger and his colleagues (2005) found that PRF was inversely correlated with disrupted affective communication; thus mothers with high PRF were highly unlikely to show signs of disrupted affective communication with their 10-month-old infants. These results suggest that PRF mitigates a parent's tendency to respond in hostile, disruptive, and frightening ways and that reflective capacities are most helpful in managing negative emotional states and interpersonally charged situations. This aligns with Beebe and her colleagues' (2010) finding that the parents of secure children remain present in moments of distress.

Finally, maternal anomalous behavior was found to mediate the relationship between PRF and infant attachment, suggesting that maternal behavior might *also* be an important vehicle for the intergenerational transmission of attachment. And, indeed, as will be clear from the following review, researchers have consistently found that *both* PRF and contingent and nonthreatening parental behavior are essential aspects of providing a secure base for the child and lay the groundwork for secure attachment, resilience, and a range of other positive outcomes (Zeegers et al., 2017). That is, both explicit (verbal) and implicit (behavioral) forms of mentalization are the *mechanisms* whereby the parent's orientation to affects, intimacy, autonomy, and people becomes an intrinsic part of the child's experience of affects, intimacy, autonomy, and people. These are likely highly reciprocal and transactional processes, such that reflection promotes sensitivity and diminishes negative affective communication and positive, reciprocal, and pleasurable interactions reinforce reflection. It is for this reason that throughout this book we emphasize that *both* should be the focus of clinical intervention. Promoting maternal synchronous and responsive behavior while ameliorating negative parental behaviors, *as well as* encouraging PRF, are thus critical to the MTB-P approach.

Research Using the PDI: Subsequent Studies

A number of studies have since replicated and expanded upon Slade, Grienenberger, and their colleagues' original findings, affirming the direct impact of PRF on a number of child outcomes, its relationship to a range of parental variables, and—perhaps most important—its role in mediating or moderating the link between both parent and child variables on the one hand and child outcomes on the other (Slade & Sleed, 2023). This literature also provides the theoretical and empirical foundation for the development of reflective parenting programs (Slade, 2002, 2007).

Child and Parent Correlates of PRF

PRF and Child Outcomes

A number of studies have linked PRF on the PDI to child attachment (Borelli et al., 2016; Stacks et al., 2014), child RF (Ensink et al., 2016), adolescent RF (Benbassat & Priel, 2012), and preschoolers' emotion understanding (Jessee, 2020). Lower PRF has been associated with child behavior problems (Ensink et al., 2016; Ensink et al., 2017a). As had been the case in our original research, PRF was found to mediate the link between adult and child attachment (Borelli et al., 2016), and the link between PRF and child attachment was mediated by maternal sensitivity (Stacks et al., 2014). PRF was also found to moderate the link between infant negative affect and toddler behavior problems (Wong et al., 2017) and to moderate the link—in both mothers and fathers—between parental warmth and adolescent social self-perception (Benbassat & Priel, 2012).

PRF and Parental Behavior and Representation

PRF and maternal behavior have been linked in several studies. Stacks and her colleagues (2014) found that parenting sensitivity was positively associated with PRF, whereas parenting negativity was associated with lower PRF. Nancy Suchman,[6] who pioneered a mentalization-based intervention for mothers with substance use disorders and their toddlers, distinguished between a mother's capacity to reflect upon her own experiences as a parent (Self-RF) and her capacity to reflect upon her child's experience (Child-RF). She and her colleagues (2010) found that Self-RF was linked to mothers' sensitivity to cues and capacity to engage in ways that fostered the child's socioemotional growth and cognitive development. Two studies have linked RF on the PDI with RF on the AAI (Crumbley, 2009; Steele et al., 2008). Researchers have also linked PRF to the quality of parental representations. Schechter and his colleagues (2005) found that PRF was associated with balanced representations of the child on the Working Model of the Child Interview (WMCI; Zeanah et al., 1986) and Huth-Bocks and her colleagues (2014) linked PRF to secure-base scripts in a storytelling task.

PRF, Parental IQ, and Executive Functioning

PRF is a form of "controlled" mentalizing that involves the use of the prefrontal cortex and a range of executive functions (Luyten & Fonagy, 2015). Unsurprisingly, then, in a major validation study of the PDI, Sleed and her colleagues (2018) found that PRF was linked to IQ. Women with higher nonverbal IQ scores were likely to have a broad range of PRF scores, whereas those with scores at the low end of the nonverbal IQ range had significantly less variability in their PRF scores. PRF has also been linked to executive functioning (EF). Two studies suggest that PRF is affected by deficits in working memory, inhibition, cognitive flexibility, and planning (Håkansson et al., 2018a; Yatziv et al., 2020). However, EF plays less of a

---

[6]We so miss our brilliant, generous, and spirited colleague, who died on December 25, 2020.

role when a parent is making quick judgments about the mind of the child (Yatziv et al., 2020). Such quick judgements are likely a form of "automatic" mentalizing (Luyten & Fonagy, 2015) that is unmediated by cortical processing, and would thus be less likely to involve executive functions. We will return to a discussion of automatic mentalizing later in the chapter.

The finding that higher levels of PRF are linked to IQ and EF must be understood within a broader context, however. Sleed and her colleagues (2018) found that mothers struggling with mental health difficulties (anxiety, depression, personality disorders) tended to have both low PRF and low nonverbal IQ. This underscores the fact that emotional problems can impair aspects of intellectual functioning. Håkansson and colleagues (2018a) also found that associations between EF and PRF were no longer significant in a sample of mothers with substance use disorders when IQ and mental health difficulties were controlled for in a regression analysis. This suggests that the capacity to mentalize and to make use of a range of executive functions are affected both by significant limitations in IQ and by mental health difficulties. Thus parents who are cognitively impaired, as well as those with significant mental health problems, will show lower levels of PRF on the PDI. As we will discuss later in this chapter, these parents' mentalizing capacities may be better evaluated by nonverbal measures such as parental embodied mentalization (PEM; Shai & Belsky, 2011, 2017), or reflective parenting in action (Ensink et al., 2017b).

PRF and Socioeconomic Risk

A number of socioeconomic risk factors have also been associated with lower levels of PRF, including level of education (Benbassat & Priel, 2012; Huber et al., 2015; Sleed et al., 2018; Stover & Kiselica, 2014), income level (Yatziv et al., 2020), marital status (Borelli et al., 2016), and maternal age, such that older mothers are likely to have higher PRF (Sleed et al., 2018). Stacks et al. (2014) found that a composite measure of socioeconomic risk (including single parenthood, maternal age of less than 21 years, less than a high school education, and annual income less than U.S. $20,000) was inversely linked to PRF. In the only study to specifically examine the relationship between race and PRF (Borelli et al., 2016), parents identifying as Latinx or Black had lower Child-RF. However, when annual income was controlled for, the link between race and PRF was no longer significant. This finding—like those we discussed in Chapter 3, in which sensitivity is linked with attachment when socioeconomic risk is controlled for—suggests that race, per se, does not affect PRF, while also making evident that, in the absence of structural supports or other strengths, the socioeconomic risks that are endemic in marginalized and oppressed populations who are living below the poverty line and exposed to a range of cumulative traumas and adversity *do* affect parental mentalizing capacities.

PRF and Clinical Risk

The most comprehensive study of clinical risk is Sleed and her colleagues' (2018) large-scale study comparing PRF outcomes across three samples with varying levels of clinical risk (*N* = 323). The researchers found that mothers in the three different risk groups had significantly different PRF levels. Specifically, the mothers in a sample of incarcerated women had significantly lower PRF than did those in the clinical and normative groups, and the clinical group had significantly lower PRF than the normative group. It is important to note that there was considerable variation across the three groups in socioeconomic and cognitive risk. Mothers in the prison sample "were younger, less educated, had more female babies and were more likely to self-identify as Black. The children in the normative group were significantly older than those in the two other samples, and mothers in the normative group had a significantly higher nonverbal IQ than mothers in the clinical group" (Sleed et al., 2018, pp. 314–315). The normative group also differed from the clinical group on a range of social exclusion and deprivation criteria, such as income support, unemployment, and so forth.

Researchers have consistently reported lower levels of PRF in parents with substance use disorders (Håkansson et al., 2018b; Levy, 2004; Suchman et al., 2010), in those who have themselves been sexually abused (Ensink et al., 2017a), and those who are victims of domestic violence (Huber et al., 2015; Schechter et al., 2005; Stover & Kiselica, 2014). Håkansson et al. (2018b) also reported that mothers with substance use disorders who had suffered high levels of adversity in childhood (emotional, physical, and sexual abuse and neglect) had lower levels of PRF than those who had less trauma exposure, whereas those who reported high levels of adaptive experiences (feeling safe, competent, and cared for) had higher PRF scores than mothers who had fewer adaptive experiences. Without exception, all of these samples were drawn from low-income populations with high levels of socioeconomic risk.

Once again, we find a conflation of risk factors in much of this research, making it virtually impossible to tease apart the effects of socioeconomic risk (poverty, minoritized status), mental health status, and IQ on the development of parents' capacity to mentalize. This brings us back to the question of context, and particularly to the question of the multiple ways that stress, be it from a lack of social, economic, and educational resources, from ongoing exposure to adversity, trauma, and systemic racism, or from the weight of psychiatric disturbance (which may stem in part from cumulative stress and oppression), profoundly affects a parent's capacity to remain curious and open to the child's experience. This might lead to the conclusion that it is not valid to use a measure like PRF in populations with high levels of socioeconomic or clinical risk. However, as we discuss later in this chapter, intervention research suggests that the *parents most likely to benefit from intervention are those who begin treatment with low levels of PRF. Parents who begin an intervention without evident capacity to imagine their child's experience are those most likely to improve over the course of treatment.*

PRF in Pregnancy: The Pregnancy Interview

The Pregnancy Interview (PI; Slade et al., 1987) was developed by Arietta Slade, Laurie Grunebaum, Mary Reeves, and Alison Ross as we began a project to study the antecedents and sequelae of infant attachment security. The interview (see Appendix II in this book), which was substantially adapted in 2003 (Slade, 2003), invites the expectant mother to reflect on her emotional experience of pregnancy, the ways it has affected her sense of her identity and experience of being parented, and the effect impending parenthood has had on her relationship with the father of the baby and with her family. The interview also invites the mother to describe her relationship with her unborn child and probes her evolving representations of the child and their relationship. Recently, in response to the large numbers of fathers participating in trials of MTB-HV in the United Kingdom and Denmark, we adapted the PI for use with fathers during pregnancy (FaPI; Slade, 2017).

Parents begin to imagine their babies well before birth and likely well before conception (Slade & Cohen, 1996; Solomon & George, 1996), and they begin to mentalize about their infants as they get closer and closer to delivery (Pajulo et al., 2012; Sadler et al., 2016; Slade & Sadler, 2019; Smaling et al., 2015; Smaling et al., 2016a). We defined prenatal PRF as the capacity to describe (1) a relationship with the fetus, recognizing that the child will be a sentient, intentional, and separate being with a mind of their own; and (2) the complexity of the parents' own experiences during the transition to parenthood (Slade et al., 2004c). We scored transcripts using a coding system that—like the PDI–PRF coding system—was based directly upon Fonagy and his colleagues' RF Scale (Fonagy et al., 1998).

Research Using the PI

To date there have been relatively few studies of PRF on the PI, as training in PI–PRF scoring has only recently become available. Hanneke Smaling and her colleagues, working with data collected as part of the Mother–Infant Neurodevelopment Study in the Netherlands, have led the way in this research. They studied a large sample of pregnant women, roughly half of whom were considered high risk (based on presence of a psychiatric diagnosis, substance use, and a range of socioeconomic risks, including low maternal age, low social support, lack of education, single status, unemployment, and poverty). In line with the point we made in the previous section, note that this definition of risk conflates socioeconomic and clinical risks. In their first study (Smaling et al., 2015), prenatal PRF in the low-risk group was significantly higher than RF in the high-risk group; in addition, the more risk factors a woman had, the lower her PRF. In their second study, Smaling and her colleagues (Smaling et al., 2016a) examined the impact of prenatal PRF and accumulated risk on mother–child interactions when babies were 6 months old. Prenatal PRF was positively correlated with more sensitivity and higher levels of positive engagement across a range of interactional contexts and negatively correlated with maternal intrusiveness during a teaching task and with internalizing–helplessness during more challenging tasks. Finally, the relationship between the parent's risk status and behavior was mediated by prenatal PRF. These researchers also found that prenatal PRF (Smaling et al., 2017) and postnatal relationship-focused PRF (Smaling et al., 2016b) were negatively associated with maternal reports of child aggression.

We found similar links between risk and prenatal PRF in our MTB-HV program (Sadler et al., 2013); very few women in our large sample of high-risk pregnant women living in an underresourced community were truly capable of stable, ongoing RF at the start of the intervention. A qualitative analysis of the PIs of 30 pregnant adolescents participating in the MTB randomized clinical trial revealed great variation in their ability to think about and describe the many emotions experienced during pregnancy and how they envisioned caring for their soon-to-be-born infants (Sadler et al., 2016). Differences in level of RF appeared to be linked to a number of factors, among them developmental factors and the quality of teens' relationships with their partners and families. Taken together, these studies make evident that, like postnatal PRF, prenatal PRF is associated with both child outcomes and parental behavior, particularly in the context of high levels of socioeconomic and clinical risk.

PRF over Time

The studies that have examined the relationships between prenatal and postnatal PRF have found PI and PDI scores to be modestly correlated (Pajulo et al., 2012; Sadler et al., 2013; Slade et al., 2019; Smaling et al., 2016b), with PRF improving over time. That PRF improves from pregnancy to the child's infancy makes intuitive sense, as the parent comes to know the child. Whether these changes continue across development is another question. In a small study of the parents of toddlers in a low-risk sample, Poznansky (2010) found that, as PRF scores on the PDI increased as the children moved from late infancy (10 months of age) to late toddlerhood

(28 months of age), the rate of change was predicted by the mother's attachment organization, with secure mothers more stably reflective across the first 28 months of the child's life, whereas insecure mothers had low scores in infancy but "caught up" to the secure mothers by the time the children became toddlers. Mothers whose attachment organization was insecure had more difficulty reading their infants' intentions, and negotiating negative affects when doing so depended on making sense of subtle, nonverbal cues. When the children were toddlers, and cues were more overt and explicit in language, insecure parents looked more reflective. However, close examination revealed that—despite such apparent similarities—insecure mothers were much more likely to focus on struggles with their own and the child's anger and aggression than were secure mothers. Thus the *content* of their reflections were different.

The Parental Reflective Functioning Questionnaire

The Parental Reflective Functioning Questionnaire (PRFQ-1: Luyten et al., 2009; PRFQ-2: Luyten et al., 2017) was developed by Patrick Luyten and his colleagues to more easily and quickly assess PRF, particularly within the context of research. There are two versions of the PRFQ—one with 18 questions and the other with 39. Both are multidimensional assessments of PRF made up of a series of statements such as the following: "My child and I can feel differently about the same thing," "When I get angry with my child, I always know the reason why," "I am often curious to find out how my child feels," "How I am feeling can affect how I understand my child's behavior." The parent rates each on a 5-point scale, from "strongly disagree" to "strongly agree." These questions were derived from the key aspects of PRF described by Fonagy et al. (1998) and Slade (2005). Although it was initially designed for use with parents of children under 3, researchers (Mazzeschi et al., 2019; Pazzagli et al., 2018, 2019; Rostad & Whitaker, 2016) have since used the instrument with parents of children as old as 11 years of age.

Factor analyses of questionnaire responses led to the identification of three distinct factors of PRF (Luyten et al., 2017): (1) interest in and curiosity about (IC) the child's mental states, (2) certainty about mental states (CMS), and (3) prementalizing modes (PM; e.g., malevolent attributions, inability to enter into the subjective world of the child). Thus, rather than yield, as the PDI does, a single PRF score, the PRFQ yields a score for each factor. As we discuss in Chapter 5, the identification of distinct aspects of parental mentalization (or the lack thereof) allows for a more nuanced assessment of how specific elements of parental mentalization affect a range of outcomes. Luyten and his colleagues (2017) evaluated the factor structure and validity of the PRFQ-39 using data from three separate studies. Factor analyses across three samples with parents from diverse socioeconomic backgrounds (N = 600) validated the PM, CMS, and IC factor structure with both mothers and fathers, with factor items loading somewhat differently for mothers and fathers. A recent validation study of the PRFQ confirmed these factors for the 18-item version (De Roo et al., 2019). Across the three validation studies, maternal PM (which we discuss more fully in Chapter 5) was most consistently correlated with indices of insecure attachment in both mother and infant and with parenting stress. It was also most associated with demographic variables such as maternal education and working hours. IC was positively correlated with infant attachment security, as well. In summarizing their work, Luyten and his colleagues (2017) underscore a point that we have made throughout this book, namely, "that genuine interest and curiosity in the mental states of one's infant, and the relative absence of prementalizing modes of reflecting about the mental interior of one's infant, is conducive to the development of attachment security in the infant" (p. 21). A number of studies lend support to Luyten and his colleagues' findings linking parent's interest and curiosity in the child's mental states and positive outcomes, on the one hand, and prementalization and negative outcomes, on the other (Condon et al., 2019a; Krink et al., 2018; Mazzeschi et al., 2019; Pazzagli et al., 2019; Rostad & Whitaker, 2016; Rutherford et al., 2015, 2017, 2018; Schulteis et al., 2019). Pajulo and her colleagues have also developed pre- and postnatal versions of the PRFQ (PPRFQ; Pajulo et al., 2015, 2018).

The Impact of Intervention on PRF

Over the course of the last 10 years, inspired in part by the mentalization-based treatment approach pioneered by Bateman and Fonagy for adults (2004, 2009, 2016), for adolescents (Bleiberg, 2013; Fonagy et al., 2014), and for children and families (Fearon et al., 2006a; Midgley et al., 2017), a number of parent–child intervention programs were developed and tested with the specific aim of raising PRF over the course of treatment. Various forms of intervention were tested, using both the PDI and the PRFQ: home visiting (Condon et al., 2022; Londoño Tobón et al., 2022; Sadler et al., 2013; Slade et al., 2019; Stacks et al., 2019), group interventions (Huber et al., 2015; Lo & Wong, 2022; Menashe-Grinberg et al., 2022; Sleed et al., 2013; Steele et al., 2018), dyadic interventions (Fonagy et al., 2016; Paris et al., 2015), intensive residential interventions (Pajulo et al., 2012), and individual parent interventions (Suchman et al., 2010, 2011, 2017). With the exception of the Anna Freud Center Parent–Infant Program (PIP; Fonagy et al., 2016), where the base rate of PRF was higher than in most of the other programs evaluated, all programs significantly raised PRF over the course of the intervention. PIP did, however, lower indices of hostility and helplessness in parental representations of the child.

There are two interesting aspects to the consistent finding that mentalization-based parenting programs appear to be successful in enhancing PRF. The first is that in a number of studies (Huber et al., 2015; Paris et al., 2015; Sadler et al., 2013; Stacks et al., 2019), PRF increased significantly from intake to graduation only in high-risk mothers. Sadler and her colleagues (2013) and Stacks and hers (2019) found that the interventions were effective in raising PRF only in those mothers who started the intervention in the prementalizing (< 3) range. Huber and her colleagues found similarly that the PRF scores of those mothers who were not yet fully mentalizing (< 5) increased over the course of the intervention, whereas those with scores of 5 and above did not. Interestingly, the PIP participants were relatively high functioning from the start; this may be one of the reasons that the intervention was less effective in raising PRF (Fonagy et al., 2016).

The second interesting aspect of these findings is that in all but the Huber et al. (2015) study, in which the range of scores was wider than in other studies, PRF scores on the PDI were generally low, even at graduation. That is, even though there were significant increases in the scores of high-risk moms across studies, scores at graduation were rarely above a 3.6. This suggests that mothers moved from prementalizing modes into having a basic awareness of thoughts and feelings, but none showed evidence of full mentalizing, which would result in a score of 5. Two of the studies (Stacks et al., 2019; Suchman et al., 2017) also recorded each participant's highest score across the interview; here, too, the highest scores were never fully in the mentalizing range. In none of the studies reviewed here did high-risk parents score in the mentalizing range after completing the intervention. This is a critical finding, for it suggests that the goal of treatment with high-risk parents should not necessarily be mentalizing, per se, but developing a language for thoughts and feelings that will hopefully pave the way for mentalizing over time.

Which to Use: The PDI/PI or the PRFQ/PPRFQ?

Choosing a measure depends, as always, on context and aims. The PDI–PI and the PRFQ–PPRFQ are very different measures; the PDI and PI are in-depth clinical interviews, and the PRFQ and PPRFQ are brief questionnaires. Although time intensive to administer and score, the PDI and PI offer clinicians an opportunity to get a deep sense of the parent and their relationship with the child, including but not restricted to their mentalizing capacities. Often these discussions can set the stage for the long conversation that is the treatment itself. As we describe in Chapters 13 through 16, these interviews can offer critical insights into the parent's psychological organization, insights that can inform supervision and direct the treatment in a number of ways. At the same time, an obvious advantage of the PRFQ and PPRFQ is their brevity. Though they are not clinical tools in the sense that the PDI and PI are, the factor structure of these questionnaires allows clinicians to identify areas that need attention and highlight strengths. For example, a mother with lower levels of prementalizing on the PRFQ is likely at less clinical risk than one whose level of prementalizing is higher. There have been efforts in recent years to build these kinds of distinctions into PDI–PRF scoring (Leroux et al., 2017), but as yet these have not been used outside of small clinical research studies. Importantly, a recent study confirms the convergent validity of the PDI and PRFQ, with the IC and CMS factors correlating with higher levels of PRF and the PM factor correlating with lower levels of RF (Anis et al., 2020). These results suggest that both instruments measure similar phenomena, albeit in different ways.

Embodied Mentalization or Mentalizing in Behavior

Recall that Grienenberger and his colleagues (2005) found that the association between a parent's reflective capacities and the child's security was mediated by parental behavior. Responsive, attuned parental behavior (as opposed to anomalous parental behavior) is one of the ways that parents communicate their appreciation of and engagement with the child's mind. In 2011, Dana Shai (Shai & Belsky, 2011) introduced the idea of implicit or nonverbal mentalizing and suggested that a mentalizing stance could be detected in a parent's bodily responses to their infant's nonverbal cues and intentions (see, too, Tortora, 2005). The assessment of mentalizing need not be confined to what parents say but can also be observed in what they do. Shai and Belsky (2011) described these phenomena as "embodied" or nonverbal mentalizing. They defined "parental embodied mentalization" (PEM), which is measured by observing parents in interaction with infants under 12 months of age, as the ability to "(a) implicitly conceive, comprehend, and extrapolate the infant's mental states from the infant's whole-body movement, and (b) adjust their own kinesthetic patterns accordingly" (p. 173). In the initial concurrent and predictive validation study of PEM, Shai and Belsky (2017) found significant correlations between PEM and maternal sensitivity, attachment security at 15 and 36 months, peer/social competence, language abilities, and academic skills at 54 months. PEM was also negatively correlated with child behavior problems. Shai and her colleagues subsequently published two studies linking PEM to other measures of parental mentalizing, specifically RF on the PDI (Shai et al., 2017), and maternal mind-mindedness (Shai & Meins, 2018), establishing the convergent validity of PEM as a measure of parental mentalization.

In related work, Ensink and her colleagues (Ensink et al., 2017b) developed a scale of "reflective parenting in action" that—like Shai's

PEM—assesses a parent's reflective capacities on the basis of their interaction with, rather than reflections upon, the child and their relationship. The scale's three factors—Reflective Stance, Affectionate Support, and Negative Parenting—were significantly correlated (in the case of Negative Parenting, negatively correlated) with PRF. The authors make the point—entirely consistent with one of the central points of this chapter—that reflective parenting can "best be seen as an orientation or stance that is both implicit in the parent's interactions with the child as well as explicit in the discourse about the child" (Ensink et al., 2017b, p. 585). In other words, it is not simply a matter of how parents consciously reflect on their child's experience but also how they behave in interaction with the child that matters in terms of the child's feeling safe in the world and in their relationships.

Action and Words: Bringing It All Together

Both conscious reflection and interactive behavior reveal the parent's mentalizing capacities. PRF, on the one hand, is an example of what Luyten and Fonagy (2015) refer to as "controlled mentalizing," namely, the "conscious, verbal, and reflective processing of social information . . . that requires the capacity to reflect consciously and deliberately on and make accurate attributions about the emotions, thoughts, and intentions of self and others." Further, it ideally reveals an "accurate and balanced appreciation of a social situation—which relies heavily on the capacity for effortful control and the subtle distinctions language allows us to make" (Luyten & Fonagy, 2015, pp. 368–369). By contrast, *mentalizing in behavior,* namely, caregiver sensitivity or embodied mentalization, are examples of what Luyten and Fonagy (2015) refer to as "automatic" mentalizing, a rapid processing of social information that "is reflexive and requires little effort, focused attention or intention" (Luyten & Fonagy, 2015, p. 368). It originates in parts of the brain that are "primarily involved in threat detection and automatic modulation and processing of (social) information" (Luyten et al., 2017b, p. 180). Such processing occurs out of awareness, a "gut" reaction that has much in common with Porges's (2011) notion of "neuroception," which we describe more fully in Chapter 7. Such automatic reading of the minds of others is our default position, and one that has, of course, considerable evolutionary value. We quickly assess whether another person is safe or dangerous and act accordingly.

Automatic mentalizing can have a positive or a negative bias. Embodied mentalizing (Shai & Belsky, 2011), reflective parenting in action (Ensink et al., 2017b), and caregiver sensitivity (Ainsworth, 1978) would be examples of positive automatic mentalizing. Likewise, an adult or child can "read the room" with the expectation of things being OK, of people in the world being generally benevolent. When stress and arousal build, however (Mayes, 2006), usually as the result of internal or external threats (intense negative feelings, painful interactions with others, larger societal assaults), the world is experienced as dangerous, and more negatively biased automatic mentalizing prevails. The prementalizing modes we describe in the next chapter are examples of negative automatic mentalizing.[7] When these modes prevail, relationships suffer, and—relevant to this book—the parent–child relationship suffers. That is, the presumption of danger or aggression or threat when there is none (or little) can be quite maladaptive, because such modes of processing information are "prone to bias and distortions, particularly in complex interpersonal situations" in which individuals are likely to be upset and aroused (Luyten & Fonagy, 2015, p. 368).

Summary

We have asked the reader to integrate a good deal of complex material in this chapter. To briefly review, the bulk of the research reviewed here focuses on PRF, which is measured by parents' narrative responses to the PI or PDI or by their responses to the PRFQ. Across studies, PRF appears in many ways to serve as the "carrier" of the parent's own history and way of being in the world, supporting Fonagy's original hypothesis that parental reflective capacities underlie—at least in part—the intergenerational transmission of attachment (Fonagy et al., 1995). Time and again, the mediation and moderation analyses reviewed in this chapter make it clear that the parent's capacity to keep the child's mind in mind and to keep their own mind in mind is what allows them to, for example, communicate their own sense of security to the child, regulate their own stress reactions so as to parent in a reciprocal, respectful way, and protect the child from experiencing the abuse that they had suffered. Taken together with the multiple links between PRF and a range of child and parent outcomes, this research makes a very strong case for the importance of focusing on enhancing PRF as essential to deep change in parenting. It also underscores the need to shift from a focus on particular parenting skills to expanding a parent's understanding of and curiosity about the child. Many of the studies reviewed here make the point that when parents are able to identify thoughts and feelings, there are positive impacts on a range of parental behaviors and the child's state of mind about people and relationships. This is the fundamental logic behind the MTB-P approach.

---

[7]As may be nonattuned responses on the maternal mind-mindedness scale (Zeegers et al., 2017).

PRF scores vary little across studies and appear vulnerable to a range of socioeconomic risks. Although this would appear to mitigate against its use as a measure and goal of treatment effects (Barlow et al., 2021), intervention studies have repeatedly shown that raising a parent's PRF even slightly can have a significant impact on the child and on the parent–child relationship. Add to this the fact that parents with the lowest PRF at baseline tend to show the greatest improvements over the course of an intervention. That is, moving from prementalizing modes toward a basic awareness of mental states has an impact on a range of positive outcomes, whereas simply becoming more able to mentalize does not. This finding suggests that mentalization-based interventions may be particularly suitable for high-risk parents whose levels of stress directly interfere with mentalizing processes. These are the parents for whom reflective parenting programs seem particularly effective.

The research we have reviewed here, particularly the work of Grienenberger, Shai, and Ensink, also makes a strong case for closely observing parental behavior, particularly in times of distress. These moments tell us so much. As we mentioned previously, many dyads find pleasure in each other. For clinicians, this can be enormously reassuring and hopeful. But *what happens* to the child, the parent, or within the dyad in moments of conflict and struggle? When there is difficulty, the parent's capacity to attend to it, address it, and ameliorate its effects are key to discovering ways to promote, rather than disrupt, the child's sense of safety, trust, and pleasure in the world. Given today's dominant focus in infant mental health practice on observing and enhancing reflective functioning (Camoirano, 2017; Lo & Wong, 2022; Zeegers, et al., 2017), the importance of watching *what happens* between parent and child can get lost. As we have learned from decades of infant research, there are the small ruptures, a signal gone unnoticed, a tease when there should have been a hug, distress that builds without comfort, a scary glance or harsh grip. These are the "actions and action outcomes" (Main et al., 1985, p. 75) that accrue and coalesce into fear and insecurity.

In sum, there are many ways to observe, measure, and enhance a parent's capacity to make meaning of the child, and of themselves, as a parent and as a person. As illustrated in Figure 4.1, it is this overarching mentalizing dimension that concerns us as clinicians and upon which so many of our interventions are focused.

Up to now, we have focused on what reflective parenting looks and sounds like. But what are the signs that a parent is having difficulty in these areas? In the next chapter, we turn to the question of impaired parental mentalizing and its manifestations. We also discuss mentalization and trauma and, particularly, the ways that developing the capacity to reflect upon traumatic experiences can mitigate some of its negative effects.

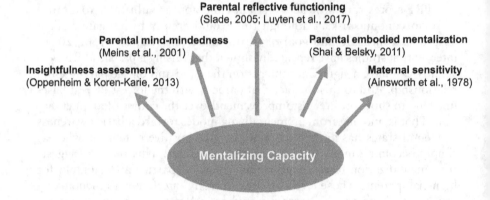

FIGURE 4.1 There are many ways to mentalize.

▲▲▲▲▲▲   QUESTIONS FOR CLINICIANS   ▲▲▲▲▲▲

Parental mentalizing is conveyed in word and deed, in curiosity and respect. As such, there are many opportunities for clinicians to observe a parent's interest in and willingness to adopt a "mentalizing stance" toward the child.

▶ When the parent is talking to or about the child, do you see evidence of an interest in and curiosity about the child's internal experience?

▶ Do parents use mental state words (describing thoughts, feelings, desires, and intentions) to describe their own experience or that of the child? For example, does the parent describe the child as angry? Sad? Or happy and content? Do they describe the child as knowing or sensing or understanding? Similarly, does the parent describe themselves as having thoughts and feelings?

▶ Does the parent appreciate that the child's behavior is a window to their internal states, namely, their thoughts and feelings?

▶ Does the parent appreciate the ways in which their own thoughts and feelings affect the child? And vice versa?

▶ Do you see evidence of curiosity and interest in the parent's bodily stance toward the child? Do they incline themselves toward the child? Do you see nonverbal turn-taking and reciprocal exchanges? Do you see warmth and affectionate support conveyed in the parent's bodily movements?

Chapter

5

Impaired Mentalizing and Trauma

In the last chapter, we made a broad case for the value of parental mentalizing in promoting a range of positive outcomes. However, clinicians are often challenged by the fact that many of the parents we see *struggle* to mentalize, to respond sensitively and reflectively, particularly in moments of distress and conflict. They may be lost in the chaos of their emotions and relationships or haunted by the past. Despite their best efforts and intentions, *seeing* and *hearing* the child may be very difficult; knowing themselves may be equally fraught. In Parts II and III we discuss a variety of approaches to addressing these issues clinically. In this chapter, we bring together the literatures on impaired mentalizing and complex attachment trauma to consider the roots of parents' mentalizing difficulties and describe their clinical manifestations. We address three broad questions: What are the relational roots of disruptions in parental mentalizing? What do impaired mentalizing and traumatized parenting look like? Finally, in what ways can the development of mentalizing capacities be therapeutic, if not transforming?

Throughout this chapter we advance the argument that the more a parent feels threatened—by the ghosts of their own relational trauma and unmet attachment needs, by the child and their needs, and/or by real, external threats to the parent's own agency and survival—the more likely they are to struggle to see and hear the child. When parents are highly stressed, namely, in fight, flight, or freeze mode, when the primitive, automatic parts of the brain are activated by *real or imagined* threats, their capacity to *give* care and fully experience the delights of intimacy will be compromised. We describe the science underlying these responses in Chapter 6, but the point we make in this chapter is that when parents are too activated—often for entirely understandable and human reasons—it is very difficult to keep the child in mind. Finding themselves in a state of "fright without solution" (Hesse & Main, 1999), they are, in whatever way, fighting for their own— and *often the child's*—survival.

The Relational Roots of Impaired Mentalizing

What are the roots of impaired mentalizing? The simplest answer to this, which is borne out by decades of research (Luyten & Fonagy, 2015; Mayes, 2006), is that threats to survival or strong emotion can disable the parts of the brain that are essential to mentalizing, specifically the prefrontal cortex. Recall the "mantra" of mentalization theory: "You can't mentalize when you're upset," that is, really stressed, angry, or emotionally overwhelmed. In the face of fear, helplessness, rage, and utter aloneness (Allen, 2013), mentalization is absent (Fonagy, 1993), paving the way for more primitive mechanisms to take over. In neurobiological terms, when the parts of the brain that register threat or danger (namely, the limbic system, including the amygdala) are highly activated, when arousal, particularly negative arousal, is at its height, the prefrontal cortex, which guides conscious reflection and reasoning, is offline (Mayes, 2006). As we have described in previous chapters, many circumstances can activate the stress response.

In this chapter, we turn specifically to relational, developmental, or attachment trauma (Allen, 2013; van der Kolk, 2014). These are all terms that refer to traumatic experiences with one's primary caregivers (such as abuse or neglect), particularly when these continue over long periods of time and profoundly alter the ability to make meaning of oneself or others. When the person meant to provide care is the "source of alarm" (Main & Hesse, 1990), the terror, rage, and sadness that are the sequelae of trauma can neither be shared nor borne. They cannot be put into words, nor can they be known or felt, leaving the sufferer little recourse other than dissociation, depersonalization, or hyperarousal. These primitive efforts to survive by fleeing, fighting, or freezing also profoundly affect the capacity to make sense of others. As we described in Chapter 4, the child learns to read the mind of the other as a function of being seen and heard. The caregiver who is either profoundly withdrawn from or actively harming the child is, by definition, not seeing the child's need or fear. What the child then sees is not a mirror; rather, they see something terrifying and overwhelming in the parents' eyes, too frightening and deadly to contemplate (Fonagy & Target, 1995). As such, the child will be prone to see the world and the minds of others as frightening and unfathomable.

How do parents' traumatic experiences disrupt the capacity to protect and support their children? Parents who have themselves been traumatized, most particularly at the hands of their caregivers, come to parenthood with two vulnerabilities: (1) They have difficulty regulating strong emotions *as a function of their own attachment trauma*, and (2) the strong emotions evoked by parenthood, and particularly their children's needs and strong feelings, can themselves trigger traumatic memories and primitive ways of coping. Both vulnerabilities predispose them to difficulties seeing, hearing, and coming to know the child. Rather than moving to modulate the child's distress by offering the comfort and safety of reflection, they default to projection or withdrawal, their responses are—as we described in Chapters 2 and 3—"too much," or "too little," frightening–frightened, or hostile–helpless. The mechanisms underlying the intergenerational transmission of insecure attachment are set in motion. As stress builds, the child feels neglected, invaded, or both; all are extremely aversive.

As we noted in Chapter 1, Selma Fraiberg's observation that adults' early relational trauma could have a profound impact on their parenting was to catalyze the infant mental health movement. Fraiberg and her colleagues (1975) argued that children who suffer at the hands of their caregivers survive by, at one and the same time, identifying with their caregivers and suppressing the affect associated with abuse, neglect, or abandonment. They survive by, in a sense, *becoming* their caregivers, thereby obliterating what it feels like to be *them*, alone and frightened. This protects them from the feelings of helplessness and terror that, without parental care, are simply unendurable. When, as parents, they are confronted *with their own* children's helplessness and distress, without access to their own childhood feelings, they are primed to repeat the past. In Fraiberg's own words:

> The key to our ghost story appears to lie in the fate of affects in child-hood. Our hypothesis is that access to childhood pain becomes a pow-erful deterrent against repetition in parenting, while repression and isolation of painful affect provide the psychological requirements for identification with the betrayers and aggressors. The unsolved mystery is why, under conditions of extremity, in early childhood, some children who later become parents keep pain alive; they do not make the fateful alliance with the aggressor which defends the child's ego against intoler-able danger and obliterates the conscious experience of anxiety. (1975, p. 420)

A parent's own relational trauma can make it difficult to recognize and respond to the child's distress. They cannot bridge the troubled waters; rather, the child is left alone with what is often unbearable pain.

Fonagy and his colleagues (Fonagy et al., 1991b; Fonagy & Target, 1997) used a mentalizing framework to expand on this idea. They argued that the child comes to know his or her thoughts, feelings, and intentions through the parent's reflections on them. The parent brings coherence to the "blooming, buzzing confusion" (James, 1890, p. 462) of the child's earliest experiences by organizing and attuning to them. In so doing, the parent gives the baby "back his own self" (Winnicott, 1967, p. 33). The child discovers themselves in the parent's eyes. But when parents are not able to "see" the child, usually because the child's negative affects threaten the defenses that the parent long ago erected against their *own* negative affects, the child must conform to the parent's view of them. This is Winnicott's (1965) "false self." The child is left with no choice but to take on "the mind of the other, with its distorted, absent or malign picture of the child" as part of their own sense of identity (Fonagy & Target, 1995, p. 494). As Winnicott (1967) put it:

> What does the baby see when he or she looks at the mother's face? . . . ordinarily, the mother is looking at the baby and what she looks like is related to what she sees there . . . [but what of] the baby whose mother reflects her own mood or, worse still, the rigidity of her own defences. . . . They look and they do not see themselves . . . what is seen is the mother's face. (p. 27)

If the parent sees the child as greedy, needy, angry, weak, or bad, *this* is how the child will come to see themselves. The child's actual internal experiences—and particularly their negative affects—will remain unnamed and unknown. When the child, in turn, becomes a parent, they may likewise struggle to see their own baby outside of the realm of their own projections.

Fonagy and Target (1995) argued that when the baby's subjectivity is lost, violence becomes possible. Ordinarily, for example, a child's fear signals the parent to protect and comfort them. If the parent does not see the child, does not see their fear or pain, these usual responses are short-circuited. Instead, for instance, the parent may become enraged, being confronted with intolerable reminders of their own childhood helplessness (recall our description of a disorganized baby). Or the parent may disappear, responding to the child's needs with helplessness. Rather than activating the parent's "caregiving system" (Solomon & George, 1996), the child's distress disables it. At the moment the child most needs to be known, they are left unaccompanied and afraid.

In the following sections, we use three different frameworks to describe the impact of trauma on parenting. We begin with research on prementalization and Luyten and Fonagy's (2017) notions of concrete and intrusive mentalizing. We then align these ideas with Lyons-Ruth's notion of hostile–helpless orientations to caregiving. Finally, we consider how the posttraumatic adaptations of complex trauma (Herman, 1992a; van der Kolk, 2014) may directly affect parenting.

Prementalizing

From the outset, Fonagy and Target (1996) concerned themselves with describing what impaired mentalizing might look like, using as their guide the primitive and limited abilities of small children to understand the mind of the other. Unfortunately, the literature on how to label, define, and classify impaired PRF is confusing, and not especially clinician-friendly. Various terms have been used to describe it, including nonmentalizing, anti- or prementalizing, maladaptive and pathological mentalizing, as well as psychic equivalence, pretend, and teleological modes. To add to the confusion, the bulk of these have been defined and categorized in slightly different ways. In a sense, none of these terms is quite accurate, because they conflate various kinds of nonmentalizing, namely, (1) the reliance on primitive forms of thinking that are manifest *before* the child develops a theory of mind (thus, *prementalizing*) and (2) pathological or antimentalizing, reflected in hostile projections and other misattributions. Here, following Luyten and Fonagy (Luyten & Fonagy, 2015; Luyten et al., 2017), we opt for the term that is used most consistently, that is, prementalizing.

Luyten, Fonagy, and their colleagues (Luyten & Fonagy, 2015; Luyten et al., 2017) describe two general types of prementalizing that align directly with the dimensions we introduced in Chapters 2 and 3. On the one hand, they describe a *deficit* in the capacity to mentalize, namely, a general lack of interest in and/or inability to enter into the child's subjective world ("too little"). On the other, they describe negatively biased, *intrusive* or excessive mentalizing, manifest in the parent's tendency to intrude on the child's experience with their own projections and distortions ("too much"). These two poles—which reflect different strategies for the regulation of arousal and threat—have also been described as hypomentalizing (i.e., not enough mentalizing) and hypermentalizing (i.e., too much and inaccurate mentalizing).

Concrete/Deficient Prementalizing ("Too Little")

At one end of the spectrum are parents who are largely absent and withdrawn from the child; in a sense, the child's experience is both unavailable and apparently immaterial as well. Not only is there little effort to make sense of the child, either at a bodily or an emotional level, but the child's experience is also overlooked and denied. Parents who tend toward this mode find it difficult to acknowledge that they or their children have thoughts or feelings, effectively obliterating any awareness of their internal, subjective experience. Thus, in the Sharon Olds poem, the imagined avoidant mother sees the baby's startle, but remarks, "You're fine," and offers a forced smile. Or more malevolent examples: "He doesn't notice when I'm high. It's all the same to him" or "She doesn't remember the time she was in foster care" or "She's too young to have feelings or understand anything. Nothing affects her." Or, when speaking about themselves: "I don't remember my brother raping me. It's in the past." There is a refusal or inability to see the self or other as a psychological being; this is manifest in an utter lack of language to describe thoughts or feelings.

Parents who tend toward concrete mentalizing may also equate what is apparent *outside* (namely, the child's behavior) with what is going on *inside*. The child who has little energy for school is "lazy," the child who has tantrums is "bad." The parent responds to what is concretely in front of them as equivalent to what the child is thinking and feeling: "What I see IS," and there is no apparent sense that anything can be gained from wondering about what's behind the behavior. This is reminiscent of the way 3-year-olds think: "What I see is what is real; there is little flexibility in considering alternatives. Rather, I cling rigidly to what I see." The reason this kind of thinking is called *hypomentalizing* is that any effort to make meaning, to remember, to consider alternative perspectives, or to understand the dynamic nature of thoughts and emotions is underdeveloped and stalled. It is not hard to imagine how lonely this experience can be for the child, how empty they might feel, and how limited a vocabulary they might have to describe their inner life when confronted with a parent who misses so much of who they are. Indeed, long-term studies link parental withdrawal in infancy to severe psychopathology, particularly borderline personality disorder in late adolescence (Khoury et al., 2019; Lyons-Ruth et al., 2013). Deficient mentalizing has much in common with what Zeanah and his colleagues (1994) refer to as "disengaged" representations of the child.

Intrusive/Excessive Prementalizing ("Too Much")

At the other end of the spectrum are relational intrusions that coopt and distort the child's experience. The parent conveys to the child in one way or another that they *know* what is in the child's mind, invariably without any interest in the child's perspective, and often far beyond what is probable. The parent's own perspective takes over in the form of malevolent or otherwise distorted projections, and they are certain of what is in the child's mind. Thus, as we described in Chapter 2, the imagined mother of the resistant baby goes overboard ("*You scared? You OK? That water is so scary!*"), overwhelming the newborn with her fears, and failing to see the child's own interest and curiosity. As another example, a mother in one of our programs insisted that her 6-week-old was "giving her the finger," attributing hostility and rage to her tiny little girl. Or, "*I know you hate seeing Daddy because he left us*" when the child has just returned from a longed-for visit with her father. A more brutal example might be the father who tells his toddler, *"I know you hate me. That's why you embarrassed me. And I'm going to get you for that."* Such intrusive mentalizing can be evident even in pregnancy: *"He's telling me even now that I will never have control over him."* All of these examples reflect varying levels of intruding into the child's mind and overattributing intent to the child. These kinds of assaults on thinking, which are by definition inaccurate, are referred to as *hypermentalizing,* in that interacting with the child (or even imagining the child) activates or overarouses the parent, such that they overwhelm the child's experience with their own projections. This form of prementalizing has much in common with what Zeanah and his colleagues (1994) refer to as to as "distorted" representations of the child (see Vreeswijk et al., 2012, for a summary of this line of research).

Mentalizing and Arousal

We again return to the arousal curve (see also Chapter 2) to illustrate the concepts of deficient and intrusive mentalizing (see Figure 5.1). The left-hand side represents little or no arousal and a tendency to hypomentalizing ("too little"). In attachment terms, we would think of this as an avoidant–dismissing stance. The right-hand side of the curve represents a high level of distress and arousal and a tendency to hypermentalizing ("too much"). We might also think of this as a resistant–preoccupied stance.

These extremes stand in contrast to the secure stance, which allows for a regulated and full expression of both positive and negative affect and for balanced and coherent mentalizing. At the bottom of the circle, falling between and below the two insecure stances toward mentalizing, is the disorganized stance, in which defenses have all but collapsed, leading to complete withdrawal or frank dysregulation (or both). This stance reflects the obliteration of mentalizing processes by fear and is akin to the freezing response to stress. In insecure relationships, the child's cues are ignored or distorted; as such, they cannot be seen and do not become fully known. As a result, the child's developing capacity to make sense of others can be distorted or—in extreme instances—atrophy altogether. And the world can feel pretty untrustworthy and dangerous. We return to this graphic again in the chapters to come.

As we so often see in the child's response—a downturn of the head, a look of quiet desperation and confusion, the collapsing of the chest and shoulders—both prementalizing modes inherently invalidate and obliterate their experience. They are left feeling unheard, alone, and afraid. As Allen (2013) put it: "Were it not for the[se] various forms of nonmentalizing . . . there would be . . . much less need for a lot of psychotherapy. We would all

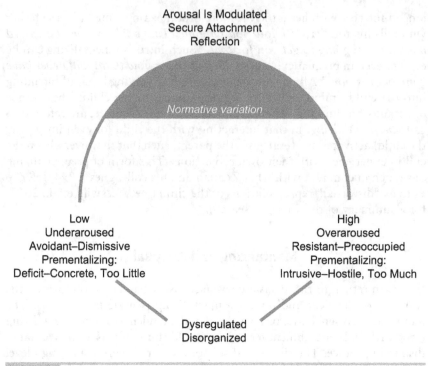

FIGURE 5.1 The arousal curve: Mentalizing.

be getting along much better, with each other and in our own minds. And we would be less likely to traumatize each other in attachment relationships or otherwise" (pp. 152–153). This is why failures of parental RF are often the direct target of MTB-P interventions.

Hostile–Helpless Parental Behaviors and Representations

In Chapter 3, we described Karlen Lyons-Ruth's work linking anomalous parental behavior to infant attachment organization (Lyons-Ruth et al., 1999b). This work set the stage for an examination of the link between a caregiver's history of relational trauma and both parental behavior and representation. What Lyons-Ruth and her colleagues found was that relational trauma confers a vulnerability to two stances toward attachment and hence toward the child, namely, the "hostile" and the "helpless" (HH) stances, which can be manifest in behavior (Lyons-Ruth et al., 1999b) or representation (Lyons-Ruth et al., 2005). Lyons-Ruth hypothesized that both stances help the parent avoid activating their own unintegrated early experiences of fear and helplessness (Lyons-Ruth et al., 1999a). Caregivers whose stance toward parenting is primarily hostile are thought to have identified with the aggressor as a way of defending against awareness of their own vulnerability and that of their infants. Caregivers who maintain an internal representation of themselves as frightened, overwhelmed, and helpless often experience others, including their infants, as malevolent and threatening. Either stance is thought to interfere with the ability to tolerate vulnerable emotions in themselves or their infants (Lyons-Ruth et al., 1999b). Lyons-Ruth and her colleagues found that the more the parent represented their own parents as hostile and/or helpless on the AAI, the more likely the parent was to behave in anomalous ways, and the more likely the child was to be disorganized.

HH classification on the AAI has been linked with severity of traumatic experiences in childhood (Byun et al., 2016; Finger et al., 2015; Milot et al., 2014), borderline personality disorder (Lyons-Ruth et al., 2007), maltreatment-related outcomes beyond infant disorganization, including disrupted mother–child affective communication (Finger, 2006; Lyons-Ruth et al., 2005). It has also been found to differentiate among parents at risk for maltreatment (Frigerio et al., 2013). Recently, Terry and her colleagues (2021) adapted the HH scale to assess prenatal representations of the child and of caregiving during pregnancy and found, in a small sample, that HH representations were linked to child removal from the home 1–2 years after the child's birth. To return to the mentalizing framework we outlined earlier, HH representations would be extreme versions of intrusive or hypermentalizing; in either case, the sense of self or the sense of the infant is distorted by defenses against intense negative affect.

Complex Trauma and Parenting

We now turn to a consideration of the way complex trauma—variously described as complex, developmental, relational, or attachment trauma—influences parenting generally and mentalizing specifically. Although mentalization theorists (Allen, 2012, 2013; Bateman & Fonagy, 2004, 2016) see trauma as one of the primary factors in mentalizing failures, the concept of mentalization has been largely absent from the literature on complex trauma (and vice versa). Nevertheless, a close look at the posttraumatic adaptations described by Herman (1992a) and van der Kolk (1994) makes clear that mentalizing deficits play a role in many of the sequelae of complex attachment trauma.

Complex Trauma

Thirty years ago, Judith Herman (1992b) made an observation that was to change the course of trauma study:

> The current diagnostic formulation of PTSD derives primarily from observations of survivors of relatively circumscribed traumatic events: combat, disaster, and rape . . . this formulation fails to capture the protean sequelae of prolonged, repeated trauma. In contrast to the circumscribed traumatic event, prolonged, repeated trauma can occur only where the victim is in a state of captivity, unable to flee, and under the control of the perpetrator. (p. 377)

Herman also suggested that certain forms of psychopathology (e.g., borderline personality disorder [BPD]) might be seen as the long-term sequelae of relational trauma.[1] Nearly 100 years after Freud rejected his own observation of the link between familial abuse and psychopathology, trauma study returned to his original (and correct!) hypothesis: that relational trauma (which is so often familial) dramatically alters the course of an individual's development.

Herman realized that the patients she was seeing had an array of difficulties that went far beyond the symptom clusters associated with PTSD. Many of them had suffered at the hands of their caregivers for years and across developmental periods, resulting in far more pervasive impairments in functioning than were typical with PTSD. These profound insights led Herman and, shortly thereafter, Bessel van der Kolk (1994) to propose a new category of traumatic stress disorders: complex trauma disorder (or complex PTSD).[2] Space limitations preclude our fully discussing their and many others' subsequent and prolonged efforts to establish the validity of this new diagnostic category (see Cloitre et al., 2019; Saraiya et al., 2021; van der Kolk et al., 2005). Instead, we focus on the pervasive impairments in adult functioning that have been linked to early relational trauma and that, in turn, profoundly affect parenting. The issue, as we see it, is not so much to determine whether or not parents fit the diagnostic criteria for complex trauma disorder (though they may; see Chapters 12 and 16). Rather, we wish to use the rich literature on complex trauma to help understand the parents we so often see as infant and child mental health practitioners and to understand the particular difficulties they may have

---

[1] Research has since differentiated the symptoms of BPD from those of both PTSD and complex PTSD (Cyr et al., 2022; Hyland et al., 2019).

[2] This disorder is at times also referred to as disorders of extreme stress, not otherwise specified (DESNOS).

managing the complex emotions of parenthood, and particularly their own and the child's distress.

Complex trauma is defined by Courtois (2004) as:

> a type of trauma that occurs repeatedly and cumulatively, usually over a period of time and within specific relationships and contexts. The term . . . extends to all forms of domestic violence and attachment trauma occurring in the context of family and other intimate relationships. These forms of intimate/domestic abuse often occur over extended time periods during which the victim is entrapped and conditioned in a variety of ways. (p. 412)

Unlike single-incident traumas, relational trauma that occurs within the context of the child's attachment relationships and across key developmental periods has the potential to profoundly disrupt basic capacities to self-regulate, trust and relate to others, think, plan, and care for one's body. The vulnerability of youth and the chronicity of fear in care-seeking together disrupt development at the level of the mind, the body, and the brain and deprive children of the kinds of experiences they need to build strong foundations for later learning, relating, and regulation across multiple domains.

The net result of such chronic disruptions is that functioning across a range of domains—relationships, affect regulation, bodily functioning, attention and consciousness, self-perception, perception of the perpetrator, and systems of meaning—is *altered*. Herman suggests that these alterations are posttraumatic adaptations designed to help the individual survive in the face of unbearable fear. As such, they are considered the chief signs of complex trauma disorder.

These alterations are often mistaken for symptoms of a particular disorder—such as anxiety or depression—when instead they are, in fact, symptoms of the individual's efforts to adapt in circumstances in which "fright without solution" occurs (Hesse & Main, 1999, p. 484). As Courtois states:

> Individuals exposed to trauma over a variety of time spans and developmental periods suffered from a variety of psychological problems not included in the diagnosis of PTSD, including depression, anxiety, self-hatred, dissociation, substance abuse, self-destructive and risk-taking behaviors, revictimization, problems with interpersonal and intimate relationships (including parenting), medical and somatic complaints, and despair. Moreover, these problems were categorized as comorbid conditions rather than being recognized as essential elements of complicated posttraumatic adaptations. (Courtois, 2004, p. 413)

As we discussed in Chapter 2, adaptation is an essential human survival function. We adapt to our "environment of evolutionary adaptedness" (Bowlby, 1969/1982) to survive. Within the context of attachment, these adaptations serve to sustain the child's primary relationships and ideally come without great cost to the child. When the child's fundamental survival is threatened, however, these adaptations cost the child (and adult) dearly (as in disorganized attachment). They are, as such, *mal*adaptations. From a clinical standpoint, mistaking the signs of complex trauma in the parent for a more circumscribed and treatable problem, such as depression, is to miss the heart of the matter. It is the fundamental alterations that must be addressed therapeutically, not their symptoms. It is like putting a Band-Aid on a skin abrasion without realizing that the life-threatening problem is internal bleeding. The Band-Aid may be important, but without more dramatic intervention, it will be of no use whatsoever.

Posttraumatic Alterations and Parenting

Interestingly, there has been relatively little empirical examination of the effect of cumulative trauma exposure on parenting (see Muzik et al., 2016). Researchers tend, for example, to study parents who were maltreated as children without distinguishing levels of trauma exposure; thus parents with complex attachment trauma and those without are grouped together, making it very difficult to determine the impact of cumulative relational trauma on parenting. Some of this has to do with the fact that there are currently few reliable and valid measures of complex trauma; another has been the tendency of researchers to focus on events (childhood maltreatment) rather than chronicity and/or whether the perpetrator was also an attachment figure. The few studies that have explored this question directly (Banyard et al., 2001, 2003; Cohen et al., 2008) consistently find that the higher the level of the parent's trauma exposure, the more likely they are to struggle in all aspects of parenting. Banyard and her colleagues (2003) found that higher rates of cumulative trauma exposure predicted low levels of parenting satisfaction, more frequent reports of child neglect, the tendency to use physical punishment, and a history of reports to child protective services. Cohen and her colleagues (2008) likewise found that cumulative trauma reliably predicted parental abuse potential, punitiveness, and psychological and physical aggression.

These reports are, of course, entirely consistent with what clinicians observe all the time. Indeed, in MTB-HV, we found that the concept of complex trauma helped us understand many of the difficulties we were seeing in our most challenged parents (Slade & Sadler, 2013; Slade et al., 2017b). Each of the posttraumatic alterations described by Herman, van der Kolk, and others helped us make sense of the particular challenges they were having *as parents.* Based on these observations, we began to think about how each of the posttraumatic adaptations intrinsic to complex trauma might affect parenting specifically. We outline some of the potential impacts in the following sections. In later chapters, we explore these issues further.

Alterations in Relationships

Early interpersonal trauma makes it very hard to trust and feel intimate with others. These are the relational "lessons of abuse" (Courtois, 2004). Attachment trauma survivors have been robbed of the experience of faith—in others, in themselves, in the world—and as such are prone to putting themselves in situations in which they are victimized or in which they themselves are the perpetrators. For those who have been violated and frightened by those meant to protect them, the minds of others are to be feared, not embraced and discovered. This may manifest in an absence of the capacity to imagine the minds of others or—in particular—to reflect upon past traumatic experiences (Berthelot et al., 2015, 2019; Borelli et al., 2019; Ensink et al., 2014; Fonagy, 1993). Prementalizing modes—too little, too much—abound. Although these struggles are likely to have an impact on all relationships, they pose special challenges for parenting, especially the ability to serve as a loving, secure, and safe base for one's child. So much of what we emphasized in earlier chapters—finding pleasure in each other, providing safety, security, and *holding the baby's mind in mind*—can be so very difficult for vulnerable parents. The baby's helplessness, need, and lovability (which serves, among other things, as the mechanism for the release of oxytocin; see Julian et al., 2018; Strathearn et al., 2009) can be threatening to the parent and readily trigger the frightening and frightened stances described by Main and Lyons-Ruth. The parent's distrust and suspiciousness of others are—within the context of parenting—antithetical to the child's feeling safe, understood, and cherished. This is the reason, as is evident throughout this book, that MTB-P focuses so directly on developing and sustaining secure relationships—between parent and clinician, between clinician and child, and between parent and child.

Alterations in the Regulation of Affects and Impulses

Traumatized individuals often have difficulty recognizing, labeling, and expressing their emotions and as such are vulnerable to emotional and behavioral dysregulation. Affective lability, or swings from high to low, from rage to hopelessness and submission, is common, as are struggles with impulse control. These are manifest in struggles with anger, self-destructive behavior, excessive risk taking, suicidal ideation or acts, and sexual difficulties (e.g., promiscuity or fear of sexual intimacy). As is shown in the case examples throughout Parts III and IV, these are the struggles of many of the parents we saw in MTB-HV. So often this is the child's experience of the parent—angry, taking risks that endanger the child, struggling with suicidal thoughts, engaged in transient sexual relationships, and so forth. This is a frightening base, one that cannot be relied on. The emotions of parenting—joy, delight, deep contentment, fear, anger—can also be intensely destabilizing for traumatized parents and can lead to episodes of dysregulation that can be disorganizing to the child. They can also find it very difficult to label and organize the child's own thoughts and feelings and thus "pass on" difficulties in affect regulation. Finally, parenting is profoundly intertwined with one's sense of self: The child, as *part* of the parent, has so much potential to gratify or disappoint. For the vulnerable parent, the inevitable narcissistic injuries of parenthood can be nearly unendurable. This is the reason, as we describe more fully in Chapter 7, that we place so much emphasis on self, bodily, and affect regulation, as these are essential to creating a more secure environment for the child and more emotional stability for the parent.

Alterations in Bodily Functioning

Traumatized adults often have a great deal of difficulty listening to and caring for their bodies; surviving abuse or neglect requires, in effect, actively tuning out one's bodily signals. The body is the "scene of the crime", one that the victim can neither escape nor acknowledge. And, as we discuss more fully in Chapter 6, cumulative, toxic stress and adversity lead to a range of poor health outcomes, likely as the result of the relative absence of parental care and proper medical care, and to the breakdown of bodily systems as the result of chronic stress. So much of parenting, particularly in the earliest years of life, involves the body: the parent's, as well as the child's. From the dramatic physical changes of pregnancy to the many moments of close bodily contact between parent and child, two physical bodies are intertwined, for fathers and mothers both. The parent's capacity to read the child's nonverbal, embodied cues is essential to security, mutuality, and safety. It is also essential to the child's physical health.

In MTB-HV, we saw parents struggle to feel comfortable with their own and their children's bodies and to read their children's cues—when they were tired, when they wanted to play, when they felt good, when they were in pain, when they were hungry. Parents who had themselves been traumatized as children often underfed or overfed their babies, missed signs that children were too cold or too hot, or overlooked evidence of physical illness. Sleep was often disrupted, and some parents had a great deal of difficulty establishing sleep schedules for their children. Seeking medical care and following medical advice for themselves or their children could be an enormous struggle. The opposite was also noted, with some parents being hypervigilant and overprotective of their children's bodies and physical safety. This is why, in our original MTB-HV model, we not only paid close attention to the quality of the parent–child interaction but also incorporated nurses and specifically a health care component into the intervention.

Alterations in Attention and Consciousness

Difficulties in attention regulation, memory, and executive functioning, as well as problems in planning, focusing on, and completing tasks, often emerge secondary to relational trauma. As a result, parents who have been traumatized are prone to dissociation, amnesia, and/or hypervigilance. Hyperactivity and distractibility may signal either or both efforts to cope with terror as well as underlying neurological impairments. These coping strategies may well compromise the parent's capacity to be emotionally present for their own child, whether manifest in the parent's withdrawal and inattention or in their high level of anxiety and vigilance. Imagine, for example, the parent who, when triggered, "disappears," becomes lost in thought (or, more aptly, *not* thinking), and cannot be roused or brought back to the present. Or another who is so attuned to potential danger that relaxed and joyful presence and contemplation is impossible. In either scenario, the parent's capacity to deploy their attention to the child in a flexible way is disrupted. Either (or both) will leave the child feeling abandoned or rattled and intruded upon, compromising their own developing capacities for attention, executive functioning, and consciousness. Parents struggling in these ways may also have difficulty organizing everyday life for the child by maintaining schedules and following routines.

Alterations in Self-Perception

Alterations in self-perception are linked to feelings of shame, guilt, aloneness, powerlessness, and damage. The feeling that "*I am damaged/damaging, worthless/useless/bad*" is common among those who have survived attachment trauma. As we discussed in earlier chapters, one of the joys of parenting is the feeling that—as Sharon Olds (1984) put it so beautifully— "*I am good for him*"; "*I can be a 'good-enough' parent*"; "*I can get you through the night, across the troubled waters*"; "*I got this.*" As Benedek (1959) noted so long ago, these experiences are important for both parent and child: The child comes to feel that they, too, are good enough, and the parent discovers that they can heal their own wounds by finding goodness in nurturing the child. Needless to say, it can be harmful and painful to both parent and child when the feeling that "*I am bad/worthless/useless*" pervades caregiving. The parent's perception of themselves as bad gives the child little to hang onto, with no safety or strength to be found in the caregiver. The self that the child discovers in the parent's eyes (Winnicott, 1965) is simply not "good enough." This will invariably have an impact on the child's own sense of self-worth. Sometimes, happily, the child can find the good in the parent even when the parent cannot.

> Steffi was lamenting the fact that her son Billy had such a "terrible" mother. Listening to this, Billy, aged 7, cocked his head to one side, looked at her directly, and said, "Mom, if you ever want to know about good mothers, come to me!" He was literally reminding her that—as damaged as she felt—he thought she was pretty terrific. And, indeed, he helped her find goodness in herself that she had not recognized.

Alterations in Perceptions of the Perpetrator

This particular category of posttraumatic maladaptation is typically used to describe the way abuse survivors idealize or denigrate their perpetrators (either parents or romantic partners) or take on the beliefs of the perpetrator ("*you are worthless/bad/useless*"). We found that many traumatized parents continued to idealize their own parents or blandly insisted that they "did the best they could." These idealizations could be quite difficult to puncture because they were, like all posttraumatic adaptations, survival mechanisms. Other parents still felt extreme rage at their own parents. In either case, parents' inability to see their own parents more realistically, and particularly to acknowledge the pain of their own abuse, often stood in the way of their capacity to do "ghosts in the nursery work" or to have any kind of realistic expectations of themselves as parents. The more entrenched these idealizations were, the more difficult it was to make therapeutic progress. Many parents were also preoccupied with abusive partners. Often this meant that children were exposed to intimate partner violence or were "lost" to the parent who was consumed by the need or wish to reunite with or punish an abandoning partner. Any of these circumstances make it very difficult for the parent to see the whole child in all their complexity; often the parent's own attachment difficulties supersede their capacity to attend to children's attachment needs. At times, children could themselves be experienced as perpetrators.

Alterations in Systems of Meaning

Prolonged trauma can deprive human beings of their fundamental sense of life's purpose and meaning (Frankl, 1946/1985). There is no meaning or joy to be found in relationships or in life, and despair predominates.

Belief in oneself, in others, or in any higher power is absent. As is evident throughout the literature on complex trauma, adults chronically abused as children struggle not to succumb to hopelessness and despair (as do the clinicians who help them; see Chapter 8). The foundation upon which relationships are built is damaged, if not broken; the hope for change is absent. This profoundly affects parenting. Ideally, bringing a child into the world offers an opportunity to find new layers of meaning both in creating and nurturing a life and in creating a human being (de Marneffe, 2004). But what we see in some parents is the utter failure to believe that anything will ever change. This hopelessness derives, of course, from their own lived experience in relationships and makes it so difficult to create a different lived experience for their child.

Mentalizing Trauma: Reason for Hope

Thankfully, many individuals with trauma histories are able to form loving relationships with others and live—to use Winnicott's (1965) term— "good-enough" lives. And there are parents who have suffered at the hands of their own caregivers but do not repeat the pattern with their own children (Madigan et al., 2019). It is possible to develop the capacity to mentalize *despite* exposure to trauma; as we discuss more fully in Chapter 6, there are individuals who are *resilient* in the face of stress and trauma. From the perspective of mentalization theory, resilience arises from having had someone *know* you, hear you, see you, and protect you; someone *trustworthy*. This need not necessarily be a parent but might be a nonmaltreating parent, grandmother, sibling, friend, teacher, or therapist.

Karin Ensink's (Ensink et al., 2014) and Nicolas Berthelot's (Berthelot et al., 2015) work on the salutary effects of mentalizing trauma brings home the importance of helping parents make sense of their traumatic experiences. Following Fonagy (1993) and Fraiberg et al. (1975), they began with the assumption that trauma often leads to an *absence* or *deficit* in the capacity to reflect upon the fear and helplessness associated with such events. Furthermore, they reasoned that the inability to reflect upon traumatic experiences and affects *in particular*, rather than a general difficulty reflecting upon attachment experiences, would affect the transition to parenthood. To study this question, they administered the AAI to 100 pregnant women with histories of abuse and neglect. They scored AAIs for the general capacity to reflect on their attachment experiences (which they termed general RF, or RF-G), as well as the level of RF when abuse or trauma was "directly probed or explicitly discussed" (Ensink et al., 2014, p. 6). Trauma RF (RF-T) was significantly lower than general RF in this group of traumatized women, suggesting that the result of childhood maltreatment was a "collapse of mentalization specific to trauma" (Ensink et al., 2014, p. 1). Neither the extent nor dose of trauma was associated with RF-T; thus it seemed the significant factor was not the amount of trauma but the degree to which an individual had been able to make sense of it. Most important, Ensink and her colleagues found that the capacity to reflect upon trauma had a number of positive effects. It directly predicted the degree to which women were emotionally engaged in and felt positively about their pregnancies and were committed to motherhood; it was also strongly associated with the quality of the couples' functioning. None of the other variables studied—RF-G, or mothers' attachment status—predicted these outcomes.

In a second study using the same sample, Berthelot et al. (2015) found that mothers who were unable to reflect upon their traumatic experiences were more likely to have disorganized children. This was true regardless of mothers' general reflective capacities on the AAI, suggesting that it is the mother's *particular* capacity to make meaning of her own traumatic experience that protects the parent–child relationship from its deleterious effects. Finally, Borelli and her colleagues (2019) examined levels of RF-T in these same parents' PDIs and found that the more mothers were able to reflect on their own trauma on the PDI, the less likely it was that their own children had been abused by either familial or nonfamilial perpetrators. Here again is evidence that the capacity to make meaning of harmful, terrifying, and disorganizing experiences in one's own childhood is essential to protecting the next generation from its devastating effects.

In light of these findings, Berthelot and his colleagues proposed that RF-T be considered a resilience factor in coming to terms with early traumatic experiences. That is, "inadequate mentalization of traumatic experiences may make mothers more vulnerable to momentarily [sic] failures in responding congruently or modulating aggression or fear in the context of mother–infant interactions where trauma-related affects or memories are triggered" (Berthelot et al., 2015, p. 209). They link this to Beebe et al.'s (2010) finding, which we first mentioned in Chapter 3, that momentary failures of maternal responsiveness in the face of distress lead to disorganized attachment. Mothers who cannot reflect upon their own trauma are particularly vulnerable to momentarily abandoning the child in moments of distress, thus failing to soothe and regulate the child. The child's negative affect evokes the parent's own unmetabolized trauma; as a result, the mother fails to mirror the child and thus leaves the child without the capacity to make sense of their own negative affect. Thus, even in pregnancy, failures in the capacity to mentalize extreme and disruptive negative affect are linked to the perpetuation of attachment disorganization and the intergenerational transmission of trauma. Once again, this reminds us of the importance of attending to what happens between parent and child when the child is in the throes of negative affect, namely, anger, fear, or sadness. It also reminds us of the therapeutic value of mentalization, particularly insofar as negative affect generally and trauma specifically is concerned.

Summary

As we have discussed over the course of this and the previous chapter, *both* internal and external threats can—in the absence of protective factors—make it difficult for parents to remain present and available to the child. The perpetual activation of the stress response—be it in response to interpersonal trauma, to hunger and/or homelessness and joblessness, and/or to being assaulted or marginalized by those in power—can make it difficult to provide a secure base, and, perhaps most important, to remain engaged with the child's distress when the child needs it most. Many families experience not one but all of these threats, and, indeed, relational, biological, and societal risks are often highly conflated in both the clinical and research literatures. In these circumstances, the risks are thus cumulative and toxic, both for parents and for their children. These challenges can severely compromise the parent's capacity to invest in and recognize the child's own subjective experience.

As clinicians, although we can work in small and large ways to remedy the larger social ills that so often paralyze and disrupt families in their daily lives and to provide concrete and emotional supports to ameliorate their impacts, we cannot undo the past. Yet—particularly when we listen and watch and engage around moments of rupture, conflict, and stress—we can endeavor to engage the parent's angels and exorcise the ghosts, to build on their strengths and hear their suffering. We do this because, as Selma Fraiberg put it so beautifully, "when [the] mother's own cries are heard, she will hear her child's cries" (Fraiberg et al., 1975, p. 396). We also do this so that the parent can slowly build and rebuild what has been hurt and repair what has been broken, find agency where there has been little, break cycles that may have persisted for generations, and open windows and doors that have been sealed shut for far too long. As we discuss in later chapters, this process can take a very long time.

▲▲▲▲▲ QUESTIONS FOR CLINICIANS ▲▲▲▲▲

Mentalizing difficulties in parents are often associated with trauma. It is thus important to recognize signs of prementalizing and to identify the particular ways that a caregiver's attachment trauma may affect their capacity to parent.

▶ Do you see signs that a parent is having great difficulty imagining what might be going on in the child's mind, or in their own? Parents may lack a language for internal experience, or they may respond to the child's behavior in very concrete ways.

▶ Do you see signs that a parent projects their own experience onto the child in an intrusive or hostile way? This can be manifest in hostile or helpless representations of the child and of caregiving or in excessive attributions to or certainty about the child's internal experience.

▶ Where would you place the parent's capacity to mentalize on the arousal curve: "too little," "too much," or "just right"?

▶ When parents report significant attachment trauma, do you see evidence of posttraumatic alterations in relationships, affect regulation, bodily functioning, attention and consciousness, self-perception, perception of the perpetrator, and/or systems of meaning?

▶ Can you identify the impact of the preceding on the parent's capacity to provide care?

▶ Do you see evidence of the parent's capacity to reflect upon their traumatic experiences?

Chapter

6

Adversity, Toxic Stress, and Resilience

There are myriad scientific foundations for the central theses of MTB-P, namely, that high levels of stress, threat, or fearful arousal disrupt the development and functioning of the body and the brain and that safety-promoting relationships are key to ameliorating these primary impacts. As we outlined in Chapters 2–5, this thesis is central to attachment, mentalization, and trauma theories. It is also central to much of the science underlying the study of adverse childhood experiences (ACEs) and toxic stress, as well as many of the basic principles of affective neuroscience (Panksepp, 2004; Porges, 2011) and epigenetics (Essex et al., 2013; Grigorenko et al., 2012; Schwartz et al., 2019). In fact, distinguishing any of these perspectives from one another is quite complex, as they are highly interrelated and complementary. Thus, for example, trauma theory emerged first as a clinical theory that was ultimately buttressed by affective neuroscience and epigenetics and by the large-scale epidemiological findings of research on early adversity (Felitti et al., 1998) and subsequent work on toxic stress (Shonkoff et al., 2012). Likewise, although studies of ACEs and toxic stress rely on somewhat different conceptual frameworks and methodologies, both are examining the biological and psychological impacts of high levels of fear and stress on infants, children, and adults. Wallace Stevens' poem "Thirteen Ways of Looking at a Blackbird" (Stevens, 1923) captures this complexity perfectly; the blackbird appears in every stanza, stable across very different contexts. The "blackbird" in this case is the long arm of deep pain in childhood, pain that cannot be or is not modulated by those meant to protect and comfort. In this chapter, we focus primarily on the science underlying many of MTB-P's clinical approaches, specifically the study of ACEs and toxic stress.

The ACE Study

The history of the ACE study is a fascinating one. Nearly 25 years ago, Vincent Felitti, an internist and director of the Kaiser–Permanente Division of Preventive Medicine in San Diego, California, and Robert Anda, an internist and epidemiologist from the Centers for Disease Control and Prevention, developed a 10-item questionnaire to assess the scope of childhood adversity and its impact on adult patients in the Kaiser–Permanente health system. The study was inspired by Felitti's observation that a number of his chronically obese patients had histories of sexual abuse. In what turned out to be one of the most extensive and significant public health studies of the 20th century, patients were given a 10-item questionnaire and asked to endorse whether they had experienced any of the following: physical or sexual abuse, neglect, domestic violence, parental absence, substance use, mental illness, or other forms of household dysfunction before the age of 18. The final score reflects the number of items that are endorsed out of a possible 10.

The ACE questionnaire was eventually administered to more than 17,000 adult patients across the Kaiser–Permanente health clinics; the results of the study were dramatic (Felitti et al., 1998). First, early adversity was significantly linked to a range of physical and mental health concerns. Second, ACEs were highly interrelated, such that having one ACE increased the likelihood of having additional ACEs. Finally, there were significant dose–response relationships between early adversity and a range of health outcomes, such that individuals who reported four or more ACEs were significantly more likely to report increased rates of smoking, severe obesity, physical inactivity, depressed mood, and suicide attempts and more likely to be alcoholic, to use illicit drugs, to have had more than 50 sexual partners, and to have a history of a sexually transmitted diseases. In addition, they were more likely to have a range of health concerns and diseases: ischemic heart disease, cancer, chronic bronchitis or emphysema, history of hepatitis or jaundice, skeletal fractures, and poor self-rated health. The likelihood of early death was associated with the highest levels of early adversity (Felitti et al., 1998).

The findings of the original study have been replicated numerous times in a range of communities, cultures, and countries. A recent meta-analysis of the impact of multiple ACEs on health (Hughes et al., 2017) examined results from 37 studies, providing risk estimates for 23 outcomes across a combined population of 253,719 participants. Specifically, they found that for individuals with four or more ACEs, there were moderate associations with "smoking, poor self-rated health, cancer, heart disease, and respiratory disease," strong associations for "sexual risk taking, mental ill health, and problematic alcohol use," and even stronger associations for "problematic drug use, and interpersonal and self-directed violence" (Hughes et al., 2017, p. e356).

Who Is Most at Risk for ACEs?

The original ACE study (Felitti et al., 1998) examined the incidence of ACEs in a largely middle- and upper-middle-class population; the overwhelming majority of participants were White and had either attended or graduated from college. In this original sample, only 6.2% of the respondents reported exposure to four or more ACES; particularly striking, then, was the researchers' report that those with the highest rates of exposure were more likely to be Black, Hispanic, or with a racial identity that was not listed. Thus, even in this initial study with a largely middle-class sample, disparities in exposure to ACEs were linked to class and race. *Interestingly, despite the significance of these disparities, they were not to be the focus of ACE research for 20 years.* In 2018, Merrick and her colleagues (2018) reported on a large (*N* = 214,157) study of the prevalence of ACEs across 23 states in the United States. The results of this study make clear the degree to which ACEs cluster in marginalized groups and are strongly associated with poverty:

> Significantly higher ACE exposures were reported by participants who identified as black, Hispanic, or multiracial, those with less than a high school education, those with income of less than $15,000 per year, those who were unemployed or unable to work, and those identifying as gay/ lesbian or bisexual compared with those identifying as white, those completing high school or more education, than those in all other income brackets, those who were employed, and those identifying as straight, respectively. (Merrick et al., 2018, p. 1038)

That same year, in a study of the prevalence of ACEs in children across all 50 states in the United States, Sacks and Murphey (2018) reported that children living in poverty had the highest level of ACEs and that Black and Hispanic children and youth across the United States are "more likely to experience ACEs than their white or Asian peers" (Sacks & Murphey, 2018, p. 15). Maguire-Jack and her colleagues (2020) reported similar results in an analysis of data from more than 50,000 respondents in the National Study of Child Health, where they, too, found Black and Latinx children to have significantly higher ACEs than their non-Hispanic White peers. In addition, Black children were more likely to endorse a wide range of ACEs than children who were Latinx or non-Hispanic White. Worldwide, ACEs have been studied only in middle- to high-income countries (Hughes et al., 2017); thus we might expect to see even higher levels of adversity among those who live in low-income countries or who have been forced by starvation, war, and other calamities to flee their homelands.

These data make clear that growing up in underresourced, low-income, marginalized, and ethnically or racially diverse communities contributes to an accumulation of toxic stress (Shonkoff et al., 2012) and a range of poor health and developmental outcomes. They also suggest that racism itself is a powerful form of toxic stress. Surprisingly, as has been the case with the attachment and mentalization literatures, this notion received relatively little attention in the literature on ACEs and toxic stress until the social justice movement erupted with such power in the summer of 2020. In a recent paper, Shonkoff and his colleagues (2021) described the multiple and *unique* impacts of institutional and structural racism, cultural racism, and interpersonal discrimination on health outcomes. This leads us back to our previous discussions of threat and the elevation of the fear system that can result from ongoing "mundane and extreme environmental stressors" (Murry et al., 2018; Peters & Massey, 1983), namely, the unrelenting and daily exposure to the range of social, economic, educational, and health disparities that are endemic to racism.

How Do ACEs Cause Such Harm?

Felitti and his colleagues (1998) posed this question in their first published report of the ACE study: "Exactly how are adverse childhood experiences linked to health risk behaviors and adult diseases?" (p. 252). Their answer, at the time, focused on health risk behaviors such as smoking, drinking, abusing drugs, and overeating, any of which can have immediate physiological or psychological benefit in coping with enormous pain, and all of which can have serious health consequences. Today, no one disputes the idea that risky health behaviors contribute to many of the outcomes associated with high ACE exposure. But science has since offered a much deeper understanding of how ACEs get "under the skin" (Shonkoff et al., 2012). Much of this work has its roots in Bruce McEwen's pioneering research on the biology of stress, and particularly his description of the complex ways in which stress directly affects brain functioning (McEwen, 2000, 2017, 2020).

McEwen (2000) defines stress as "a threat, real or implied, to the psychological or physiological integrity of an individual" (p. 108). Human beings—like most living things—are born with the capacity to adapt to and, in fact, grow from challenges. However, when allostasis, the capacity to maintain stability or homeostasis through change, is challenged, either by too much stress or because the stress regulation system is not working properly, there is a significant cost to functioning across a number of biological and psychological systems. McEwen (2000) terms this "allostatic load," or the cost to the body when it is forced to "adapt to adverse psychosocial or physical situations" (p. 111). At certain levels, stress is protective; at higher levels, it is damaging. The biological systems that respond to stress, namely the autonomic nervous system (which triggers flight, fight, and freezing responses in the face of danger) and the adrenocortical system (which triggers the production of stress hormones, notably cortisol, adrenaline, and norepinephrine) protect the body in the short run but cause disease when stress is chronic or prolonged.

Toxic Stress

In a now-classic paper, Jack Shonkoff and his colleagues—who formed the National Scientific Council on the Developing Child at the Harvard Center for the Developing Child (HCDC)—used this framework as the basis for their theory of toxic stress (Shonkoff et al., 2012). They distinguished three types of stress responses—positive, tolerable, and toxic—the severity of each determined both by the extremity of the stress *and* the availability of a caring and responsive adult who can help the child manage and process stressful experiences (the echoes of attachment theory here are unmistakable). The distinction between the levels of stress responses reflects "postulated differences in their potential to cause enduring biological disruptions" (Shonkoff et al., 2021, p. 116). The more disruptive the stress response is, the more long-term damage is possible, across multiple levels of functioning. A positive stress response is one that occurs in the face of mild, normative stress (the first day in day care) that is modulated by caring adults in the environment. A tolerable stress response occurs when the stressor is more threatening (e.g., the death of a family member) but again is modulated by the presence of at least one supportive adult caregiver.

Toxic stress results from "strong, frequent, or prolonged activation of the body's stress response systems in the absence of the buffering protection of a supportive adult relationship" (2021, p. 116). Shonkoff and his colleagues (2012) note that ACEs and other forms of trauma are prime examples of the situations that might provoke a toxic stress response:

> The essential characteristic of this phenomenon is the postulated disruption of brain circuitry and other organ and metabolic systems during sensitive developmental periods. Such disruption may result in anatomic changes and/or physiologic dysregulations that are the precursors of later impairments in learning and behavior as well as the roots of chronic, stress-related physical and mental illness. (p. e236)

As we detail later, these disruptions occur at the very level of "brain structure and function," such that the "developing architecture of the brain can be impaired in numerous ways that create a weak foundation for later learning, behavior, and health" (Shonkoff et al., 2012, p. e236). More specifically, they note that "toxic stress in early childhood not only is a risk factor for later risky behavior but also can be a direct source of biological injury or disruption independent of whatever circumstances might follow later in life. In such cases, toxic stress can be viewed *as the precipitant of a physiological memory or biological signature* that confers lifelong risk well beyond its time of origin" (Shonkoff et al., 2012, p. e238; emphasis added).

As is evident from these basic definitions, as well as the literature on social buffering and resilience that we review later, the availability of a caring adult figure is one of the primary antidotes to toxic stress.[1] And although genetic variability may also account for individual differences in stress reactivity, there is ample evidence that "the ecological context modulates the expression of one's genotype. It is as if experiences confer a 'signature' on the genome to authorize certain characteristics and behaviors and to prohibit others" (Shonkoff et al., 2012, p. e235). Recent research also suggests that family factors (Schwartz et al., 2019), as well as the timing of adversity, may play a significant role in determining its impact (Dunn et al., 2019; McEwen, 2017).

As we describe more fully later, Shonkoff and his colleagues saw the multiple impacts of toxic stress as a clarion call to practitioners to shift their mode of practice. In particular, they called upon family care providers to develop interventions that "strengthen the capacities of families and communities to protect young children from the disruptive effects of toxic stress" as a means to promoting "healthier brain development and enhanced physical and mental well-being" (Shonkoff et al., 2012, p. e239). These would optimally prevent the "embedding" process whereby stress disrupts the brain and body. Clearly, MTB-HV, MTB-P, and many of the other interventions we described in earlier chapters are reflective of such efforts.

The scientific basis for Shonkoff's theory of toxic stress is extensive, and only the basics can be reviewed here. For more detail, we refer the reader to the series of working papers created by the HCDC (*https://developingchild.harvard.edu/resources*). But let us briefly discuss the biology of the stress response, which is mediated by the autonomic nervous system and the adrenocortical system. The adrenocortical system is part of the hypothalamic–pituitary–adrenal (HPA) axis, which plays an essential role in regulating a number of bodily systems, including the metabolic system, the immune system, and the central nervous system, along with a range of others. Ideally, the activation of the HPA axis leads to an adaptive stress response; in situations of chronic stress, however, HPA axis functioning

---

[1] Attachment researchers would, of course, describe this as a stronger and wiser adult whose job it is to protect the child and ensure their survival.

is disrupted, leading to cascades of stress hormones that result in multiple malfunctions in critical bodily systems. Prolonged disrupted HPA functioning can also lead to aberrant patterns of stress hormone production and release (e.g., blunted or abnormal diurnal cortisol patterns; Young et al., 2021). Today, a multitude of studies link the multiple physical and mental health sequelae of ACEs to chronic dysregulation of both the autonomic nervous and neuroendocrine systems (Hughes et al., 2017).

One of the most pronounced impacts of sustained activation of the HPA axis in childhood is the modification of neural structures—in particular, the amygdala, which regulates the fear response, and the hippocampus, which is largely responsible for learning and memory. In their review of the relationship between adversity and amygdala and hippocampal functioning, Tottenham and Sheridan (2010) make the point that "negative social environments become biologically embedded as changes in *neural structure and function*, and, ultimately, the behaviors that lead to mental illness" (p. 1, emphasis added). That is, the structure and function of these two critical brain regions are fundamentally changed by unregulated threat and fear early in life. These changes are mediated through the HPA axis, which "is one of the major pathways through which the effects of stress can shape brain development. The amygdala and hippocampus are rich with receptors for cortisol and are therefore major targets of the HPA axis" (Tottenham & Sheridan, 2010, p. 1; see also Loman & Gunnar, 2010).

The amygdala is part of what is known as the "limbic system," the part of the brain that regulates emotion. In both animal and human models, stress—particularly early stress—disrupts amygdala function, leading to either a heightened fear response or a lower threshold for the experience of fear (Cohen et al., 2013). Although this response is adaptive in dangerous situations, an overly active amygdala leads to what LeDoux (1996) refers to as "fear conditioning," namely, that fear becomes the conditioned response to a wide range of situations, even those that are not necessarily fear-inducing. Once established, this hyperreactive response to threat and stress is very difficult to change (LeDoux, 1996; Tottenham & Sheridan, 2010). That is, even when stressors are removed and individuals are placed in much more positive environments, changes in the amygdala do not typically reverse (Lyons-Ruth et al., 2016; Vyas et al., 2004; Yang et al., 2007). From a clinical standpoint, what these data suggest is that intervening early, when the amygdala is most plastic, is of utmost importance. They also provide a way of understanding some of the structural and functional reasons for the fact that bringing about change in traumatized individuals can be so very challenging (and slow!).

The hippocampus plays an important role in the encoding of memories and of learning; thus, for instance, the capacity to retain and access episodic memories is a hippocampal function. The hippocampus also plays a critical role in stress regulation in that it has a negative feedback mechanism that can modify or decrease HPA axis activation. In other words, the hippocampus can calm things down in stressful situations. Like the amygdala, the hippocampus is highly vulnerable to early life stress and to parental care. Brown and her colleagues (2007) found that high levels of ACEs in adulthood were associated with childhood autobiographical memory disorder, with memory for childhood events decreasing as the number of ACEs increased. Again, these data make abundantly clear the impact early adversity can have on critical brain functions and how long-lasting and pernicious these effects can be. They also shed light on the particular challenges of working with individuals who struggle to remember and to make sense of what happened to them.

Researchers have also documented relations between early adversity and the length of an individual's telomeres, biological markers of cellular stress and aging, with shorter telomeres linked to greater degrees of cellular stress. High levels of early adversity have been linked in two meta-analyses to shorter telomeres in adulthood (Li et al., 2017; Ridout et al., 2018). A recent report also links prenatal maternal reports of childhood ACEs to shorter telomere lengths in 4-month-old infants and to infant externalizing problems at 18 months (Esteves et al., 2020). In addition, telomere attrition between 4 and 18 months mediated the relationship between maternal adversity and child externalizing behaviors at 18 months.

The work of Katie McLaughlin and her colleagues exploring the long reach of adversity on the developing brain is also relevant here. In 2014, McLaughlin and colleagues proposed that different forms of early life adversity (ELA) have different downstream effects; specifically, that ELAs involving threat to the child (e.g., violence exposure) have different neurobiological consequences than those involving deprivation (e.g., neglect, institutional rearing). Subsequent work provided ample support for this hypothesis (McLaughlin & Sheridan, 2016; McLaughlin et al., 2016; McLaughlin et al., 2017). Most recently, in an extensive meta-analysis and systematic review of more than 70 studies (with a combined sample size of nearly 120,000 participants), Colich, McLaughlin, and their colleagues (Colich et al., 2020) were able to document that threat in early life was linked to accelerated biological aging, as measured by pubertal timing and cellular aging (manifested in telomere length and DNA methylation age). Threat was also linked to cortical thinning in the ventromedial region. By contrast, they found no associations between deprivation and biological aging; rather, neglect and SES were linked with thinning in the frontoparietal, default, and visual networks (Colich et al., 2020). These data make manifest, once again, the impact of early life adversity on biological markers of stress across the lifespan and of the intergenerational effects of parental adversity on their offspring.

The Intergenerational Transmission of ACEs

The original ACE study focused only on adult retrospective accounts of abuse, neglect, and parental and household dysfunction. More recently, however, researchers and epidemiologists have focused on the prevalence of ACEs in children (Sacks & Murphey, 2018). The results have been sobering. Overall, 1 in 10 children in the United States have experienced three or more ACEs, placing them at particularly high risk. The prevalence rates are even higher in more impoverished and less resourced states.

Clinicians working with underresourced and marginalized families understand that parents with high levels of ACEs are likely to have children who themselves will come to have high ACEs. Researchers have explored this question from various angles. Some studies have examined the relationship between maternal ACEs and infant physical and socioemotional health. McDonnell and Valentino (2016) found that maternal ACEs, and particularly childhood maltreatment experiences, were linked to both pre- and postnatal depressive symptoms in mothers and to socioemotional risk in the infant at 6 months, as measured by the Ages and Stages Questionnaire (ASQ; Squires et al., 2002). The following year, Madigan and her colleagues (2017) published a study that asked the question in a more complex way: To what degree did the intermediary mechanisms of biomedical risk (e.g., pre- and postnatal health complications, such as gestational diabetes, low infant birth weight) and psychosocial risk (e.g., maternal depression, single and/or adolescent parenthood, marital conflict) account for the impact of maternal ACEs on infant health? They found, unsurprisingly, that a history of four or more maternal ACEs greatly increased the likelihood of biomedical and psychosocial risk during the perinatal period but also that these types of risk had differential effects on later outcomes. Maternal ACEs (measured when the infants were 2 months old) were linked to later infant health (at 18 months) only in contexts of high biomedical risk; that is, mothers who had high ACEs and high biomedical risk were more likely to rate their infants' health as poor. And mothers who had high ACEs and high levels of psychosocial risk were more likely to rate their children as having behavioral and emotional problems. Thus health and psychosocial risks in mothers played different roles in the intergenerational transmission of adverse outcomes.

Many researchers have explored the relationship between maternal maltreatment (that is, a particular form of early childhood adversity) and child maltreatment. In a recent meta-analysis of the findings from 142 studies, Madigan and her colleagues (2019) found that mothers who had themselves been maltreated were twice as likely to maltreat their own children. That is, a mother's history of maltreatment puts her child at risk for maltreatment, with the mother herself a likely perpetrator. Studies have also linked a mother's history of maltreatment with child psychopathology, particularly externalizing disorders (see Plant et al., 2017). And yet the question remains: *How* are ACEs transmitted intergenerationally? What are the mechanisms of transmission from parent to child? Madigan and her colleagues' 2017 study suggests that poor maternal health and socioeconomic risk most certainly play a role. Research over the last decade also suggests two other broad (and certainly interrelated) mechanisms of transmission. The first is the impact of ACEs on parental functioning. The second is the mutual dysregulation of the stress response system.

Parental Functioning

As Lomanowska and her colleagues (2017) note in their extraordinary review of the science linking parental adversity with parental functioning: "parenting begets parenting" (p. 120). Parental functioning can, of course, be described in a number of ways. One is to look at how parents *behave*, that is, are they supportive or harsh, emotionally available or rejecting? To date, only one study has examined the relationship between mothers' ACE scores and parenting behavior (Kolomeyer et al., 2016). The study sample ($N = 230$) was predominantly White, and the majority of women were college educated and married; the study was conducted entirely online. ACE scores were correlated with negative–inconsistent and punitive parenting behaviors and with parental RF, which mediated the relations between ACE score and parenting behavior. There is a much broader literature on maltreatment and parenting behavior, however. In a meta-analysis of 32 studies involving nearly 18,000 participants, Savage and her colleagues (2019) reported a significant association between maternal history of maltreatment and parenting behavior. These effects were most apparent with measures of negative— that is, punitive, hostile, coercive, and intrusive—parenting behaviors. These effects were particularly strong when the children were boys. In other words, harsh parenting practices and disruptions in the parent–child relationship are likely sequelae of a mother's maltreatment history. In their systematic review of 12 studies involving a total of 3,758 participants, Hughes and Cossar (2016) found that a mother's history of emotional abuse and neglect was associated with a range of negative parenting outcomes, including disrupted parent–child relationships, parenting stress, maltreatment potential, lower empathy, and greater psychological control. However, the authors note that, because of the methodological limitations of the studies reviewed, these conclusions are necessarily tentative. Even more important is their observation that the "deficit focus" of the research they reviewed obscures the fact that many parents who were maltreated in their own childhoods (perhaps as many as 80–90%) *do not* maltreat their children. Thus, although a mother's experience of emotional abuse and neglect in her own childhood poses a *risk* for later parenting and relational difficulties, it does not, in any sense, *ensure* it.

There is also a fairly substantial literature linking maternal maltreatment history and child psychopathology. In their review of 12 studies (N = 45,273), Plant and his colleagues (2017) report strong, consistent associations between them, with childhood externalizing disorders being the most strongly linked to mothers' abuse history. Crucial mediators of this relationship were maternal psychological distress (anger, depression, anxiety, etc.) and harsh and punitive parenting practices. In a separate analysis of longitudinal data from the Avon Longitudinal Study of Parents and Children (N = 9,397), Plant and his colleagues (2017) found similar associations, namely, that maternal maltreatment predicted both externalizing and internalizing disorders, with prenatal and postnatal depression, as well as child maltreatment, mediating this link.

There is also an emerging literature on associations between overall level of parental ACEs and *parenting stress*, namely, the degree to which parents report negative feelings regarding their parenting role. Researchers have known for years that parenting stress is a risk factor for a number of negative outcomes, such as maltreatment and trauma exposure (Gonzalez & MacMillan, 2008), negative parenting practices (Crouch et al., 2019), and chaotic family environments (Coldwell et al., 2006). Recently, researchers have linked high levels of maternal ACEs with parenting stress (Ammerman et al., 2013; Steele et al., 2016), with higher levels of ACEs contributing to higher levels of parenting stress (Lange et al., 2019). What these data suggest is that parenting stress mediates the link between high parental ACEs and problematic parenting, such that parental adversity coupled with parenting stress is likely to result in harsh, rejecting, or disrupted parenting. In line with this, Crouch and her colleagues (2019) analyzed data from more than 50,000 parents who participated in the 2016 National Survey of Children's Health and found that high levels of parenting stress were strongly associated with high ACE prevalence (four or more ACEs) in children. A number of variables contributed to high parenting stress: having a male child, an older child, or a child with special health care needs; caring for a nonbiological child; being a single parent; being Hispanic; and living in a household with income below the federal poverty level. The most prevalent ACEs were economic hardship, parental separation or divorce, household mental illness, and substance abuse. Although an obvious clinical implication to be taken from these data is that parenting stress should be a target of intervention, the fact that parenting stress is so clearly related to socioeconomic hardship and class and racial inequality makes this a daunting task for individual clinicians and clinical programs.

Parental mental illness also appears to play a role in the process of transmitting adversity from one generation to the next. Letourneau and her colleagues (2019) examined child behavior outcomes in light of maternal ACEs and found that maternal depression and anxiety mediated their impact. In other words, when mothers were depressed or anxious prenatally, maternal ACEs were associated with behavior problems, but if they were not depressed or anxious, their experiences of adversity had less of an impact on their children. These effects were—once again—particularly pronounced for boys, who were especially vulnerable to the effects of maternal depression and anxiety. These findings highlight the importance of addressing maternal depression and anxiety in early intervention.

At the same time, as we discussed in Chapter 5, depression and anxiety could well be proxies for the maladaptations that flow from early relational trauma. In a recent review paper, Narayan and her colleagues (2021) make the point that understanding a parent's own early childhood history and appreciating the role of trauma symptoms, explicitly PTSD, is particularly important in understanding and preventing the intergenerational transmission of ACEs. Early adversity also interferes with the development of mentalizing capacities in parents (Condon et al., 2019a, 2019b; Kolomeyer et al., 2016; San Cristobal et al., 2017; Schechter et al., 2008), which also appear to play an important role in the intergenerational transmission of ACEs. Thus enhancing parental mentalizing provides yet another pathway to modulating the impacts of early adversity.

Mutual Dysregulation of the Stress Response System

As we noted earlier, another potential pathway for the intergenerational transmission of ACEs and toxic stress is the mutual dysregulation of the stress response system, such that parents' own tendency to resort to fight, flight, or freezing and to be highly stressed and thus either hyper- or hyporeactive creates threat and thus stress in the child. Support for this thesis comes in part from the literature on social buffering, which documents the myriad ways that supportive relationships buffer or block the overactivation of the HPA axis. As noted by Shonkoff and his colleagues (2012), loving and supportive relationships have the potential to mute the stress response. Megan Gunnar and her colleagues have been pioneers in this area for the past 25 years. Their initial work examined links between a child's attachment (as a proxy for the parent–child relationship and the child's relative adaptability) and HPA axis activation in a stressful situation. They found that the activation of the HPA axis was substantially blocked in toddlers who were securely attached, as compared with those who were insecurely attached (Gunnar et al., 1996; Nachmias et al., 1996). Thus, even though secure toddlers were distressed and frightened, their cortisol response was blocked. It was later discovered that HPA axis blocking occurred in secure toddlers only when their mothers were present; when their mothers were absent, HPA axis activation levels were similar to those of insecure toddlers (Ahnert et al., 2004). Parental presence continued to block the activation of the HPA axis through early puberty, at which time parental presence no longer inhibits cortisol rise (Hostinar et al., 2015). That is, "early in development attachment figures as social buffers may be capable of operating fairly directly on the HPA axis to reduce or prevent cortisol elevations to threatening stimuli" (Hostinar et al., 2014, as cited in Gunnar & Hostinar, 2015, p. 481), whereas by mid-puberty adolescents must rely on their own capacities for stress regulation (Hostinar et al., 2015).

Coming from a somewhat different angle, the Alberta Pregnancy Outcomes and Nutrition (APrON) Study Team at the University of Calgary has done key work investigating the relationship between maternal and infant HPA axis reactivity during the transition to parenthood and the particular role played by social buffering in mediating and moderating this link. Building on the prior research of Bublitz and her colleagues (2014) that linked maternal ACEs with maternal HPA axis functioning in pregnancy, the study team first established that prenatal maternal HPA axis functioning and postnatal infant HPA axis functioning are highly correlated (Giesbrecht et al., 2017); thus a mother's prenatal stress reactivity is associated with her infant's stress reactivity. Thomas, Letourneau, and their colleagues (2018) then examined whether maternal stress reactivity might be the mechanism whereby maternal ACEs were linked to infant stress reactivity and found that the effect of maternal ACEs on infant reactivity was mediated through maternal HPA axis function during pregnancy. That is, the effects of ACEs were transmitted to the infant via prenatal maternal HPA axis activation. Finally, they found that maternal social support both mediated and moderated the intergenerational transmission of ACEs. Prenatal social support moderated the link between maternal ACEs and maternal stress reactivity, such that maternal ACEs did not affect stress reactivity when mothers had high levels of social support. Likewise, maternal HPA axis function was unrelated to infant cortisol reactivity when mothers had high levels of postnatal social support. Thus, like Gunnar and her team at the University of Minnesota, the APrON study team identified social buffering, that is, positive, supportive relationships, as key to breaking the cycle of the transmission of adversity from parent to child.

There has also been some work done on the relationship between early adversity and the production of oxytocin, a neuropeptide strongly associated with social affiliation, bonding, maternal behavior, attachment, and trust (Londoño Tobón et al., 2018). It is also believed to decrease amygdala activation and thus modulate the stress response (Kirsch et al., 2005). Heim and her colleagues (2009) found that mothers who had been maltreated as children had lower levels of circulating oxytocin than did mothers who had not been maltreated, suggesting that early adversity disrupts oxytocin production. In recent work, Julian and her colleagues (2018) reported that oxytocin may actually function differently depending on a mother's level of early life stress. Specifically, they found that in mothers with low ACEs, oxytocin secretion was—as expected—linked to positive parenting. By contrast, for mothers with high ACEs, oxytocin secretion was linked to less sensitive parenting. Thus, within the context of harsh early rearing, oxytocin may support "more defensive behaviors and harsh parenting" (Julian et al., 2018, p. 375). These findings provide yet another layer of evidence for the endocrinological disruptions that flow from early adversity and that have a powerful impact on the parenting process. They are also reminiscent of Lyons-Ruth's (Lyons-Ruth et al., 1999b) notion that responding to the child's needs for closeness and comfort may be very triggering for vulnerable mothers and heighten their defenses and thus negative parenting practices, such as hostility or withdrawal.

Boys May Be More Vulnerable

There is considerable evidence from animal models that stress differentially affects males and females across "brain regions and multiple functions" (McEwen, 2017). Some of the studies cited earlier suggest that boys appear to suffer the consequences of maternal stress and trauma more acutely (Crouch et al., 2019; Letourneau et al., 2019; Savage et al., 2019). In addition, positive maternal memories of loving caregivers appear to be protective only for female children (Narayan et al., 2019). Although there are too few data to generalize from these studies, it seems possible that boys may be more triggering for mothers. They tend to be quite active and more aggressive than girls, and often they mature later than girls. Also, the perpetrators of violence in women's lives were often men. For these reasons, boys may be more frightening for mothers and thus elicit more hostile or helpless maternal responses. They may also be particularly challenging for traumatized parents who—when in survival mode—tend to be hypervigilant, self-protective, easily frightened, poorly regulated, and quick to anger. These are clearly questions for future research.

Protective or Resilience Factors

Developmental psychologists have been studying resilience—defined as the capacity to adapt, recover, or transform in the face of adversity (Narayan et al., 2021)—for nearly 50 years, with Garmezy (1974) and Rutter (1985) taking the lead early on. Later, Masten (2014), in particular, but also Cicchetti (Cicchetti & Garmezy, 1993; Masten & Cicchetti, 2016) and Luthar (Luthar et al., 2000) fully established the study of resilience within mainstream academic psychology. Key to resilience are factors that counteract or mitigate risk, either by promoting positive developments or by protecting the individual against risks. Children's resilience—which is not rare (Masten, 2014)—is to a large extent dependent on the family system in which they live, namely, their parents' health and behavior under conditions of adversity (Masten et al., 2015). And in some instances, where adversity is prolonged or severe and the relationships and resources that support resilience are unavailable, recovery and adaptation can be very difficult (Masten et al., 2015).

Interestingly, despite the considerable developmental literature on resilience and Gunnar and her colleagues' decades of research on the power of social buffering in mitigating the stress response (Gunnar & Hostinar, 2015), there has—relative to the study of ACEs—been little study of the factors that "increase the likelihood of successful development" in the face of considerable risk (Bethell et al., 2019, p. 2). Among the first to examine the role played by positive childhood influences in countering the impact of ACEs were Chung and her colleagues (2008). These influences were defined as being loved and supported by primary attachment figures. In a sample of nearly 1,500 single, pregnant, low-income African American women, ACEs were associated with higher levels of maternal depression, whereas positive childhood influences had a protective effect and were associated with lower levels of depressive symptoms.

In the second wave of the ACE study, which was conducted between 1996 and 1997, respondents were asked not only about ACEs but also about factors that might mitigate the impact of early adversity, specifically, family strengths. These were defined as family closeness, support, loyalty, and protection; feelings of being loved and important; and responsiveness to needs for health care. When these factors were analyzed in relation to ACEs, Hillis and her colleagues (2010) reported that family strengths do, in fact, buffer the impact of early adversity on the psychosocial consequences of adolescent pregnancy. In this largely White, college-educated sample of more than 4,500 women, they found, first, that those reporting high levels of family strengths (6 or 7 out of a possible 7) were significantly less likely to report a history of ACEs. They also found that the more family strengths a woman endorsed, the less likely she was to have been pregnant as an adolescent, the later she became sexually active, and the less she suffered the long-term psychosocial consequences of adolescent pregnancy, such as problems with family, jobs, or finances. These effects were seen across all ACE exposure levels, suggesting that family strengths buffer the impact of ACEs on adolescent development.

Since then, a small literature has evolved focusing on factors that mitigate the impact of ACEs on a range of outcomes. On the one hand, there are the large population studies by Christina Bethell and her colleagues and, on the other, the smaller clinical studies by Angela Narayan and hers. Bethell and her team first conducted a large population study in which they combined data from various governmental surveys in order to assess the impact of a range of factors on the prevalence of emotional, mental, and behavioral problems (EMBPs) in 9,417 children (Bethell et al., 2016). In line with other studies, they found that a child's level of ACE exposure was strongly predictive of EMBPs. They also found that children with high ACEs and no resilience factors had an even higher chance of developing EMBPs than children who had resilience factors. The resilience factors most associated with attenuating the impact of ACEs on the child's mental health were (1) child resilience, namely the capacity to stay calm and in control when faced with a challenge (i.e., emotion regulation), and (2) family protective factors, particularly a parent's capacity to manage stress and be involved in a child's daily life. These two forms of resilience are, unsurprisingly, correlated with each other.

In a second large population study, Bethell and her colleagues (2019) used data from the 2015 Wisconsin Behavioral Risk Factor Survey administered to more than 6,000 adult respondents to create a composite measure of positive childhood experiences (PCEs). This measure assessed how often adults felt supported, safe, and able to connect with their families, friends, and the larger community. They found that when adults reported higher childhood PCEs, they were less likely to suffer from depression and other mental health problems and more likely to have higher levels of social and emotional support, regardless of their level of exposure to ACEs. They conclude:

> Even as society continues to address remediable causes of childhood adversities such as ACEs, attention should be given to the *creation of those positive experiences that both reflect and generate resilience within children, families, and communities.* Success will depend on full engagement of families and communities and changes in the health care, education, and social services systems serving children and families. A joint inventory of ACEs and PCEs . . . may improve efforts to assess needs, target interventions, and engage individuals in addressing the adversities they face by leveraging existing assets and strengths. Initiatives to conduct broad ACEs screening . . . may benefit from integrated assessments including PCEs. (Bethell et al., 2019, p. 8, emphasis added)

In related work, Narayan, Lieberman, and their colleagues have focused on the role of benevolent childhood experiences (BCEs) in offsetting the impact of ACEs. As described in Chapter 1, this work emerged out of Lieberman and her colleagues' (Lieberman et al., 2005a) observation that even the most traumatized mothers could, at times, report memories of positive, loving interactions with caregivers. Unlike memories of "ghosts in the nursery," of terror, rage, and utter disorganization at the hands of their caregivers, these memories of "angels in the nursery" had the potential to provide hope and opportunities for resilience and healing in the face of enormous pain (Lieberman et al., 2005a). On the basis of these observations, Lieberman and her colleagues developed the Angels in the Nursery Interview (Van Horn et al., 2008), which is a simple, seven-question interview that asks a parent to describe memories of feeling loved and safe as a child. The interview takes only 10–15 minutes to administer and, with training, 10–15 minutes to code.

Narayan, Lieberman, and their colleagues (Narayan et al., 2017) evaluated whether "angel" memories might offset the impact of ACEs on the development of PTSD. They administered the Angels Interview to 54 mothers and rated angel memories from low to high on dimensions of positivity, specificity, and elaboration. They also noted the presence of "ghost" memories—recollections of frightening, traumatic, or emotional childhood events. Ghost memories were scored for the degree to which they overwhelmed or dominated positive memories, with the highest score reflecting an inability to describe angel memories without triggering negative and traumatic memories at the same time. Mothers' childhood trauma and current PTSD symptoms were also assessed. Narayan and her colleagues found that for mothers who had low levels of angel memories, childhood maltreatment strongly predicted PTSD symptoms in adulthood. If the mothers had even fleeting angel memories, however, the association between childhood maltreatment and adult PTSD was nonsignificant. That is, if a mother could remember ever feeling loved and safe, even within the context of abuse, she was less likely to develop PTSD symptoms. Importantly, Narayan and her colleagues noted that, for mothers who had suffered high levels of emotional and physical abuse, being asked to recall angel memories often triggered ghost memories. Mothers with high angel *and* ghost memories had the highest level of PTSD in the sample. In light of this, they speculated that recovery may be especially complex for individuals whose ghosts and angels vie internally for supremacy (Lieberman et al., 2005a), leaving them at the mercy of "continued psychological and emotional unrest in the form of elevated PTSD symptoms and an intermixing of high positive and negative affect" (Narayan et al., 2017, p. 472). Thus clinicians may find that the process of uncovering angel memories may also provoke other, more painful memories.

In a subsequent replication study (Narayan et al., 2019), the Angels Interview was administered to a group of 185 predominantly Latina, low-income mothers, most of whom had not completed high school and a quarter of whom spoke only Spanish. A large proportion (80%) of the mothers reported at least one type of maltreatment, and 13% reported all five subtypes of maltreatment measured. Positive childhood memories were again found to be protective against the impact of childhood trauma; that is, as in the original study, mothers with more positive memories had lower levels of PTSD and comorbid psychopathology, even in the face of considerable maltreatment. In addition, the *daughters* (but not sons) of mothers who were able to recall positive, loving memories from their childhoods had less trauma exposure themselves, even when mothers reported high levels of maltreatment. For mothers with few angel memories, childhood maltreatment predicted current PTSD, comorbid psychopathology, and child trauma exposure.

These studies provided the impetus for Narayan and her colleagues to develop the BCE scale (Narayan et al., 2018) as a counterpoint to the ACE scale. Like the ACE scale, the BCE scale has 10 items. The BCE scale incorporated questions used in prior studies of positive childhood experiences, including the work by Chung, Hillis, and their colleagues (Chung et al., 2008; Hillis et al., 2010). But in an attempt to redress some of the limitations of prior instruments, particular attention was paid to a range of cultural factors in constructing the scale, such that it could be used in multicultural and multilingual settings (Narayan et al., 2018). In a sample of 101 ethnically diverse, low-income pregnant women, the scale was found to have high test–retest reliability and to be suitable across ethnic and racial groups, in both Spanish and English languages. High levels of BCEs were inversely correlated with prenatal depression, PTSD symptoms, perceived stress and prenatal stressful life events (SLEs) and mitigated the effects of childhood ACEs on prenatal PTSD and SLEs, over and above ACEs. In other words, BCEs appeared to offset the impact of ACEs on prenatal trauma symptomatology and prenatal stress. These findings once again underscore the importance of benevolent caregiving experiences in offsetting or buffering the impact of trauma and other sources of stress. In addition, initial reliability and predictive validity studies suggest that the BCE scale may be particularly suitable for inclusion in population studies of the impact of PCEs in offsetting early trauma and disruption.

Collectively, these studies suggest that angel memories may well buffer the impact of maternal ACEs on the child. Although a small percentage of mothers did not report any angel memories, for some mothers, angel memories were observed even in the face of severe maltreatment. Narayan and her colleagues (2018) suggest that a certain level of BCEs may be necessary to offset the effects of traumatic events: "Having only five of these 10 total BCEs across one's childhood may signal risk for future impairment," leaving mothers "more susceptible to the harmful effects of their childhood adversity" (p. 27). They also suggest that every effort should be made to access angel memories in therapeutic work with mothers, beginning in the prenatal period. Over time, treatment may help soften defenses in ways that allow the emergence of more positive memories that may, in a variety of ways, offset the impact of and allow the working through of more traumatic and deeply painful ones.

Summary: The Big Picture

The multiple associations we described here make evident the fact that high parental ACEs not only affect the parent's own physical and mental health but that of their child, as well. Parenting stress, socioeconomic risk, maternal mental health, and stress reactivity all serve as mediators of this association, as may the fact that the child is male. Needless to say, all of these mediators are likely highly intercorrelated. But how can we understand these associations at a deeper level? Why are parents who were exposed to highly adverse circumstances so vulnerable when it comes to parenting? At one level, to return to some of the points we made in earlier chapters, marginalized and oppressed populations with significant exposure to systemic racism, high poverty, and very limited resources are much more likely to report high ACEs. That is, ACEs are in large part a marker of a range of threats that can make living and loving very difficult. A parent raised in circumstances that are threatening and frightening may not be able to relax the hypervigilance and self-protectiveness that allowed them to survive in dangerous situations but that now impair their ability to respond sensitively and accurately to their child's signals (Narayan et al., 2019; Savage et al., 2019). In other words, being on high alert for danger may be antithetical to a parent's ability to provide a loving, secure base for the child and to openly, flexibly, and accurately make meaning of the child's experience. Along similar lines, the child, their needs, and particularly their negative affects may trigger the pain, fear, and threat associated with the parent's trauma, such that both maternal behavior toward and maternal representations of the child are laced with feelings of helplessness and rage (Lyons-Ruth et al., 1999b; Lyons-Ruth et al., 2005).

"Angels in the nursery" (Lieberman et al., 2005a), however, protect. "Mothers who are able to retain memories of feeling safe, protected, and loved within an overall context of adversity" (Narayan et al., 2019, p. 183) may be less prone to primitive ways of thinking and of defense. Positive memories may allow them to better protect their children from their own angry impulses, to more accurately detect threats in the environment, and to protect their children from these threats. Thus, to return to the point made at the start of this chapter, namely, that high levels of stress, threat, or fearful arousal disrupt development, they particularly affect the development of the caregiving system, specifically a parent's capacity to protect, comfort, and sensitively respond to their child.

When the ACE study was published in 1998, it received surprisingly little attention in the developmental, clinical, or policy literature. This despite the fact that its findings were consistent with much of what researchers, health care providers, therapists, and epidemiologists knew about the impact of early experience on later outcomes. The study also confirmed the basic principles of dynamic psychology, namely, that early relationships matter. Why, we might ask, did it take so long for these critical findings to make their way into health and mental health practice and policy? Why did this study, which, one could argue, is—along with the discovery of penicillin, statins, and several lifesaving vaccines—among the most important public health studies of the 20th century, languish for so long? There are a number of possible explanations, of course. We have, for a number of generations, preferred to focus on changing behavior (which can devolve into blaming the victim if change is difficult) rather than on truly understanding "what happened to this person" and attempting to remedy the larger ills facing us as human beings. Thus, to a certain extent, the findings of the ACE study challenged the notion that we are responsible for our own destiny.[2] Many cultures link "good" behavior with "good" outcomes and place considerable emphasis upon individual responsibility and action. The failure to behave in a certain way is often viewed as a moral failing. Thus, if you brush your teeth every day, you will prevent tooth decay. If you have a lot of cavities, you must have failed to brush your teeth regularly. But what if your family had no money to purchase toothbrushes, toothpaste, or healthy, fresh food? What if there was nowhere in your neighborhood to buy fruits and vegetables? What if you were raised on a diet full of added sugar because the only food available in the local convenience store was junk food and your family did not have a car to drive to the supermarket? What if your parents did not have the resources to see a dentist regularly and learn about proper dental hygiene themselves? The first question often asked of a person who has the enormous misfortune of being diagnosed with lung cancer is, "Did you smoke?" But what if you had been raised in a home where everyone smoked cigarettes, and you were exposed to secondhand smoke for 20 years? And what if the tobacco industry particularly targeted your racial or ethnic group and your community? And let us not forget those individuals whose genetic makeups predispose them to tooth decay and cancer!

The multiple studies of ACEs shatter the notion that "good" behavior is necessarily an individual choice. The links between early adversity and racial, ethnic, health, and economic disparities are extraordinarily compelling. They also make abundantly clear how difficult it is to prevent early childhood adversity unless we can begin to address the profound social,

---

[2]Trauma and attachment theories similarly disrupted the status quo.

structural, and economic inequities that—in the bulk of cases—lead both to high ACEs and low PCEs or BCEs. And yet we are, in the third decade of the 21st century, singularly focused on assessing and quantifying ACEs. Collecting ACE questionnaires has become the holy grail of social and medical science. Knowing that a child has been exposed to adversity or that an adult was exposed to more abuse than we can even contemplate does tell us something very important about their level of risk. And assessing protective factors tells us something about the resources they can call on to heal. But such assessments are *only the first step*. There are no treatments or approaches guaranteed to diminish the impact of ACEs or prevent them altogether (Finkelhor, 2018), although interventions such as home visiting, which provide a range of supports for parents, certainly help (Garner et al., 2013). The problem is made more complex by the degree to which ACEs are embedded in the complex social and economic fabric of individual lives. At the broadest level, we can only change inequities through massive shifts in social and economic policy, shifts that most societies seem loath to make.

And yet, as we try to make clear throughout this book, we can make change at the individual and family levels by witnessing, holding, and hearing families' stories, by calling on their strengths, by providing them with resources and information, and by helping them navigate health and social service systems that are overstretched, underfunded, and—at times—impenetrable. Asking "what happened to you, and how can we help?" is the first step in helping "right the boat" at the individual level. And it engages us in some of the most profound social, cultural, racial, economic, and human questions we can imagine. And so it is not hard to understand why progress in asking these questions was initially slow, nor is it hard to understand why—even when many professionals now ask them all the time, and vigorously seek solutions—progress is painstaking and full of frustration.

QUESTIONS FOR CLINICIANS

▶ What do you know about a parent's history of adversity?

▶ What do you know about a parent's more benevolent childhood experiences?

▶ In what ways are you able to ameliorate some of the impacts of adversity and toxic stress?

  ▷ Provide a safe relationship that can help buffer the effects of adversity and toxic stress.

  ▷ Help interrupt the intergenerational transmission by limiting adverse experiences in the child's life.

  ▷ Provide a range of resources and concrete support to ameliorate the impacts of systemic oppression, deprivation, and racism.

▶ Do you observe the sequelae of attachment trauma, particularly the posttraumatic adaptations that are intrinsic to ongoing experiences of maltreatment and other forms of extreme adversity?

▶ How do these directly affect parenting?

▶ Is the parent able to reflect upon their experiences of childhood adversity so that these can be integrated and their effects more readily regulated?

Part

II

Establishing the Relational Foundations of Reflection

In Part I, we laid out a series of ideas that form the theoretical and scientific bases for MTB-P. The development of secure, loving attachment relationships during the first years of life is critical to a range of later outcomes, including physical and emotional health. The development of secure attachment in the child is at least partially dependent upon a parent's capacity to reflect upon and make meaning of the child's desires, intentions, thoughts, and feelings, as these are expressed in action and language. Parental mentalizing capacities (as well as child attachment) emerge within the context of safety and regulation, whereas threat and fear powerfully disrupt these processes. Higher levels of adversity and trauma profoundly affect an individual's capacity to trust others and to make sense of them in a loving and positive way.

The core aim of MTB-P is to support the development of loving, reciprocal relationships between children and their caregivers by promoting reflective capacities in parents, helping them make loving sense of their children's bodies and minds. Trauma and adversity impede parental mentalizing, largely because they make it hard both to tolerate the negative emotions of parenthood and to find pleasure in intimacy and close connection. As such, parents who are struggling with adversity and its sequelae are more likely to default to what we defined in Part I as deficient ("too little") or intrusive ("too much") mentalizing. They may also be more prone to seeing their children and themselves (as caregivers) in hostile and helpless ways. How do we, as clinicians, support the development of positive mentalizing capacities? As we hope to make clear in the next three chapters, we start by developing the *foundations of reflection*, namely, safety, regulation, and relationship, first in clinicians, and then in parents and children. Without careful attention to each, true reflection is not possible. If we wish to help young, stressed families develop the capacities that we believe ensure success across a number of domains, we must begin by creating safety, promoting regulation, and establishing secure, supportive relationships. In Chapter 7 we fully describe the relational foundations of reflection (RFR) model at the core of MTB-P; in Chapter 8 we apply the model to clinicians, and, in Chapter 9, to parents and children.

Chapter

7

The Relational Foundations
of Reflection

The finding that secure attachment in the child was linked to the parent's mentalizing abilities was fundamental to the development of MTB-HV. As such, we saw building a parent's reflective or mentalizing capacities, beginning in pregnancy, as crucial to the development of secure attachment, as well as a range of positive health and mental health outcomes in the infant, toddler, and child. To that end, a primary focus of training and supervision was—from the beginning—on developing clinicians' skills in recognizing and enhancing parental reflective functioning (PRF). However, as we trained more and more practitioners, we noticed that clinicians ended up paying *too much attention* to PRF and not enough attention to its antecedents. That is, they spent too much time focusing on outcomes and not on the steps necessary to their achievement. This had several unintended consequences. For all the reasons described in Part I, mentalizing may often be difficult for vulnerable parents, and it may develop very slowly when it begins to appear. As we describe more fully in Part III, even when parents are making progress, their capacity to reflect can come and go with the impact of strong feelings or other triggers. Nevertheless, MTB clinicians sometimes felt that they had failed because parents weren't particularly reflective. Worrying about the absence of parental mentalizing, they would inadvertently create subtle tension by asking parents to do what they could not, namely, reflect. Their frustration was palpable in the question we heard many times over: "How can we *get* them to be more reflective?"

We slowly realized that we needed to help parents *and clinicians* start from the ground up, to help them build the foundations of reflection. As we described throughout Part I, the development of mentalizing depends first upon safety or—conversely—the relative absence of threat. We cannot think about anything or attend to our feelings when we are in survival mode. Second, mentalizing depends upon regulation, the relative quieting of the body and mind that allows us to move toward others (and, in a sense, toward ourselves). Third, it depends upon trust and the support and holding of a secure relationship (Allen, 2022; Fonagy & Allison, 2014; Fonagy et al., 1995). That is, the capacity to mentalize evolves within the context of safe, secure relationships. Threat and dysregulation profoundly distort relationships and preclude mentalizing and reflection.

When clinicians focus on the parent's capacity to mentalize *before* they have established safety, regulation, and a relationship with the parent (and often the child as well), the effort to develop a parent's reflective capacities falters. Therefore, we begin here with a focus on building the relational foundations of safety, regulation, and relationship. We think of these as *relational* foundations because they are established within the context of relationships. These foundations are also dynamically connected; each has to be reestablished when disrupted by threat, and all three reciprocally influence each other through rupture and repair, progression and regression. As we reiterate throughout the book, progress is never purely linear, although it is always our hope that, with time, repeated safety, and regulation, relationships will stabilize.

Although parental mentalizing can take quite a long time to develop, particularly in traumatized parents, it is critical that the *practitioner* be able to maintain a mentalizing stance from the start. Of course this may falter under the press of strong emotions and chaotic circumstances; hopefully, however, this capacity is fairly resilient and can rebound readily with supervision and support. Our capacity to maintain a mentalizing stance even in the face of acute distress and danger serves as the model and scaffold for parents' own efforts to trust and to see and hear themselves and their children.

Finally, as is evident throughout the rest of the book, particularly in our case examples, maintaining a reflective stance does not mean abandoning *doing*. For many of the families seen in infant mental health and health practice, providing concrete support is an essential part of the work. It is impossible for parents to move out of survival mode without food or shelter or the most basic of resources. As such, it often falls to practitioners to help families gain access to these fundamentals. We believe that the MTB-P approach offers a way of providing these supports that is respectful and empowering. We call this the "dance of directing and reflecting." When clinicians are called upon to be active, to provide information and guidance, or intervene directly and immediately, such "directing" is always offered within the larger framework of the clinician's reflectiveness. "Doing" *before* reflecting short-circuits our understanding, and we run the risk of taking charge, telling parents what to do, and robbing them of their autonomy and the grace of being listened to as the basis of collaboration. In addition, "doing" without reflection can run the risk of feeling like another form of oppression to the parents, one almost certain to provoke defensiveness and a breakdown in the relationship.

The Relational Foundations of Reflection Pyramid

The relational foundations of reflection (RFR) pyramid visually represents the theory and science we presented in Part I, specifically, the idea that mentalizing or reflectiveness depends first upon safety and regulation, which in turn makes a trusting relationship possible. This relationship, in turn, provides the foundation for mentalizing. So many of the families we see struggle with threat and dysregulation much of the time and resort to the prementalizing modes we described in Chapter 5. Thus we must begin where they are and gently bring them into relationship and potentially to a stance of curiosity and meaning making. In the following sections, we fully describe each of these relational foundations and the ways they are interconnected and build on each other. In so doing, we hope to bring home the point that clinicians need to focus not just on the top of the pyramid but also on establishing and reestablishing the foundations, as necessary. As we discuss in Chapter 8, this process begins with the clinician and their sense of safety, degree of regulation, and openness to relationship. These are the foundations for the parent's and ultimately child's capacity to feel safe, regulated, and heard.

Safety and Regulation

The theory and science we reported throughout Part I make evident that threat is bad for the body, the brain, and the soul. As such, we (and all living things) are evolutionarily primed to detect threats to our survival. Threats—to the parent or child—take many forms: (1) *external* threats to literal survival: predators, environmental risks (a car barreling down the road, poisonous substances, deadly illnesses, etc.); (2) *internal* threats: strong feelings or memories that threaten one's equilibrium or disrupt relationships; and (3) *relational* threats: threats within the caregiving relationship to relational or literal safety, namely, *to* the relationship from *within* the relationship (a frightening or dissociated parent). These circumstances have the potential to initiate a cascade of physiological and behavioral responses, which—when they persist—undermine neural and neuroendocrine functioning and affect development in a myriad of ways. The child or adult is in "limbic system overdrive" (van der Kolk, 2014), and higher order functions are compromised, if they are available at all. The parts of the brain that register fear, primarily the amygdala, remain in a state of arousal. The HPA axis, a critical stress response system, is activated. Mentalizing is impossible.

Happily, not only are we primed to detect threat, but we are also primed to *seek safety*, the antidote to threat. For all humans (and indeed all mammals), what makes threat manageable and keeps it from disrupting development and relationships is the experience of safety. This dynamic serves as the basis of the attachment relationship; the child is evolutionarily primed—in situations of threat—to seek care from one who is stronger and wiser and who thus can protect them and ensure their survival. This is their secure base. Threats to safety are part of everyday life and activate the attachment system. In infancy and childhood, it is the parent who manages threats to the child's physical or emotional safety; what keeps fear and threat from being traumatic is the parent's readiness and availability to provide safety and to reestablish balance with soothing, comfort, and regulation. Restoring safety and countering fear take place in the smallest moments and recur over and over.

Threat leads to dysregulation, and safety leads to regulation (see Figure 7.1). As such, safety and regulation are deeply interconnected, the relationship between them reciprocal and dynamic. Optimally, when safety is threatened (and it regularly is, even in the most benign developmental

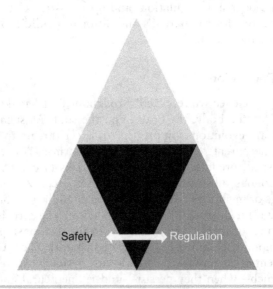

FIGURE 7.1 The foundations of safety and reflection.

circumstances), regulation restores. These dynamic forces constitute the basic components of the attachment system: namely, the detection of threat, the activation of the attachment system, and the search for safety in regulation.

When the child's fear is met by the parent's reassurance and comfort, threat barely registers, fear is regulated, and life goes on; eventually, parental ministrations become internalized and lead to self-regulation. This is what Winnicott (1965) meant by the parent ensuring the child's "going on being." The baby in Sharon Olds's poem, at first fearful, feels the calm enter him when gently reassured by his mother's holding. His attachment system, briefly activated, is quieted by her presence, and he can explore. Regulation allows the child to experience the world outside of their own fear/anxiety, to—within a framework of safety and containment—know themselves, see the other, and function as a thinking, perceiving being. Remaining in an even relatively minor state of fearful arousal disrupts development and keeps the child in a state of dread, protecting the self rather than turning outward to others and the world. As we saw in Gunnar and her colleagues' early work on social buffering (Gunnar et al., 1996), when a child who is securely attached is threatened, their cortisol or stress levels remain low. When a child feels threatened within the context of an *insecure* attachment relationship, however, their cortisol levels show greater reactivity, and they remain—in one way or the other—fearful. This is also one of the key points of the literature on toxic stress (Shonkoff et al., 2012). Protective, reciprocal, and loving relationships can protect the child from the negative effects of stress and fear. When fear persists, in part because of the caregiver's inability to protect the child, its effects color the world.

We find the work of the neuroscientist Stephen Porges (2003, 2004, 2011) particularly helpful in thinking about the reciprocal relationship between safety and regulation. Human beings, he proposes, are born with the capacity for "neuroception," namely, a mechanism that allows individuals of all ages to evaluate threat and—conversely—safety. This evaluation takes place through the senses—sight, hearing, smell, taste, and touch—and engages neural circuits that—without our conscious awareness—allow us to distinguish "whether situations or people are safe, dangerous, or life-threatening" (Porges, 2004, p. 19). When danger is detected, self-protective defenses are activated, whereas, when the environment is experienced as safe, social engagement is activated, and defenses are inhibited. Without such a mechanism—which has the dual function of evaluating threat and promoting social interaction—our species would not have adapted and survived.

Porges (2003) defines these self-protective defenses in terms of biologically based mechanisms for stress regulation, namely, fight, flight, and freezing. The level of disruption or dysregulation depends on the level of threat. When situations are life-threatening, our most ancient mechanism of self-protection is initiated, namely, "death-feigning." The body starts to shut down, blood pressure drops, the heart slows, and breathing slows. Behaviorally, this fear manifests in freezing and immobilization. When threats are less dire, the sympathetic nervous system and HPA axis are engaged, and the body moves into action: metabolic activity, cortisol, and cardiac output (i.e., faster heart rate, greater ability of the heart to contract) increase. The body is on alert. Behaviorally, one of two potential defensive strategies is employed: flight or fight.

By contrast, when an individual feels safe, these defensive reactions and the activation of the sympathetic nervous system are inhibited. Oxytocin is released. The stress response is mitigated, and social engagement is possible. This is behaviorally manifest in facial expressions (smiling, open eyes), vocalization, and listening. When the social engagement system is activated, immobilization *without* fear (which is necessary, for example, in nursing infants or in adult intimacy) is possible. Humans have the capacity from birth to signal readiness for social engagement. Pathways between the cortex and the brain stem regulate the muscles of the face and head, so that we can "gesture with our heads, put intonation in our voices, direct our gaze, and . . . distinguish human voices from background noises" (Porges, 2011, pp. 14–15). Infants can initiate social interaction by making eye contact, vocalizing with an appealing inflection and rhythm, displaying contingent facial expressions, and modulating the middle-ear muscles to distinguish the human voice from background sounds more efficiently. When we feel safe, we can make eye contact, we smile, we respond contingently to others, and our bodies are open and relaxed.

By contrast, the perception of danger leads to reduced tone in these critical muscles, at which point "the eyelids droop, the voice loses inflection, positive facial expressions dwindle, awareness of the sound of the human voice becomes less acute, and sensitivity to other's social engagement behaviors decrease" (Porges, 2011, p. 15). We would add to this the many signs that the individual (and their body) is closed to communication: The chest and torso are collapsed, movement in the arms is constricted, and the head is dipped or slightly turned away (Shai & Belsky, 2011; Tortora, 2005). Porges also draws attention to the "gut" reaction we can have in response to threatening situations, a reaction that may be the only sign we have that something is amiss.

We return to the arousal curve (see Figure 7.2) to illustrate how these defensive strategies map directly onto categories of insecure attachment (Porges, 2003, 2004) and prementalizing. The "flight" stance is consistent with avoidant–dismissing attachment and deficient–concrete prementalizing (too little), whereas the "fight" stance is consistent with both the resistant–preoccupied stance and the intrusive–hostile category of

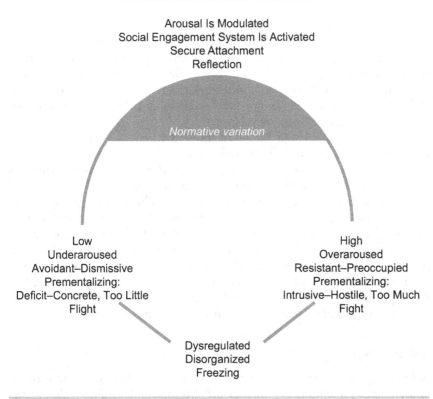

Arousal Is Modulated
Social Engagement System Is Activated
Secure Attachment
Reflection

Normative variation

Low
Underaroused
Avoidant–Dismissive
Prementalizing:
Deficit–Concrete, Too Little
Flight

High
Overaroused
Resistant–Preoccupied
Prementalizing:
Intrusive–Hostile, Too Much
Fight

Dysregulated
Disorganized
Freezing

FIGURE 7.2 Arousal: Fight, flight, and freezing.

prementalizing (too much). And "freezing," the most ancient and lifesaving of defensive maneuvers, is aligned with attachment disorganization and a complete collapse of mentalizing.

The critical thing to remember is that these defenses or adaptations are *activated* by threat and the need to find comfort and solace in whatever way is possible. The curve's apogee marks the activation of the social engagement system, with defenses softened and, perhaps, abandoned—that is, when the infant or parent (or clinician!) feels safe and regulated, open to relationship, and able to reflect. The individual's eyes, ears, and facial muscles are open and relaxed, their chest is open and relaxed, their voice has a soothing intonation and prosody, and the gut is quiet. This is the optimal state for social interaction and meaningful reflection: alert and attuned, the child is tuned into the outside world, and both their gaze and facial movements are quiet as they fully take in people and objects around them. As the infant develops, they can remain in this state for longer and longer periods and engage in interaction in a way that is hugely pleasurable to their parents (and to the infant as well!). Importantly, the activation of the social engagement system allows for the activation of reciprocal systems *in one's interactive partner* (Porges, 2011). Thus the parent's openness to relationship has a reciprocal effect on their child; smiles, openness, warmth, and other indications of safe connection trigger the same circuits in the child. Likewise, a clinician's openness to social engagement can allow for co-regulated interactions with the parent.

What does this mean for clinicians? In MTB-P, we often think of our work as moving the parent (and, ultimately, the child) from one pole *toward the curve's apogee*, becoming either more able to tolerate emotion or more able to regulate it, with the goal being openness to relationship and the activation of the social engagement system. This requires us to always begin by assessing our own, as well as a parent's, level of threat and dysregulation. There is such a tendency, particularly when clinicians are expected to implement a particular curriculum module or realize a particular goal, to jump to the goal without attention to the *process*. Are we feeling threatened? Are we dysregulated? And the parents? Are they feeling threatened or dysregulated? If so, neither we nor the parents will be ready for or open to the social engagement that is critical for any therapeutic success.

Relationship

Safety and regulation lay the foundations for the relationships that make *living* beings the *human beings* they are. Infants, children, and adults need love, comfort, and emotional connection to thrive as human beings. Relationships offer the connections and closeness that help the child (or adult) feel safe, known, and understood and provide a basic remedy for fear—of loss, of annihilation, of psychic emptiness. Relationships with our nearest and dearest help us discover how we feel, what we want, what we see, and what we know—or, conversely, cannot know, think, or feel (Bowlby, 1979; Stern, 1977, 1985). For better or for worse, we each bear the unique imprint of the care we received (or didn't) as children. Relationships also teach us about the *other*. It is through relationships that infants and children learn what is in the hearts and minds of those closest to them. In part, coming to know the other is a function of the instinct to survive (we seek care from those who can provide it, and we must know our enemies to survive them), but at the same time it also allows for deeper and more meaningful intimacy and closeness, a feeling of connection that is one of life's ultimate and most human pleasures.

In the RFR model, the development of trusting and reciprocal relationships, of full social engagement, *depends* upon the (relative) achievement of safety and regulation (Porges, 2011). Once the child or parent feels safe and regulated, they can fully engage with the other, and a real relationship—in which two people truly come to know one another—is possible (see Figure 7.3). When threat and dysregulation persist, however, relationships are in some fundamental way distorted. van der Kolk (2014) makes a similar point when he argues that trauma treatment must combine "top-down approaches (to activate social engagement) with bottom-up methods (to calm physical tensions in the body)" (p. 86).

Reflection

From the perspective of MTB-P, when a clinician, parent, or child feels safe, trusting, and understood, they can begin to discover the world and the people in it. Together with another, they can discover the world, the child with the parent, the parent with the clinician, the clinician with the supervisor. They can become a "we," exploring in collaboration (Fonagy et al., 2021).

> A toddler finds a daisy on his daily walk with his father. He squats to examine it more closely. Dad says simply, "Oh, is that a daisy? You wanna' see the daisy?" The child continues his intense examination, deep in thought. Dad says, "That's so pretty. You like that, don't you?" In that simple exchange, the child's curiosity, as well as his interest and pleasure, are mirrored and supported.

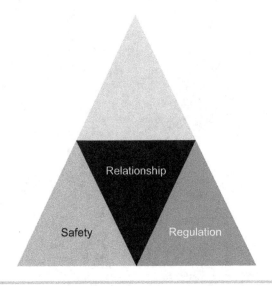

FIGURE 7.3 Safety and regulation support the relationship.

They are also amplified and highlighted. The child is discovering a daisy by contemplating it with his father, who is providing the frame or scaffold for his observations and pleasure. This is how he comes to know his inner world and, eventually, to know the inner world of others.

From the safety and regulation of key relationships, infants and toddlers can begin to think, to reflect upon their own experience and on the experience of the other. This, in turn, leads to the affective correlates of reflection, namely, empathy, compassion, and "fellow feeling."

Children come to trust the knowledge and information imparted by caregivers; adults come to trust the knowledge and information imparted by the clinicians working with them (Fonagy & Allison, 2014). These are all forms of what Fonagy and his colleagues (2021) call collaborative or "relational mentalizing." Werner and Kaplan (1963) called this the "primordial sharing situation," and Winnicott (1971) the "playspace" between parent and child that gives rise to the symbol, understanding, and knowledge. From the safety of their relationships, children and their parents can begin to contemplate and make meaning of people and things in their universe, namely, to reflect and to learn. The richness of this process is entirely contingent on their foundational experiences of feeling safe, contained, and known by the other (see Figure 7.4).

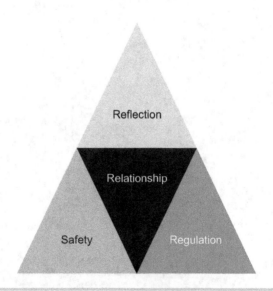

FIGURE 7.4 The relational foundations of reflection.

Clinical Use of the RFR Pyramid

The RFR pyramid provides a way of practitioners' locating themselves in a clinical encounter.[1] Clearly, as the levels of the pyramid build on each other, the clinician always begins at the bottom and starts the work where there is difficulty. We discuss the process in a range of contexts across the next two chapters, but, as a general rule, if the parent feels safe (judging by their bodily posture, the nature of their speech, the coherence and authenticity of their narratives) and seems regulated (showing no signs of fight, flight, freezing, or their correlates), they are then open to social engagement, and to the power of the clinician–parent relationship. Can intimacy deepen, can more powerful thoughts, memories, and feelings be shared? Is the "we mode" possible? From there, can the parent genuinely imagine—in word and in deed—the child's experience, as well as their own? Of course, ruptures and disruptions are normal. It is important to remember, therefore, that all the forces in the pyramid are *dynamic* (see Figure 7.5). Safety and regulation will need to be established again and again, and trust and connection restored over and over.

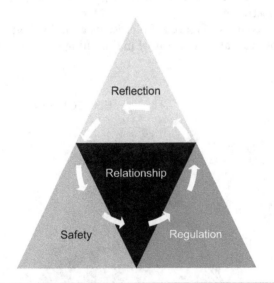

FIGURE 7.5 The cyclical and dynamic aspects of reflection.

---

[1]As we discuss more fully in Chapter 8, this concept has much in common with Gilkerson's FAN approach (Gilkerson & Imberger, 2016).

Distortions in the RFR Pyramid

In this section, we use the pyramid graphic to illustrate how the three general defensive strategies we have emphasized throughout this book (too little, too much, and disorganization) distort the relational foundations of mentalizing and mentalizing itself. In many ways, these illustrations are simply another way of representing what we have been saying throughout this chapter. Nevertheless, we hope that for those readers who appreciate graphics, these will add another dimension to their understanding.

We begin with Figure 7.6, which represents an individual who over-regulates; the experience of threat (so important to survival and emotional health) is atrophied, overwhelmed by regulation. Relationship and reflection are constrained and restricted. Think of the baby we described in Chapter 2, managing his fears by suppressing them so as not to upset the mother.

This is someone who has learned that the best way to survive in relationships is to down-regulate and contain one's affects, including anxiety and fear. This inhibition limits the degree to which the they can experience their inner life and deeply connect with others. As a consequence, reflection is thin and constrained.

By way of contrast, Figure 7.7 represents an individual who maintains a high level of arousal as a means of maintaining closeness (and perceived

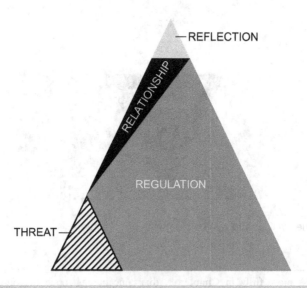

FIGURE 7.6 Overregulation/avoidance/flight.

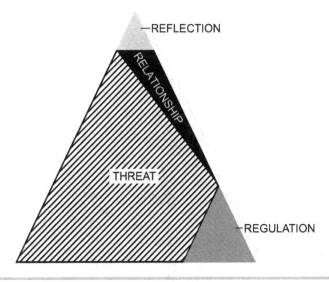

FIGURE 7.7 Underregulation/resistance/flight.

safety) (Cassidy & Berlin, 1994). Regulation is fleeting and unsuccessful; as a result, the relationship is distorted and reflection is minimal. Think of the resistant version of the baby we described in Chapter 2, who keeps fussing, cannot settle, and maintains the relationship through a fraught closeness.

Finally, in Figure 7.8, continuing or perceived threats in the disorganized individual's experience of others inhibit regulation and relationship. Reflection is all but impossible.

In Table 7.1, we summarize the various threads described throughout this chapter and their relationships to each other. Although these graphic representations greatly simplify complex, layered processes, we hope that they provide a road map for clinicians to begin to identify where a parent or child (or they themselves!) are struggling and thus where to begin.

Summary

When we think clinically about establishing safety, regulation, and relationship, we begin at the bottom of the pyramid, by establishing safety, reducing threat, and supporting the development of regulatory capacities. As we describe throughout this book, and particularly in Part IV, the provision of safety in the context of helping inhibits fight, flight, or freezing and allows the development of the healing relationship and thus the healing

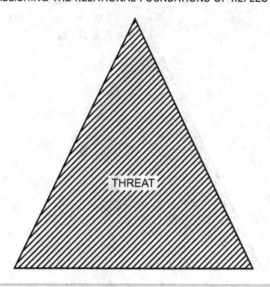

FIGURE 7.8 Dysregulated/disorganized/freezing.

TABLE 7.1. Threat, Stress, and Their Sequelae

Level of arousal	Defensive strategy	Attachment classification	Mentalizing
Low (too little), stress response system is deactivated	Flight	Avoidant–dismissive	Concrete, deficient prementalizing (hypomentalizing)
High (too much), stress response system is hyperactivated	Fight	Preoccupied–resistant	Intrusive–hostile prementalizing (hypermentalizing)
Extremely high, stress response system alternates between de- and hyperactivation	Freezing	Disorganized–unresolved	Dissociation, derealization, highly inaccurate attributions

work. Badenoch (2017) puts it simply: "Safety *is* the treatment" (p. 73). Without safety and regulation, the social engagement system cannot be activated, and the relationships that support reflection, and the trust that supports wondering, play, and imagination, cannot develop. The more vulnerable the individual, the more intensely threats are registered, the more readily defense or dysregulation will follow, necessitating a move back to the bases of safety and regulation and to the reestablishment of trust and connection, so necessary and important for reflection. In the following chapters, we apply this model first to the clinician's experience (Chapter 8) and then to the experience of the parent and child (Chapter 9).

Chapter

8

The Relational Foundations
of Reflection in the Clinician

We begin our discussion of the clinical applications of the RFR model by focusing on the establishment of safety, regulation, and relationship in the clinician; in Chapter 9, we turn to the parent and child. We begin with the clinician because their sense of safety and capacity to regulate, to engage with the parent and child, and to mentalize makes the work possible. This is illustrated by the nested mentalization model (Figure 8.1; Slade et al., 2017a), which represents the layers of "holding" (Winnicott, 1965) that are necessary to support parents and their children. The clinician, who

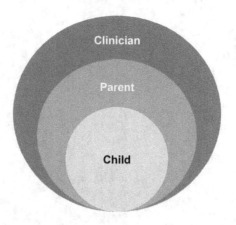

FIGURE 8.1 Nested mentalization model.

has the biggest "arms," holds the parent, who is then able to use their *supported* arms to hold the child. This graphic makes clear how essential it is that the clinician feel safe, regulated, and able to fully engage if they are to create safety and diminish threat, promote regulation, and build (and *re*build and *re*pair) a trusting attachment relationship with the parent (and child). This, in turn, will make it possible for the caregiver to fulfill the essential and evolutionarily programmed parental role of ensuring the child's safety, regulating and organizing the child's experience, and providing a "bigger, stronger, wiser, and kind" secure base that ensures the child's humanity and capacity for discovery (Bowlby, 1969/1982; Hoffman et al., 2017; Powell et al., 2013; Solomon & George, 1996).

Threats to Safety in the Clinician

We begin with threats to the clinician's sense of safety. Recall that in Chapter 7 we discussed Porges's (2004) concept of "neuroception," namely, the way that individuals of all ages use their senses to process information from the environment to continually evaluate risk. *Naturally, these processes occur in clinicians.* We, too, assess danger, and, when threatened, we, too, can mobilize our defenses to fight or flee. Sometimes, when overwhelmed, we may freeze. Whether or not we are consciously aware of it, when we are threatened, we have difficulty making eye contact, our smiles fade, our vocal intonations flatten out, we stop listening. Our hearts pound, or we feel sluggish and unresponsive, we disengage, we dissociate. Our bodies stiffen and tighten, the chest collapses, we look down or away. Our "gut" tell us something, and we are wary, uneasy. By contrast, when we feel safe, we can make eye contact, we smile, our intonation is textured, we respond contingently, and our posture is open and relaxed. "Social communication can only occur during states when we experience safety, because only then are the neurobiological defense strategies inhibited" (Geller & Porges, 2014, p. 181). And *social communication is at the heart of any clinical encounter.* If we communicate openness and presence, we signal to the parent and the child that they are safe, and that we—and any help we provide—can be trusted. But if we are threatened, we cannot create safety.

In Chapter 5, we discussed the ways that threat can inhibit mentalizing, or the ability to communicate effectively and coherently. This can happen to clinicians, too: We get concrete, overwhelmed; we are certain, not curious. We cannot think straight, we cannot find the words to say what we want to say, we lose our train of thought, we can't remember what we meant to say. The narratives we offer don't quite make sense, we can't find the thread, we are vague, or just plain confusing. Our usual abilities to imagine the other's experience, to identify our own thoughts and feelings, to think clearly, to organize our thoughts, to remember, and to get our message across are a little (or a lot) scrambled.

Although it is common to observe these phenomena in the behavior of caregivers and their young children, recognizing them in ourselves and appreciating their relevance to our own clinical practice is crucial. As the psychoanalyst Harry Stack Sullivan (1947) put it, "We are all much more simply human than otherwise" (p. 7); we, too, experience the gamut of human emotions; we, too, can be threatened. These experiences tell us something very important about the clinical situation and teach us something important about ourselves. They also turn us to the important task of reducing threat in the clinical encounter. We now turn to the three levels of safety we described in Chapter 7: physical safety, internal safety, and relational safety, and consider their impact on the clinician's capacity to fully engage with the parent and child.

Threats to Physical Safety

It may seem unnecessary to begin with the obvious, which is that clinicians cannot work reflectively when they are in literal danger. They, as human beings, will fight, flee, or freeze in the effort (conscious or not) to survive. And yet this is a complex issue, for a number of reasons. Home visitors often work in neighborhoods where there are high levels of crime and violence. Violence or threat of violence to a child or family member may be the reason practitioners are in the home to begin with. In MTB-HV, it was extremely rare for clinicians to fear for their safety; as they got to know neighborhoods, neighbors, and families, they felt reasonably safe and protected. But this did not mitigate the need to be careful and thoughtful about physical safety and to find other ways to meet with families when it was too dangerous to be in the home. In these circumstances, they often had to help families find ways to be safe, as well. Office-based mental health and health practitioners, teachers, and other educational therapists can sometimes feel physically endangered, too. This may have to do with the location of the clinical space, the safety of the building, or—more directly—the level of agitation or disturbance of a child or parent in acute crisis.

Threats to Internal Safety

The Clinician's Feelings

As has been well described in the literature on reflective supervision (see Fenichel, 1992; Gilkerson, 2004; Gilkerson & Imberger, 2016; Heffron, 2005; Heffron & Murch, 2010; O'Rourke, 2011; Parlakian, 2001; Simpson et al., 2018; Tomlin et al., 2014; Watson et al., 2016; Weatherston

& Osofsky, 2009) and vicarious trauma (McCann & Pearlman, 1990; Saakvitne et al., 2000), the clinician's sense of internal safety can be and often is disrupted by the feelings, sometimes complex and urgent, that are stirred up by working with vulnerable young children and their caregivers. Children reveal their pain in their nonverbal behavior or in their play. Parents suffer with the weight of everyday life and the weight of their own traumas; they may feel angry, despairing, desperate, frightened, and sometimes so sad they are frozen. In whatever ways they defend themselves against the impact of their experience, by blocking it out or being consumed by it, it is always there. Sometimes caregivers' pain is so great that they project it onto clinicians, potentially perceiving the clinician as yet another perpetrator. As we described in Chapter 1, Selma Fraiberg and her colleagues (1975) proposed that once a parent is able to experience the *affects* associated with their own traumatic childhood experiences (and—as often as not—current trauma), they are able to parent their own children in more benevolent, loving ways. In order to enable this process, clinicians must hold and feel the trauma, too, and experience the feelings the parent cannot. As such, clinicians can find themselves swamped by a range of negative reactions: fear, anger, dread, a sense of deadness, boredom, judgment, and helplessness. Even despair.

> An experienced clinician learned that a young parent she had been working with for over 2 years had been arrested for speeding and driving without a license while accompanied by her toddler son. The clinician was very upset; their years of work together might now be upended by the involvement of child protective services or criminal prosecution. She was angry and disappointed with the mom: "How could she put her son in danger? What was she thinking? She should've known better." The subtext was clear: "Hasn't our work meant more to her than this?"

Feelings of anger and disappointment can be jarring and unwelcome: "*I am a helper. What 'good' person would feel this way?*" Clinicians can also find themselves jumping into action, trying to *do* something as a means of regulating their own distress.

This can be very tough work. Clinicians try to contain complex feelings, to meet what can be overwhelming demands, and to calm themselves enough to help parents regulate and attend to their babies. And they aim to do this with compassion and without judgment. They put in long hours and try to keep thinking and feeling, to formulate appropriate responses, and make observations, assessments, and clinical decisions. And sometimes they fail and have to right themselves, again and again. As Osofsky (2009) points out, the weight of such "empathic strain" can lead "clinicians to shut down emotionally, terminate the case prematurely, or leave the field" altogether (pp. 673–674). Without attention to clinicians' inner lives, to their understandable responses to families and to the great difficulty of the work, these intense emotions remain threatening and cannot be metabolized. In the next sections, we discuss the particular threats of vicarious trauma and implicit bias.

Vicarious Trauma

One of the potential sequelae of such emotional intensity is *vicarious trauma* (McCann & Pearlman, 1990; Pearlman & Saakvitne, 1995), "the cumulative transformative effect on the helper of working with survivors of traumatic life events" (Saakvitne et al., 2000). Vicarious trauma involves many of the sequelae of trauma exposure: preoccupation with the parent or child's trauma, helplessness, fear, reexperiencing, emotional numbing, anger, irritability, isolation, disrupted sleep, and physical illness. Such experiences can lead clinicians to question their identity, to find their worldview subtly changed by feelings of uncertainty, emotional numbing, depression, anxiety, and despair. The clinician's "inner self" is transformed by their empathic engagement with the client's pain, and as such they become traumatized as well; these are the "risks in connecting" (Saakvitne, 2002). In many ways, we can see vicarious trauma as the sequelae of prolonged threat to the clinician's sense of safety.

Writing to her long-term supervisor, Kim, an experienced nurse clinician (herself the parent of a young toddler) eloquently describes what this can feel like.

Dear Denise:

     Yes . . . I'm on vacation. ☺ But, as you can see, since I'm sending you this email at 3:05 A.M., sleeping is not always my forte. I've been grappling with how to handle the stresses of the job that I will be returning to next week after my vacation . . . been thinking a lot about vicarious trauma and just wanted to share something that hit me as a truth because maybe this will help someone else struggling as I am. Part of the vicarious trauma for me is not only feeling and experiencing the pain of what these girls endure and/or have endured in the past. It's also that working with them has increased my own awareness of life's realities, and of the potential for traumatic events in everyday life. It's given me a heightened awareness of my own vulnerability to the horrible things that can happen . . . to me, to my baby, to my family. This makes me feel helpless and fearful and contributes to my nightmares, which often lead me to being awake

at 3:05 A.M. ☺ The "what if's" of life have increased
dramatically for me. Staying away from the news used
to work for me, but now, this job IS the daily news!
We go into the areas with the shootings and the
poverty and hunger, and they're sharing those stories
with us. Sometimes, they share things my mind never
knew existed. I can't change the channel.
   Also, the girls we work with have not only been
through awful individual life experiences, but they
also live everyday lives of just mere existence and
poverty. So, I'm also realizing that seeing the daily
despair just does something to me, and it's then
a struggle to not bring that sense of despair and
hopelessness into my own personal life.
   Thanks so much!

There are so many threads in this letter. First, Kim is describing the weight
and pain of hearing about tragedy and traumas so deep that they are nearly
unfathomable. She is also describing the sense of helplessness she feels
in being unable to remedy so much of what ails the families she is seeing. These struggles in turn provoke her fear for her own and her family's
safety, as she is now aware at a different level of how random and devastating danger can be. She finds herself in an existential crisis, struggling
with even larger feelings of despair and powerlessness. This brings to mind
the despair and loss of meaning that can accompany exposure to chronic
complex trauma (Courtois, 2004). What is so important, though, is that
Kim is aware of these feelings, and thinks—even in the dead of night—to
reach out to her supervisor. As we describe later in the chapter, vicarious
trauma requires us to be aware of and attend to our own vulnerabilities,
to take care of ourselves, and to continue to look for ways to find meaning
and community in a lonely and sometimes desolate time. We all have our
own "shark music" (Hoffman et al., 2017; Powell et al., 2013); what's most
important is to listen to it.

Implicit Bias

Implicit bias—which pervades both the health and mental health care systems (Hall et al., 2015; Merino et al., 2018)—poses another kind of threat
to clinicians' sense of safety. Racism is baked into the basic structures of
our society. It is also one of psychoanalytic theory's "ghosts in the nursery," implicitly and explicitly sanctioned by Freud from the start (Holmes
et al., 2023; Stoute, 2017). Prejudice, in its many forms, has the potential
to interrupt our capacity to be fully open with and trusting with families
who we see as different from us, and it affects families' capacity to trust us.
Racist or other forms of bias can make us afraid, and our judgments and

assumptions can harm families and rightly make them fearful or mistrustful of us.

There has been an enormous push within the field of infant mental health (St. John et al., 2013) to investigate the multiple ways that bias can limit and distort work with infants, children and families. The "diversity informed tenets of infant mental health" (*www.diversityinformedtenets.org*) are now an essential aspect of infant mental health training and practice. These include—on both individual and community levels—working to cultivate awareness of our own and other's biases, champion children's rights globally, acknowledge privilege and combat discrimination, recognize and respect nondominant bodies of knowledge, honor diverse family structures, understand that language can hurt or heal, support families in their preferred language, allocate resources to system change, make space and open pathways, and advance policy that supports all families. Clearly these tenets are applicable to a range of health, mental health, educational, and other services, and encourage us to interrogate our responses to families at multiple levels.

Anton Hart (2017), a multiracial psychoanalyst, suggests that we engage with "otherness" in a radical, open way:

> The heart of the matter is learning how to become increasingly undefended around matters of diversity and otherness such that you can be open: open to the other person who will be, in some significant ways, most certainly different from you. . . . Genuine openness can only emerge in the context of an unscripted dialogue, one that involves making contact with and participating in an exchange that will, necessarily, threaten the dialogic participants' understandings, identities and perceptions. (p. 12)

Though Hart doesn't use the term *mentalization*, he describes "radical openness" as a "stance of attempting to notice, question, and relinquish presumptions about the self and the other" and the "receptivity to that which is unexpected in relation to oneself and in relation to the other" (p. 13). This is the "not-knowing," curious reflective stance. If you can manage not to be afraid, to let your defenses down, to let go of threat, the "we" space described in Chapter 7 becomes possible.

Program or Curricular Demands

Program or curricular demands can also threaten clinicians' sense of comfort and ease in the work. Interventions vary in the degree to which they follow an established curriculum and expect close adherence to that model. Nevertheless, all have curricular expectations or demands of one sort or another. They provide clinicians with a vital road map for how to proceed.

At the same time, they can create stress for the clinician. In MTB-HV, for example, we inadvertently inserted enhancing PRF as an implicit demand upon clinicians. Similarly, clinicians working in very structured interventions may feel pressured by curricular demands that they cannot, for the moment, meet. Imagine a situation in which the nurse/clinician was supposed to discuss the dangers of co-sleeping, but the parent had been completely undone by an eviction notice and the very real threat of imminent homelessness. The clinician has no choice but to deal with the crisis at hand. Or the practitioner has been asked to screen a parent for depression by administering a short questionnaire. The baby is sick, however, and the clinician has to accompany parent and child to the clinic. The data manager is not going to be happy. Or the clinician has been trained in a model but finds herself simply overwhelmed by the clinical situation. She wants to just listen to the parent, but she's not sure that's OK. She really wants to help but has no idea where to begin.

These experiences are common ones for clinicians, no matter whether they are implementing a structured program or working privately in dynamically oriented practice. They may deviate from a program protocol in the face of clinical need or do something they feel compelled to do (even though it might upset their supervisor) or find that they simply do not have the tools they need in a particularly difficult situation. The anxiety over such struggles can leave the clinician feeling conflicted, unprepared, and unable to be fully present or that they have, in a big or small way, failed. Or that they are helpless. This may lead them to defensively tune out or to cling rigidly to one position or another. These are critical issues for supervision.

The Frameworks of Discipline

Discipline, while providing vital professional "holding" to the work, can also constrain us in important ways. We all bring our training to the work: "I am" a social worker, nurse, psychologist, early childhood specialist, speech therapist. This is *how* I work, *what* I work on, what I *know* best, and what I *know* works. These invaluable frameworks provide us with maps for the journey, without which we would simply not know where to begin or end. They provide safety. And yet as containing and organizing as these frameworks can be, they can also be limiting, crutches we cling to in the face of overwhelming circumstances, especially when we are new to the work. "Despite this dyad's distress, I have to finish the physical exam, and get on to my next patient." "This parent has missed three sessions. I'm going to have to discontinue services." "I've given her the paperwork for housing assistance so many times. Until she fills it out, I can't help her." In other words, "I have a job to do, and if I can't do it, there's no other way that I can help."

As clinicians become more experienced and comfortable in their clinical roles, these frameworks can become more flexible (although, admittedly, many health care delivery systems allow little flexibility); veteran clinicians have a sense of when to adhere to frameworks and when to loosen them a little bit, to slow down, ask questions, take a deeper look. At times, less experienced clinicians can chafe at frameworks and challenge them; sometimes these are healthy challenges, and sometimes they are not helpful and potentially destructive. Ideally, the frameworks of one's discipline are never so binding that they interfere with the ability to respond to a person in the moment, as a *human* being, to listen, to provide the help (concrete or otherwise) that is needed. But when circumstances are overwhelming, cleaving to one's discipline is completely understandable, particularly when we see it as a natural (though not particularly helpful) response to threat.

Relational Safety and Relational Threat

Clinicians can feel *relationally* threatened by parents and, on occasion, children, as well. This can occur when a parent is rejecting or hostile to a clinician or a child lashes out. Other subtle experiences of relational threat occur when a clinician feels invaded or violated in some less tangible way by the parent's unmetabolized aggression. Often these experiences are difficult to recognize and name but might best be described as a kind of "gut" reaction, or a subtle awareness that "this person feels psychologically dangerous *to me.*" For instance, the parent might use or manipulate the clinician in a way that feels pernicious and dangerous. The feeling of being relationally threatened is certainly an uncomfortable feeling, but it is useful to recognize. For one, it alerts the clinician to powerful feelings in the parent and what are likely frightening experiences for the child. More important, perhaps, it helps the clinician identify processes that can be fruitfully discussed in supervision and that will help soften (or, if necessary, strengthen!) the defenses that are triggered in interaction with the parent. It may also help identify a caregiver who needs a different intervention or treatment.

Any and all of these experiences—grappling with the intensity of one's own feelings and reactions, feeling the demands and expectations of one's program or discipline, coping with the reality of uncertainty, ambiguity, or lack of preparedness—can be challenging for clinicians. They may find themselves closing off their minds to new solutions, to alternative options, and—at times—to just allowing deep human contact. As such, these threats must be addressed at multiple levels—by the clinician, by the team, and by the supervisor, who can hear and organize such threats, reduce those that they can, and at least soften those they can't change. We can never create a model that will work in all circumstances, and we can never be fully prepared and without uncertainty. Threat is inevitable, but awareness helps.

Regulation

Many of the responses described in the preceding section on threat and safety are manifestations of the dysregulation that follows threat to the clinician's capacity to feel safe in the work. In the following section, we try to tease apart different types of dysregulation, understanding that—although they often happen at once—distinguishing them within oneself has direct clinical utility and guides self-care and supervision. Where do I need attention and help, and what will be most restorative for me?

Bodily Dysregulation

The experience of threat in the clinical situation is often registered in the clinician's body. The heart races, breathing accelerates, muscles tighten (in the face, shoulders, and arms), and palms sweat. Alternatively, clinicians may find themselves in a torpor, bored, slowed down, lethargic, sleepy, unable to move effectively, chilled, and unresponsive. Any of these variations of fight, flight, or freezing are signs of bodily dysregulation, triggered by seen or unseen threats. Ideally, these states remind the clinician to wonder about their own triggers or to consider whether their body is "speaking" for the parent or child. Why is their sympathetic nervous system on high alert? What is going on?

This first step in regulating such states is recognizing them. This may involve attuning to our bodies in ways that are unfamiliar and perhaps foreign. But, for clinicians as well as families, "the body keeps the score" (van der Kolk, 2014). Identifying our own bodily experiences helps us more fully experience what we are thinking and feeling. This makes it possible to take steps to regulate these bodily disruptions. If we are hyperaroused (elevated heart rate, rapid breathing, etc.), we need to take steps to settle ourselves and find our way back to a more regulated state. Pausing in the moment to take a series of deep breaths, with the length of the outbreath longer than the inbreath, can be very helpful, as can a regular practice of meditation, deep relaxation, yoga, or other bodily-based techniques. Indeed, many studies confirm the value of such practices for a range of health and mental health professionals (Baldini et al., 2014; Bruce et al., 2010; Shapiro et al., 2005). When families are chaotic and dysregulating, such techniques can help us "stay" in the room.

If we are sleepy, lethargic, bored, or shut down, however, relaxation techniques are likely to be less effective. We need to "wake up" our nervous systems. Standing up, moving energetically, taking some deep breaths, or having a drink of water will help us reengage. Often, unfortunately, it is not until after the session that we realize that our shoulders are aching from the tension of holding them at attention, that our teeth are gritted, that we haven't taken a real breath in 30 minutes, or that we feel utterly wiped out. In any event, we need to think about what might be provoking our response and try to address it both in the moment (perhaps just by naming it) and later in supervision. As clinicians become more experienced with the work, and more comfortable listening to their bodies, it becomes easier to recognize signs of dysregulation during a session.

Emotional Dysregulation

As we mentioned earlier, we often find ourselves having intense feelings about a parent or child, feelings that alert us to the fact that, again, something clinically relevant and important is going on, either within ourselves, within the family, or both. Such feelings can be very dysregulating and threatening, potentially leading us to become either highly activated and distressed or shut down and tuned out. Clinicians, too, can inhabit the "too little" and "too much" ends of the arousal curve. In the following example, the clinician moves between being flooded and being shut down as she copes with a live and very difficult situation.

> Juliana reported to her social worker that her husband was threatening her in front of the baby. She was a petite, fragile woman, and the infant was quite young; in addition, the mother had a chronic medical condition that was poorly managed. The clinician was very alarmed. At first, triggered by her fear for Juliana, the clinician escalated her efforts to get the mom to tell her husband to leave. Juliana protested that her husband was a good man; the clinician insisted that he was dangerous. Juliana felt unheard and overwhelmed and canceled several sessions in a row. When they met again, Juliana seemed very withdrawn and remote. She refused to discuss the situation, which was, of course, ongoing. Hitting the wall of Juliana's defenses, the clinician then found herself disengaging and shutting down, feeling hopeless and powerless. Both the clinician's becoming activated and her shutting down were responses to the fear she felt for Juliana and the baby and the anger she felt toward the husband. Both also drove a wedge between the clinician and Juliana and disrupted Juliana's sense of safety in the clinical situation. It was not until the clinician discussed the situation with the team and her supervisor that she realized how activated she had been.

Here we see the clinician and mother "swapping" states of dysregulation: The clinician gets highly aroused (too much), and the mother then withdraws (too little) and avoids the clinician. The mother's withdrawal eventually leads the clinician to withdraw herself (too little) as she grapples with her helplessness.

Other signs of dysregulation signal the disruptions of vicarious trauma—thinking about a family constantly, feeling judgmental about them, feeling hopeless, powerless, or despairing. The first step in attending to intense, dysregulated, and dysregulating feelings is recognizing them and talking them out, likely in supervision. Such feelings can be very threatening to our sense of ourselves as clinicians, and it is thus easy to minimize or deny them. We don't want to think of ourselves as having anything but good and helpful feelings toward our families. But of course we do—we are humans, they are humans, and typically we (and they) are dealing with very challenging *and arousing* situations. When faced with complex and sometimes seemingly insoluble problems, *we* (and they) are going to be activated, on alert, and thus less able to contain, regulate, and reflect upon our feelings. If we are able to recognize and acknowledge these feelings, we will be less inclined to act on them in ways that can be destructive and shaming (e.g., confronting a parent) and more able to come up with alternatives that will protect the child, although sometimes there are simply no good ones.

Relationship

The psychotherapy outcome literature has long placed great value on the *quality* of the clinician–patient relationship, noting that this matters more than just about any other factor in predicting outcome, including the type of therapy (Allen, 2022; Holmes & Slade, 2018; Wampold & Imel, 2015). The same proviso can readily be applied to other professions. A midwife's willingness to take the time to address the parent's anxiety, to hear how frightened she is of labor and delivery (particularly when she has a sexual abuse history), and to help her develop a plan for her labor (Simkin, 1992; see Chapter 11) will very often result in a smoother, less traumatizing birth. Likewise, it probably doesn't matter as much whether a teacher uses phonics or whole-word approaches to teach reading as it does that they are able to engage the child in a trusting relationship in which they can play, learn, and gain confidence in safety. To put this in the terms of attachment theory, a secure attachment provides the foundation for exploration and discovery (Ainsworth et al., 1978). Fonagy and Allison (2014) use the term "epistemic trust" to describe the trust that derives from a secure attachment relationship: "*I trust in the information/knowledge/perspective that you offer because I trust in you and feel safe with you*" (see also Fonagy et al., 2019, 2021). In Porges's terms, the absence of threat and dysregulation *allows* for social engagement.

That the quality of the clinician–parent–child relationship *matters* is a given in infant mental health and other forms of relationship-based practice. Yet, though much stress has been placed on the importance of the practitioner–parent–child relationship in promoting change, there has been surprisingly little attention paid, in the training of psychotherapists, social workers, nurses, doctors, teachers, infant mental health specialists, and other child care professionals, to how to develop and maintain a therapeutic relationship. As we describe in this section, this first depends upon the clinician's feeling safe and regulated enough to be emotionally open to and present for the parent or child. It also depends upon the degree to which the clinician is experienced by the parent or child as *trustworthy*.

Safety and Regulation: Contexts for the Therapeutic Relationship

The RFR model is grounded in the notion that all relationships—including the therapeutic relationship—flourish within the context of safety and are distorted by fear and threat. What this means concretely is that the clinician's sense of safety and regulation is a necessary prelude to truly connecting with the parent or child. Without these foundations, practitioners are likely to be too activated and dysregulated to engage with the parent or child in a meaningful way and are less likely to be experienced as trustworthy. When we struggle with our own fears, feel threatened, or are hijacked by our bodily reactions, we can become an unreliable base, unable to transcend our own stresses to really hear and see the other, be it parent, child, or colleague. The more sensitive a parent is to rejection or abandonment, the more acutely they will feel our moments of disconnection and absence. This is why attending to what we are experiencing, on a multiplicity of levels, is so important. Sometimes it can be as simple as doing a quick body scan or taking a series of deep breaths before a session; sometimes the work must be deeper. But we must bring the whole of ourselves to the work.

Our Trustworthiness

In his remarkable book *Trusting in Psychotherapy*, Jon Allen (2022) notes that, rather than focusing on method—that is, *what* we do—"we should shift the balance of our efforts from developing *therapies* to developing *therapists*" (p. xxvii). Rather than focusing on *how* to deliver a particular treatment, we should focus on therapists' capacity to be *trustworthy*, to be fully present, authentic, and engaged. If trusting the therapist is the foundation for change (Fonagy & Allison, 2014), then the therapist (or nurse, home visitor, or other provider) needs to be someone the parent can, in fact, trust. "What I have in mind here, in the psychotherapy relationship and other relationships, is the experience of *presence, living engagement, the sense of the other person, the sense of self in relation to other, and the feeling of understanding and being understood*" (p. 28, emphasis in original). For Allen, it is the "skill in being human" (2013) that is so essential to any therapeutic relationship. The deep social connection is what is mutative. Jeree Pawl, one of the founders of the infant mental health movement, put it simply: "How you are is as important as what you do" (Pawl & St. John, 1998). *In other words, who you are matters.*

An infant mental health supervisor or trainer could well argue that the importance of the clinician–parent and clinician–child relationships are front and center in training. Nurse and physician educators could, as well. At face value, all of this is true. We train practitioners in the importance of reliability, consistency, predictability, acceptance, and resisting judgment. We train them to join the parent "where they are at," to listen, to be patient. And we train them to adopt "a basic helping orientation: Be authentic, non-judgmental, genuine, accepting, respectful, responsive, present, empathic and supportive" (Midgley et al., 2017, p. 84). However, much of this guidance is behavioral: Show up when you say you're going to show up, be on time, be a good listener, slow down and be patient, and so on. And much of it focuses on method: This is what you should *do*.

In many ways, these descriptions skirt a key, *human* element, one that has been emphasized again and again in the psychotherapy literature: warmth, empathy, and positive regard. As Allen (2022) notes, it is our own "uniquely human capacity for social connection and cooperation . . . our implicit (nonverbal) capacity for relating" (p. 46) that makes the difference. Particularly for those individuals whose capacity for trust has been savaged by attachment trauma, "the cultivation of trust and an intimate bond will not be the foundation for therapy or the vehicle for therapy; it will be *the work of therapy* and the ideal *outcome* of therapy" (p. 22). Courtois (2004) likewise sees the establishment of trust and safety as the primary goal of trauma treatment, with trauma *processing* possible only after safety is ensured. Trusting and being trustworthy is at the heart of what we do. From a position of trust, we can support, listen, and even challenge the parent or child.

Our humanity and—more so—our willingness to be human is mutative. It is striking that even today experienced psychotherapists feel the need to make this point forcefully and repeatedly. Although some of this has to do with the current obsession in the psychotherapy literature with what to "do" rather than how to "be," these authors are also taking on one of the more pernicious legacies of classical psychoanalysis, in which acknowledging the importance of a meaningful, emotional connection to one's patients was, in effect, forbidden. In particular, the analyst's feelings *toward* the patient were regarded as a manifestation of their own conflicts and needs. Most feelings about the patient were considered "countertransference" and were seen as having great potential to disrupt and derail treatment. Although the field's understanding of transference and countertransference has changed dramatically over the past 100 years, vestiges of these attitudes remain in subtle ways. In particular, there remains a caution against acknowledging feeling *too* connected to the parent, of caring for and about them. It is viewed as transgressing a boundary that is necessary for treatment to proceed. Such cautions may lead the clinician to create distance that confirms some the parent's most difficult and disappointing relational experiences. For mental health practitioners, in particular, it is time to lay to rest the notion that our compassion, concern, care, warmth, and deep concern for families is *countertransference*, a pejorative label that inherently devalues the clinician's humanity. The human qualities that promote closeness, trust, and emotional intimacy have a central and important place in any therapeutic process, regardless of the practitioner's discipline. *These are the agents of therapeutic action.*

The notion of therapeutic neutrality (which Freud himself rarely practiced!) is another holdover from the early days of psychoanalysis. Part of our caring is that we are *not* neutral. And yet we must manage our opinions and our observations carefully. Take the previous case example: The parent was choosing to stay with an abusive partner, which the clinician had *very strong* feelings about. She cared about the parent and the baby. And she felt righteous rage toward the father. When triggered like this, however, the clinician had a great deal of difficulty *protecting her relationship with the mother* from her own distress and anxiety. In these circumstances, it can be so challenging to remain curious and open to understanding the parent's perspective—neither neutral (which could easily feel uncaring) nor overly intrusive (which can also feel uncaring and humiliating). It is a very tough balance; nevertheless, the goal is to leverage the therapeutic bond to help the parent protect herself and the child.

We recognize, of course, that the use of the term *care* raises a number of issues, just as "love" did for Bowlby decades ago (as it also did for psychoanalysis!). What do we mean by *care*? What kind of care is appropriate and helpful? What is the "right" balance? Clearly, caring in this context is different from the care we feel for our children, close family, and friends. At the same time, we do *care*, about the families' losses, their setbacks, and their joys. And not only do we matter to *them*, they matter to *us*. As we discussed in Chapter 3, *mattering* to another is what gives the child a sense of belonging in the world. The practitioner's *willingness* and *openness* to *care* for and about families, to truly become a secure base (and thus, to some extent, an attachment figure) for the parent and child is a critical "active ingredient" of any relationship-based intervention. The child or parent's capacity to hear and use and make meaning of what the practitioner has to offer depends upon their experience of the practitioner as safe, regulating, *emotionally available*, and *caring*.

Let's return to Porges's example of the unthreatened infant who communicates a willingness to engage socially with their eyes open and up, chest open, language clear and communicative, intonation and prosody marked. We can all think of practitioners who meet a parent for the first time with a smile, a physical stance of interest, and a kind tone of voice. We can also imagine many other iterations of the same exchange: the clinician who quickly defaults to a question-and-answer format, who makes only fleeting eye contact, who uses a clipboard or folded arms as an interpersonal shield (Tortora, 2005). We can also imagine clinicians who are presumptuous and overly familiar. Both stances can be inherently threatening to the parent: "*Why is this person not hearing me/so interested in me? Why is this person crowding me? Putting words in my mouth? Violating my personal space without permission?*" Clearly, the balance is a delicate one that must be negotiated again and again. There are certainly situations in which our warmth or concern will raise hackles or trigger distrust. When that is the case, we respect the parent's feelings, their fears of trusting a professional or a person of a different color or sexual orientation, their fears of intimacy of any kind. So we move more slowly; we do not, however, abandon the personal qualities that invite trust and closeness. We titrate these, observing the parent's defenses, and responding accordingly. But the point we wish to make strongly here is that being present, being yourself, being engaged, and letting the child and the parents *matter* to you is essential. Our clinical stance is necessarily saturated with our humanity.

Reflection

The next and final stage in the RFR pyramid is reflection, which is supported by safety, regulation, and relationship. Even when these are well established, it will often take time for parents to pause and wonder and be curious about their own or their child's bodily experiences or inner life. Giving space to this new way of watching and listening can be very challenging. Clinicians, by contrast, are called upon to be reflective from their first meeting with parents. Indeed, the clinician's capacity to maintain a mentalizing stance—to wonder and not assume—is the crux of the reflective parenting approach. That this can be difficult is the reason we have placed so much emphasis on developing clinicians' capacity to listen to their own fears, to register whether they feel threatened, and to engage with families as fully as they can. *Their capacity to mentalize depends upon it.* A mentalizing stance makes it possible to follow Sally Provence's advice: "Don't just *do* something. Stand there and pay attention. The *parent and the child* are trying to tell you something." *What* are they trying to tell us? We understand that behaviors *mean* something, that they communicate something, and that our job is to make sense of what that might be. Rather than taking these at face value (or trying to change them), we approach behavior as indicative of underlying feelings and thoughts that we have to *discover*. And the discovery is a mutual process, with us always checking our understanding against that of the parent. When threats abound, mentalizing can be an enormous accomplishment, even for an experienced clinician. We return to the particular ways clinicians can enhance a parent's mentalizing capacities in Chapter 10.

Supervision

As pictured in our expanded nested mentalization graphic (Figure 8.2), the supervisor provides a critical holding environment for the clinician, so that they can, in turn, hold the parent and child in all their complexity. And just as the clinician provides safety, regulation, and a trusting relationship to the parent and child, the supervisor does the same for the clinician, supporting the clinician's capacity to reflect upon their own and the family's experience and to build a range of critical clinical skills and competencies.

Supervision has been a mainstay of dynamically oriented mental health practice since the beginning of the psychoanalytic movement, where it has long been assumed that having a regular opportunity to discuss the complexities of the work with supervisors and peers is essential. As such, regular and ongoing supervision was an integral part of MTB-HV and is likewise an essential aspect of MTB-P. In MTB-HV, we adopted a blended supervision model across both disciplines that combined what is commonly

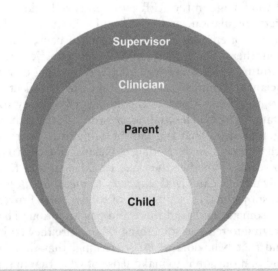

FIGURE 8.2 Expanded nested mentalization model: Supervision.

called "reflective" supervision with "clinical" supervision. *Reflective* supervision, which typically refers to helping a clinician process their own strong feelings about the work, as well as those of the parent and child, is a multidisciplinary practice for professionals working in a variety of settings. This form of supervision—which is today considered best practice for practitioners working with families and young children—has been well described in the infant mental health literature (Fenichel, 1992; Gilkerson, 2004; Gilkerson & Imberger, 2016; Heffron, 2005; Heffron & Murch, 2010; O'Rourke, 2011; Parlakian, 2001; Simpson et al., 2018; Tomlin et al., 2014; Watson et al., 2016; Weatherston & Osofsky, 2009).

One of the most popular reflective supervision models, the FAN (facilitating attuned interactions) model (Gilkerson & Imberger, 2016), has much in common with the RFR model. Initially developed by Linda Gilkerson for use in training paraprofessionals, it is now widely used in training and supporting multidisciplinary practitioners across a range of early intervention programs, particularly the Nurse–Family Partnership (NFP). The model is aimed at promoting attunement and providing a structure for engagement, as well as a guide for reflection. Like the RFR pyramid, the FAN approach begins with the establishment of mindful self-regulation in the clinician, which then sets the stage for exploring feelings, thinking, doing, and reflecting with parents. The model's arc of engagement makes clear that regulation is essential to engagement and that forward and backward movement under the press of threat or dysregulation, either in the clinician or the parent, is normal and expectable. When used as part of reflective supervision, the FAN model places a premium on observation rather than action and thus helps clinicians focus on regulating rather than doing, taking the time they need to breathe and not simply jumping into action.

Clinical supervision has received less attention in the infant mental health and early-intervention literature. This is a form of *discipline-specific* practice in which a supervisor serves as a teacher and a guide, deepening the clinician's capacity to assess the parent and child, to make clinical formulations, and to develop a broad and rich clinical repertoire. Some view clinical supervision as an essential aspect of reflective supervision, and, indeed, these two processes are highly intertwined. Nevertheless, we wish to be clear that developing the clinician's skills in their particular discipline is critical to professional practice. For instance, we can see in Fraiberg et al.'s classic paper (1975) how the synergy of Edna Adelson's and Vivian Shapiro's years of clinical experience and skill, their deep understanding of development and psychopathology, as well as the expert guidance provided by their supervisor, Fraiberg, made it possible for them to arrive at the *essential* diagnostic question: "*Why doesn't this mother hear her babies' cries?*" (p. 392). This led them to try to understand how and why the mother had so profoundly turned away from her baby. And this question was what led—ultimately—to the discovery of Mrs. March's particular ghosts and to activating the angels of hope and promise as the work proceeded. Faced with Mrs. March's "resistance," they searched for a different way of working that would minimize Mrs. March's terror and shame and that would protect the baby and the family unit. This led the team to modify the parameters of psychoanalytic psychotherapy so as to create a new clinical approach to working with parents and young children: infant–parent psychotherapy.

Although a good deal of learning takes place during the didactic phase of clinical education, clinicians really learn the "tools of their trade" through supervision. For therapists, this means learning the tools of dynamic formulation, of clinical technique, and of developmental assessment and diagnosis. As such, a supervisor or consultant's expertise in dynamic psychology, in evaluation and diagnosis, and in the *processes* of psychotherapy (resistance, ambivalence, and transference) is essential. Likewise, nurses and other health professionals rely on a supervisor's expertise when faced with developmental and health challenges and the need for evaluation, diagnosis, formulation, and treatment. And when a particular intervention, such as child–parent psychotherapy or NFP, is being implemented, the supervisor plays a critical role in maintaining fidelity to the model. Across disciplines, the supervisory experience itself provides a vital training ground and offers a myriad of opportunities for learning and synthesis.

Safety and Regulation in the Supervisory Relationship

A supervisor is a teacher and a guide, with areas of expertise of tremendous relevance to the clinician's work. The degree to which the supervisee can take in and hear what the supervisor has to offer has much to do with the supervisor's capacity to create a safe place for the clinician, to remain open, curious, and willing to listen in a nonjudgmental way. Although there are certainly times when supervisors may challenge clinicians or use their expertise to guide and reframe clinical process, threat is antithetical to the supervisory relationship. As obvious as this might seem, it is not especially uncommon for clinicians to feel unsafe in supervision and to experience the supervisor as critical, uninterested, disengaged, or disapproving. Or as too busy and distracted.

One practitioner reported that—in her second year of training—her new and very senior supervisor threw up his hands after hearing her present the case of a suicidal mother with a young infant and exclaimed, "Do you have any idea what you're doing?" Needless to say, she never felt safe in her supervisory work with him. And within a few weeks the mother pulled out of treatment.

Although this is an extreme example, the supervisor in this case was subscribing to an "old" model of supervision: I am the expert here to show you the way. And, in this case, unfortunately, the supervisor seemed to need to shame the supervisee as part of asserting his dominance and expertise. This put the clinician on the defensive and certainly precluded the development of a trusting supervisory relationship. Aside from the fact that the supervisor might have invited the clinician to reflect on her own fears and sense of helplessness, he could have used this moment as an opportunity to share his knowledge and experience working with severe depression, suicidality, and potential lethality. He might also have offered his reflections on what might be going on for the mother dynamically. This was something the clinician clearly needed to know in order to help this particular mother with her hopelessness and despair *and* build her clinical repertoire for the wide range of patients she was going to encounter over the course of her career. Although some of this might well have been addressed in her didactic training, the actual application of what she had learned to the clinical context would have been greatly enhanced by the hands-on learning that optimally takes place within the supervisory relationship.

Even benign supervisory efforts can be experienced as threatening.

A home visitor found herself unable to say no to an adolescent mother's repeated requests that the clinician drive her to school and buy her a sweet tea on the way. The school bus left very early; the young mother, who was up late cooking dinner for her partner, who worked the late shift, simply could not get up in time. So many mornings the home visitor's phone would ring well before she had gotten her own kids on their school bus. Off she would go, leaving her husband in charge. She faithfully reported this to her supervisor, who gently tried to engage her in thinking about why it was so hard for her to say no and whether she might be able to help the mother find other ways of getting to school. The home visitor would shrug, look guilty, and acknowledge that this wasn't such a great idea. But she just couldn't say no, and so the calls and the rides to school continued. The supervisor grew frustrated. The home visitor grew to dread yet another reflective conversation (or, in this case, nonreflective conversation) with her supervisor. Somehow the supervisor and supervisee just couldn't create enough of a reflective space for the clinician to wonder about her need to gratify the mother and take care of her in ways that—from the larger view of the treatment—failed to promote the mother's autonomy. And so the supervisee's behavior continued, unreflected upon. As did the supervisor's annoyance.

Here the supervisee and supervisor were unable to collaborate. Although one might well argue that both have a responsibility to remain self- and other-aware, the power differential in these relationships makes it very hard for the supervisee to feel open to collaboration without the supervisor having laid the foundation for safety. Otherwise, the "supervision" part of the experience ("*I have some thoughts about how you might think about or address this situation*") will be experienced against the background of defensiveness. For these reasons, it falls to the supervisor to monitor their own reactions and to carefully observe the supervisee for signs that they are feeling threatened and defensive. For example, the supervisor might have said, "*I can see that we're kind of at an impasse here. I wonder whether you're feeling guilty, and like you've been 'bad.' I know that I've been getting annoyed, which certainly doesn't help you! Let's try to back up a little and think about what's going on with mom, with school, and with you. I'm going to set aside my concerns about your driving her to school. I'm sorry if I made you uncomfortable. Let's try this again.*"

Obviously, supervisors also need to provide a safe space for the intense and overwhelming feelings that are part and parcel of working with traumatized parents and children, though not all supervisors are prepared or inclined to hold the depth and breadth of these reactions. Just as there is "risk in connecting" (Saakvitne, 2002) for the clinician, so there is risk for the supervisor, the possibility of feeling vulnerable when trying to maintain both professional boundaries and their role as a *supervisor*. And yet often it can be so helpful to a clinician to realize that they are not alone in their pain, or to hear that the supervisor, too, is deeply moved, confused, or overwhelmed. They can be safe together in the completely human position of not knowing what to do.

Another layer of regulation is provided by the supervisor's providing regularly scheduled private time and space for supervision. That is, for the practitioner to truly feel safe in supervision, they must also know that they will—without fail—have time that is protected and consistent to discuss their work. This is essential to the development of the supervisory relationship. Sadly, in busy, stretched settings it is often the case that scheduled supervisory sessions are canceled, often because the supervisor is overwhelmed by various clinical, training, and administrative responsibilities.

The Development of the Supervisory Relationship

As the supervisee comes to feel safe, a "playspace" (Winnicott, 1965) for mutual exchange and understanding can develop. As such, the supervisee becomes more and more able to trust the knowledge and wisdom the supervisor has to impart; again, Fonagy and Allison's (2014) notion of epistemic trust—which literally means "trust in knowledge"—is relevant here. Within the framework of a secure supervisory relationship, the clinician can explore options, think creatively, and allow themselves to consider a range of issues and possibilities. Clinicians come to trust not only that they can fully collaborate with the supervisor but also disagree, question, and learn from a mutual dialogue. It is important to note, however, that one of the inherent complexities in the supervisory relationship is that the supervisor may well be tasked with the job of evaluating the clinician's progress and performance. This can leave the supervisee feeling vulnerable and exposed. Here, again, the degree to which the supervisee trusts the supervisor and trusts the safety of their relationship will determine how well such inevitable feelings can be processed and managed.

Reflecting Together

Safety, regulation, and a trusting relationship serve as the bases for reflection. On the one hand, this means that the practitioner's evolving reflective capacities allow them to reflect upon their own internal experiences, as well as those of the children and parents with whom they are working. But it also means that the practitioner has the capacity to *learn* from the supervisor (Heffron et al., 2016). Reflection, as we have described elsewhere, is an executive function of the prefrontal cortex. That is, it is one of a range of functions that allow the individual to think, take perspective, make sense of complex information, integrate, and plan. As such, safety in the supervisory relationship supports not only reflective functioning, per se, but also learning, creativity, synthesis, exploration, and development. Another "we" space is created. These integrative processes are key to the practitioner's developing clinical hypotheses and formulations that—as we discuss further in Chapter 10—are essential to change and reorganization. These processes are also key to developing the skills of a particular discipline, be it—as in the case of MTB—mental health care, relationship building, support for child and adult development, or health care and promotion. The blended supervision model we have described here not only has the benefit of reducing the stresses inherent in the activating and distressing aspects of the work but also of helping clinicians develop as professionals. These skills reduce vicarious trauma, build confidence, and increase their trustworthiness to families, who themselves are reassured by and benefit from the clinician's expertise (Allen, 2022).

Self-Care

"Are you taking care of yourself?" is a common trope among clinicians, with "self-care" trumpeted as a panacea for much of what ails stressed clinicians (and families). Self-care—which is so important when threat is such a central part of our work—has been defined in many ways. There is the first, most obvious layer: getting enough sleep and rest, eating healthily, staying fit, and so on. There is the layer of finding out what is personally replenishing—a warm bath, a yoga class, a run, a catnap, a phone call with a friend, a giant Starbucks mocha, a pause in the park in the sun, or binge watching something escapist on TV. There is the layer of maintaining a balance between work, play, and rest, setting reasonable and clear boundaries to help manage the threats that are intrinsic to working with trauma. And then there are a myriad of other ways to respect how difficult our work is, making choices that protect and nurture us. These include having fun, "making room for you and sensual pleasure. . . . To balance the cost of bearing witness, we need opportunities that allow us to turn away, to escape from harsh reality into fantasy, imagination, art, music, creativity, and sheer foolishness" (Saakvitne, 2002, p. 448). And, indeed, we all take care of ourselves in unique and individual ways; the critical thing, however, is to fully leave the arena of pain.

Self-care can be and often is very difficult; so often practitioners do not practice what they preach (Allen, 2022; Osofsky, 2009). Many of us regularly mutter that we need to take some time off, that we have to "practice self-care," but we pretty consistently fail to do so. Sometimes it seems that those who most need to take care of themselves are those who can't or won't. Very experienced clinicians and supervisors who have simply become accustomed to putting in very, very long days without a break rationalize this as necessary. Why is this? Although the answers are undoubtedly complicated and individual, shame often appears to play a role. "Our unrealistic expectations for ourselves and each other about professional detachment and 'neutrality' can create a barrier of shame that prevents the honest disclosure of the pain and anxiety of the work. We need to be willing to speak the language of feelings, rather than constructs, and to express fears and doubts, rather than . . . formulations" (Saakvitne, 2002, p. 446). Acknowledging vulnerability can be shameful. For some practitioners, the mission to help others becomes distorted to the point that they come to believe that their contribution is so essential that they *cannot* take a moment away, that they don't need it, that they are, in a sense, different from everybody else in their superhuman powers. One supervisor described this as being a kind of "oxytocin junkie": *"I'm being so helpful and so good."* Sadly, some agencies reinforce both the shame of vulnerability and the necessity of invincibility by failing to support clinicians in their efforts to take care of themselves. Time off is discouraged, caseloads are large, time and supervision is scarce. It is so important to combat "should-talk" (as opposed to self-care) and to challenge administrative and other barriers toward nurturing our own needs, because, unless we can take care of ourselves, we can't take care of each other.

There is also the self-care that comes from community. Vicarious traumatization is best transformed by focusing on meaning, perspective, and community (Saakvitne, 2002). We examine our work together, we find hope, we see progress, we laugh, we surround each other in comfort, and we name our losses and fears for each other. This is how we find meaning, and this is how we create a "we" space to hold the pain of what we see and feel every day. When the core group of MTB-HV clinicians began meeting regularly as a team more than 20 years ago, one of us started bringing chocolate to the meetings. Quickly it became a necessary staple, and soon it was jokingly listed on our PowerPoint slides as an "essential ingredient" of MTB-HV. Sometimes it was a candy bar that we'd pass around the table, each of us breaking off a hunk the size of which spoke to our affect hunger that particular day. Sometimes it was a container of our favorite peanut butter cups. Occasionally someone would bring in "fancy" chocolate and we'd feast. And even more occasionally, there was chocolate cake. We'd all protest that we *shouldn't* really eat it, that we should only have a tiny piece; sometimes the more disciplined of us would pass altogether. We would laugh about it, making light of what felt more and more like an important ritual. But we needed it. We met toward the end of the day, we were tired, we were depleted, and we were talking about such hard things. We also caught up with each other at these meetings: whose child was off to school, who had hit terrible traffic on the way into work, who was taking care of an ailing parent, whose case was keeping them up at night, and so on. We would listen, laugh, comfort, and then—sometimes grudgingly—get to "work."

We have not met in person for more than 3 years. Our offices were shuttered as the pandemic dragged on, and the team scattered across the state. We meet online, but somehow there is less laughter, less time for news, commiserating, or just companionable sitting around. Our chocolate stash at the office dried up and had to be thrown out, and although we likely all have our private stashes, it's not the same. We've lost a vital form of self-care, the self-care of community. The pandemic has made this particularly difficult. Cynicism, exhaustion, resignation, and hopelessness remind us that connection and collective meaning making is a powerful antidote to suffering.

Summary

The relational foundations of reflection begin with the clinician, with their sense of safety, their capacity to regulate, and—finally—to fully engage with the children and parents they are working with. These are the conditions that make it possible for clinicians to take a reflective stance, regardless of their discipline. And these are the conditions that allow the development of clinical formulations and clinical skill. Both reflective and clinical supervision play a key role in this process; together, they provide a safe playspace to both make meaning and learn from the supervisor's expertise. And just as the parent–clinician relationship should provide safety, regulation, and relationship as a means to reflection and learning, so should the supervisory relationship. Self-care and community support provide additional layers of safety and self-regulation.

QUESTIONS FOR CLINICIANS

The following questions orient clinicians to developing the capacity to observe "where" on the RFR pyramid they are in their work with parents and children. In a given clinical encounter:

▶ Do you feel physically safe? Safe with your own feelings?

▶ Do you feel relationally safe?

▶ Are you experiencing vicarious or shared trauma?

▶ Are you struggling with the expectations of the intervention(s) you are delivering?

▶ Are you too bound by your discipline?

▶ Are you feeling regulated or defensive?

▶ Do you have ways of regulating yourself and remaining in touch with sensation?

▶ With the families you're seeing, do you, in your physical and clinical stance, convey a willingness to show up emotionally?

▶ Is this a risk you can or will take?

▶ Are *you* someone they would be inclined to trust?

▶ Are *you* able to be bigger, stronger, wiser, and kind (Hoffman et al., 2017; Powell et al., 2013)?

▶ Most important, as painful or risky as it may be, can you let yourself *care* for them?

▶ Do you regularly "check" your own capacity to mentalize? (See Chapter 10 for clinician mentalizing self-assessment checks.)

▶ Does your supervisory relationship provide safety and regulation, as well as the opportunity for reflection and clinical learning?

▶ Are you able to take steps to care for yourself?

Chapter

9

The Relational Foundations
of Reflection in Parents and Children

As represented by the nested mentalization model we described in Chapter 8, the caregiver's safety, regulation, and openness to relationship are the clinician's next concern. Recall that—as we discussed briefly in Chapter 2—just as the attachment system is built into our evolutionary heritage, so is the caregiving system, namely, the reciprocal biological system that ensures that parents care for and protect their young (Bowlby, 1969/1982). That is, parents and other caregivers are primed from the moment of the child's birth (and likely from early in the pregnancy) to do what is necessary to make sure that infants survive and thrive. We see this in the simplest acts: the way a pregnant woman protects her belly, the way a mother wraps her arms around an infant when a loud noise sounds, leans in close so the baby can see her, elongates vowels so that the baby can discriminate sounds, modulates her voice to soothe and contain, exaggerates her facial expressions so that the baby can get the message, and so forth. And of course we see it in the monumental and courageous acts of desperate parents who feed their children first when food is scarce, throw themselves over the child to protect them from danger, and—in some instances—sacrifice their lives to save the child's. Unfortunately, the caregiving system can also be distorted and coopted by the caregiver's own history, needs, and anxieties. Thus, in a number of ways, the trio of threat, dysregulation, and relational difficulties can profoundly shape a parent's capacity to provide a secure and loving sanctuary for the child. This is where Selma Fraiberg and David Olds began nearly 50 years ago, and that is where practitioners working with young families find themselves focused and challenged as they work with caregivers to regulate and diminish threat and allow for the emergence of less disrupted and more open relationships.

In this chapter, we begin with the parent's sense of safety and then continue on to regulation and relationship, the relational foundations of reflection. We then turn to these same foundations in the child. We begin with the parent for the reasons we described in Chapter 8—namely, that we are hoping to influence the child's relational environment. If we focus too directly on the child, the parent can easily feel overlooked and disrespected. It is easy to forget this, particularly when we are worried about the child or discouraged in our efforts to connect with the parent. But unless the situation requires us to protect the child directly, the parents are our conduit to *their* child.[1]

The Caregiver

Safety

When working with a parent, we first ask, "Do they feel safe?" Just as we look to the body and to the quality of thought and language in detecting threat in ourselves, we do the same with parents. Sometimes, it is quite easy to tell when caregivers are threatened. Usually, however, the signs are more subtle. Are they open to social communication—making eye contact, smiling, speaking clearly and with intonation, listening—or are they avoiding our gaze, facial expressions flat and almost deadened, speech also flat and without inflection, closed to dialogue of any sort? Do they communicate wariness and distrust? Are they physically shut down, torso collapsed, head down or turned away, movements constricted? When caregivers speak, do they avoid or resist us by rejecting, minimizing, denying, or arguing with what we have to offer (Talia et al., 2014)? Is their speech flat or pressured? Are their narratives—even about the most basic aspects of their daily lives—coherent and communicative, or are they incoherent, vague, contradictory, flooded, disorganized? Do caregivers stay on the topic at hand, or do they change focus, shift to another idea? Are they able to think straight and make sense? Do they tend to speak—as we described in Chapter 4—in prementalizing modes? Do we see evidence of hostile or helpless representations of the child? Recognizing certain features of speech and

---

[1]Beginning in March 2020, many aspects of infant mental health and health practice were moved online due to the pandemic. Today, as we discuss in Chapter 17, this continues, albeit to a much lesser extent, though in certain rural communities it has become the norm. When we are working with families using a telehealth platform, observing the subtleties we describe in this chapter can be quite challenging, as can establishing the direct personal connection that is at the heart of face-to-face work. And yet we do the best we can under these very difficult circumstances.

their defensive and interpersonal functions (Talia et al., 2014) allows us to again ask the question: *"What is the threat that is provoking these particular defenses, and how can I address it?"* What is the nature of conversation and communication when painful memories, interactions, and emotions come to the fore? In the sections below, we consider potential threats to the parent's sense of safety.

Physical Safety

Recall the discussion of adverse childhood experiences and toxic stress in Chapter 6 and the profound layers of impact that flow from exposure to assaults on the body, whether in the form of interpersonal, community, or societal violence. Whether a caregiver is physically threatened by a partner or family member or by the very real potential for physical harm when simply walking down the street or by the overt assaults and microaggressions (Sue, 2010) that are part and parcel of systemic racism and classism, the fear system is on alert, at the level of the body and the brain.

What does this mean for us as clinicians? At the most basic level, if the caregiver's literal, physical safety is threatened, our job is to make sure they are as safe as possible. Thus, if the parent is worried that a violent partner may return shortly, the clinician's job is to secure their physical safety, that is, help them find a place to stay, contact the police, and stay with the parent until they are safe. We make sure the parent or caregiver is protected. If, on the other hand, we are reasonably sure that the caregiver is safe in their home or our office, then a different level of work can proceed. But we can never ignore real threats to physical safety. Although this may seem self-evident, clinicians can—under the threat of their own anxieties—overlook threats to physical safety and try to proceed according to their clinical plan.

What about less immediate, but no less real, threats to physical safety in the form of community or societal violence? Here, we provide safety by hearing these fears, holding them, and acknowledging their force and reality. And we help parents think through the various ways they can protect themselves. We try to build agency by helping them plan—to avoid certain neighborhoods and situations, to develop emergency plans, to eventually move to a safer neighborhood. We can try to help parents develop ways of insulating themselves against racist assaults and of reclaiming their agency in ways that are meaningful and not self-destructive. Developing a perspective and having a plan go a long way in managing fear and threat.

Internal Safety

Whereas some dangers are overt, such as threats to physical safety, other dangers are less palpable. But they are no less powerful. Parents (like clinicians) can be threatened by their internal experiences. We must never underestimate how dangerous feelings can *feel*. By virtue of our training, of our interest in feelings, we can often forget how scary it can be to feel *anything*: excitement, joy, delight, anger, fear, sadness, or despair. Or even just interest. And our simple and basic assumption as clinicians that a person *has* feelings can be threatening as well; for many caregivers, particularly those who have struggled to overcome early traumas and adversity, some feelings are associated with bad outcomes and cannot be acknowledged, even to themselves. That is one good reason to avoid the therapeutic trope "What are you feeling?" unless we are fairly certain this won't be disruptive in and of itself.

We have learned over and over again from such infant researchers as Daniel Stern and Beatrice Beebe or such clinicians as T. Berry Brazelton and D. W. Winnicott that the parent–child interaction determines the fate of the child's affects; that is, the child can learn early on that there can be bad outcomes from having feelings. How do we imagine that the adult's caregivers met their delight, their trepidation, their anger, their sadness? Were these opportunities for communication, for attunement, for closeness? Or were they moments of disappointment and fear? For some adults, these entirely human, communicative, critical early experiences were met with scorn, rejection, humiliation, hostility, rage, or, worse, no reaction at all. These responses implicitly signal that the child is bad or worthless or invisible and elicit powerful feelings of shame. Thus the experience of simply *having* a feeling can be linked to shame, a feeling so difficult to tolerate that it must be avoided at all costs. We must be alert to those feelings that are experienced as safe and those that are experienced as dangerous (Haft & Slade, 1989).

In our work, we continuously gauge the caregiver's level of threat by registering the many physical, behavioral, and linguistic cues to their withdrawal or agitation and trying to diminish threat in whatever way we can. For instance, a clinician working with a pregnant woman might ask at a first meeting how she is feeling about her pregnancy. This may be, in fact, a very important question or simply an icebreaker. But the woman immediately turns her eyes to the side and then shifts her gaze down. She covers her belly with her hands, slumps down in the chair, and mumbles a few words that the clinician can't hear. This is a clear signal that the mother-to-be is threatened. Our job at these moments is to restore safety to the degree that we can. If we have threatened the parent with a discussion of feelings, we need to find a way to diminish the sense of threat. In this instance, the pregnant woman may not be ready to talk about her feelings about the pregnancy. She doesn't know or trust the clinician yet. The clinician has to find a less threatening way to engage. This might mean focusing on her physical experience of pregnancy: "How are you sleeping? What do you feel like eating?" Or the clinician might simply say, "Oh, sorry, that's such a big question. . . . When did you find out you were pregnant?" and slowly break up the inquiries into more manageable bits. Or, as we discuss more fully later in the chapter, if the therapeutic relationship is well established, the recognition of threat may lead to processing it and understanding it more deeply.

Another example: The clinician begins a dyadic session by asking a simple question: "How've things been going?" The mother responds sharply (and in front of the child), "Oh, things would be just fine if it weren't for this little jerk. He just loves to mess with my head." This is an example of intrusive–hostile prementalizing (too much). The clinician thus knows right away that the mother is feeling threatened by something. In this instance, she may be frightened by a recent visit from child protective services, or she may be frightened by domestic violence. It could be anything, but slipping into both these primitive projections and a hostile caregiving stance signals immediately that there are feelings and potentially circumstances that are very threatening to her.

Relational Safety

Another of our assumptions as clinicians is that we will form a relationship with the parents and caregivers we see. This, too, can be threatening for caregivers, for a variety of reasons. It is hard to think of ourselves as potentially threatening, of frightening parents (or children, for that matter), but—especially for parents with complex relational histories—we have to be alert to this possibility. To begin, parents who may not have found even the most basic safety in relationships may well find our attempts to connect with and come to know them threatening. Why would we be any different from those who betrayed and hurt them? Why should they let their defenses down? And to circle back to their sense of internal safety, why would they want to discuss feelings with *us*?

The problem of relational safety is compounded by the circumstances in which we meet families. We are often employed by agencies that they have little reason to trust and that have the authority to take their children away. We are mandated reporters. Respect and humanity are often sorely missing in care delivery systems, governmental agencies, and even educational systems. And, given the fact that there are still few BIPOC clinicians working in underserved communities, there are likely to be racial and ethnic differences that will likely be, in and of themselves, threatening. And even when the clinician and family are of the same ethnic, racial, or cultural background, there are often enormous class differences between families and clinicians. Privilege takes many forms. In all of these instances, safety is something that has to be achieved, rather than assumed.

Finally, the negative feelings, anxieties, and judgments that clinicians routinely struggle with in this challenging work can have a direct impact on parents, despite clinicians' best intentions. Whereas—as we described earlier—overt judgments and other negative reactions clearly affect parents, there are many more subtle instances in which a parent picks up on the clinician's anxiety and reacts to and against it, shutting down, becoming irrational, argumentative, and so on.

The following passage—an exchange between Sandy, age 22, and her very familiar and trusted home visitor, Lisa—provides a clear example of a negative spiral in which the clinician's (understandable) anxiety further threatens an already threatened and agitated mother. Lisa has been working with Sandy and her daughter, Joni, for more than 2 years, beginning when Sandy was pregnant. The subtext in this clinical vignette is that Lisa is worried that Sandy—who is in a fury at a friend and threatening to go out and fight with her—is going to get herself in trouble with the police and, potentially, child protective services. Each time that Lisa voices any version of that concern, Sandy feels threatened and becomes concrete, irrational, and defensive. Prementalizing modes abound: Sandy is certain that her interpretation is correct and insists that there would be no legal consequences for her actions. Her feelings (rage, need for revenge, humiliation) dominate any assessment of reality. She is also quite unable to see her child's distress and fear and sees her only in the light of her own intense affect. The threat seems multilayered: "I am not being heard!" "I have to fight for my dignity and you don't get it." "You are trying to get me to calm down and I am not there yet. This feels shaming." When Lisa can just mirror her distress, her shame, and her rage, Sandy's speech is more fluent and expressive and she relaxes. Her thinking clears up.

In the following transcript, those comments of Lisa's that seem to threaten or trigger Sandy are <u>underlined</u>. Instances of prementalizing are labeled "PM."

When Lisa arrives, she finds Sandy spitting mad. Joni is walking around the room looking at toys. Throughout the visit, the child picks up toys again and again and brings them to Sandy. Joni looks apologetic and seems to be muttering "I'm sorry."

LISA: What's going on? How have things been?

SANDY: Bad. Terrible. I'm raging. I found out yesterday that this so-called friend, not even, just an acquaintance, has been going around telling people that I have crabs. I couldn't believe it. I was so mad when I found out! I just spent the whole afternoon walking around her neighborhood, hoping to run into her so I could kick her butt.

LISA: Oh, that's terrible! Why would she do that? Sounds like you were really mad—furious, in fact.

SANDY: Yeah, exactly, why would she do that? You best believe when I see her I'm going to kick her butt. I don't understand. I mind my own business.

I don't do nothin'. I just stay in the house and clean and take care of my daughter—and she feels like she can just spread this stuff around about me. You'd best believe she's got somethin' coming to her and I told everyone in the neighborhood to tell her to watch out 'cause if I see her I'm going to kick her butt. (PM)

LISA: I get it. You're so mad you want to really hurt her. What do you think that would be like for Joni to see?

SANDY: Well I wouldn't do nothin' if she was with me.

LISA: Oh, well, that's good, but if she wasn't with you, would you fight her?

SANDY: Oh yes! You best believe I'll kick her butt! She can't just go around talking crap like that. She needs to know she can't just get away with that. I'll look like a punk if I don't do nothin' about it. (PM)

LISA: I can see how angry you are that she's been spreading these rumors about you and you think that she's messed with your reputation

SANDY: No, I don't think she has, she has. (PM)

LISA: Oh, OK, sorry, she's messed with your reputation. I'm just worried about you and Joni if you fight her. What do you think it would be like if, for instance, you started a fight with her and she pressed charges against you or someone called the police and you were arrested?

SANDY: Oh, that wouldn't happen. I truly believe that if I were to fight her, any police officer or lawyer or judge that heard the story would take my side and understand that she lied and spread rumors and I had to defend myself and my reputation and they would not let anything happen to me. They wouldn't do nothin', as in getting arrested or going to jail, nothin', because they'd know I was in the right and I didn't do nothin' wrong. (PM)

LISA: Hmmm, well, you know, even if they did understand and take your side . . . that is, feel that you were in the right, there are written laws on the books and in court that might say essentially, "If Sandy started this fight then she has broken the law and she will be arrested," and if you are arrested that might even mean you'd have to spend time on probation or, worse yet, in jail.

SANDY: No, I don't believe that would happen. (PM)

LISA: You don't? OK, let me just make sure I get where you are coming from. You are really mad, furious, raging mad, and maybe hurt, too—so mad that, for a while, it was the only thing you could think about. And so mad that the only thing you feel will make it right is if you fight this woman.

SANDY: Yeah, exactly—that's about right.

LISA: OK, so you are so angry and hurt you feel like you need to fight her. But, I'm just curious, what do you think about when you think about what you want Joni to learn about feeling hurt and angry and what to do with those feelings?

SANDY: (*smiling slightly*) *I* know what you mean. I don't want her to fight in the streets or nothin' but this is not the same, I have to do something or I look like a punk. (PM)

LISA: It's not the same? What would you want her to do?

SANDY: I don't know. She'd probably do the same thing. (PM)

LISA: But what you are saying is that you don't feel like you could just ignore it—communicate to this woman somehow by not fighting, that she's not even worth the time or effort to fight??

SANDY: No!! She told people I have crabs, you best believe she's gonna' get hers when I see her.

LISA: It seems like a really hard position to be in. You are so mad and hurt and you feel like your only way to feel better is to hurt the person who hurt you.

SANDY: Yeah, exactly.

Lisa: I get how mad you are but I'm still worried because I don't want you to do anything that ends up getting you hurt or in trouble. That would hurt Joni too. I'd hate to see that happen.

SANDY: That wouldn't happen.

(*Lisa feels stuck and pauses to think about where to go from here. She observes what else is going on in the room, pausing to reflect and buy some time.*)

LISA: Hmmm, so it seems like we see things differently. Hey, I was just noticing Joni. I was wondering, does it sound to you like she's saying, "I'm sorry" when she brings the toys over to show you? I was just curious, wondering if she might know you are angry but doesn't know you're not mad at her. Maybe she's trying to make you feel better by bringing things over to you and saying "I'm sorry"?

SANDY: No, she knows I'm not mad at her. I always talk like this. She's not saying "I'm sorry"— I don't know how she could say "I'm sorry" because she's never heard that before.

LISA: Oh.

Each time Lisa attempts to do anything other than simply acknowledge and echo Sandy's experience (and thus hint that there are other ways to see the situation, asking her to mentalize), Sandy defends herself, with the result being impaired mentalizing and frightening behavior: She becomes concrete, she contradicts herself, she becomes irrational ("no judge would find me guilty," etc.), and she acts and talks in ways that would be frightening to the child (who is very close by). One example of impaired mentalizing occurs when Lisa says that Sandy "thinks" that her friend has "messed with her reputation." This is an attempt on Lisa's part to get Sandy to think of other possible explanations for the friend's behavior. But Sandy is having none of it, even though she seems to realize that Lisa is suggesting that the friend's behavior could mean something other than what she (Sandy) thinks it does. Sandy instead sticks to her *concrete* interpretation: *What I see is what is.*

By contrast, when Lisa simply mirrors her intense affect, Sandy relaxes and acknowledges it and provides a sensible explanation for her feelings (someone went around saying bad things about me and I am mad). But Lisa's job, as a clinician, is also to protect the child (who is clearly aware of her mother's anger) and to protect Sandy from herself. This puts Lisa—who sees that Sandy is frightening Joni and is genuinely worried that Sandy is going to go out and do something dangerous—in a very difficult position. Unfortunately and unavoidably, Lisa's observations and concerns are triggering for Sandy, but—in the moment, with Sandy enraged and threatening—Lisa finds them difficult to contain. Had Lisa been able to sit with her anxiety internally, Sandy—after blowing off steam and raging for a while—might have calmed down and been able to think more clearly. But Lisa's feelings, totally understandable and important, derail Sandy and her ability to process what *she* is feeling. Although we certainly cannot avoid situations in which our and the parent's aims are at cross-purposes, we can try to remain attuned to their consequences and try to both acknowledge and repair ruptures. Thus, as in this example, Lisa returns to Sandy's feelings and just stays there. She might also try to repair the situation further, saying—either in the moment or at the next meeting—"*You know, I realize that I'm not quite hearing you, and that must feel pretty bad.*"

A more complex and sadly common example is provided by situations in which the clinician must report the parent to child protective services. The moment parents learn that they are being reported, their fear system is likely in the state of highest alert: They feel terrified (at the thought of losing the child), enraged (at the clinician), humiliated (by the clinician), and truly unable to react in any but the most self-protective ways. The clinician must then (often over days and weeks) take on the mammoth task of first addressing these fundamental and human reactions by providing comfort, empathy, and understanding of the parents' feelings and then working to gently activate the parents' concern and desire to protect both themselves and the child. But above all, the clinician must remain alert to signs that the parents are threatened and try to address the fear, either in the moment or when it is clinically possible. It is here that supervision and therapeutic maturity are so essential.

Regulation

As we described in Chapter 3, the experience of safety is regulating. Thus threat and dysregulation often go hand in hand. Even if no active threats to the parent are evident to us, we can readily infer that a parent feels threatened by the extent to which they are dysregulated and disrupted. This can manifest itself in many ways.

As we have described in previous chapters, parents can, on the one hand, actively or unconsciously suppress their feelings, resulting in over-regulation (too little). They may be shut down and unresponsive and fail to make eye contact. Their shoulders may collapse into the chest, their speech may be flat and inexpressive. They may speak in short sentences and respond to our questions in monosyllables. Getting them to engage in the most basic conversation may be like pulling teeth: *"I don't know," "Nothing," "I'm fine," "I don't remember"* are the hallmarks of this stance. What we are seeing in these instances (and its less dramatic iterations) is the use of down-regulation or "shutdown" to defend against threat.

On the other hand, parents may also be hyperaroused and affectively flooded, as Sandy was in the preceding example. They, too, resist contact, but in different ways (Talia et al., 2014). We cannot get a word in edge-wise, our words and our observations are overridden or rejected, their speech is pressured and noncommunicative (too much). There are few opportunities for dialogue, for the "serve and return" (National Scientific Council on the Developing Child, 2012, 2020) that marks true exchange. Here, too, eye contact is fleeting, the body is in motion. They are closed to us by virtue of their extreme arousal and distress. Again, we can see these phenomena in degrees or as fluctuating, depending upon the level of threat and defense.

van der Kolk (2014) makes the very important point that when individuals are highly threatened and dysregulated, words (observations, interpretations, etc.) may have little value and can, in fact, be highly activating. To a parent in a self-protective, defensive mode, they can feel assaultive. To use a different terminology, when a parent is in "limbic system overdrive," they likely have little capacity to do anything but react in ways that make them feel safest. And so, what can we do? We can introduce activities that calm the autonomic nervous system so an individual can return to the present and to the possibilities of human connection. van der Kolk (2014) calls this "limbic system therapy" and describes two avenues to regulation in the face of flight, fight, and freezing: bodily regulation and social engagement. Typically, we begin with the former, as the parent is not ready to really engage in the therapeutic relationship. Social engagement only becomes possible when threat is diminished.

Bodily regulation—helping parents modulate arousal or become more connected and open—can be accomplished in a variety of ways. On the one hand, there are the time-tested Eastern practices of meditation and deep relaxation and, on the other, techniques inspired by the arts. Whether it is pausing to engage in deep relaxation, encouraging a parent to take some long breaths with longer exhalations, to briefly meditate on the breath, to tap out rhythms on a drum, to make a drawing, sing a song, stretch the body, take a short walk, or even write a poem, all provide well-documented routes to achieving calmer and less dysregulated states.

Mindfulness practice has been the most thoroughly studied of these approaches and has been linked in several studies to "mindful parenting" (Bögels et al., 2010). The term was coined by Kabat-Zinn and Kabat-Zinn (1997) and refers to the practice of paying attention to the child, and to parenting, intentionally, here and now, and nonjudgmentally. Interventions that train parents in mindfulness techniques influence the parent–child relationship by attempting to (1) reduce parenting stress and reactivity; (2) reduce parental preoccupation or negative bias in relation to the child and parenting; (3) improve parental executive functioning, particularly in impulsive parents; (4) break the cycle of intergenerationally transmitted dysfunctional parenting; (5) increase self-nourishing attention and self-compassion; and (6) improve couple and marital functioning and coparenting (Bögels et al., 2010). Cultivating presence and compassion, the cornerstones of mindfulness practice, invite the parents to adopt a curious, open, accepting, and loving (Siegel, 2007) stance toward their own thoughts and feelings, as well as those of the child.

MTB-P is not a mindfulness intervention, per se, although remaining present, compassionate, curious, open, accepting, and caring is intrinsic to our approach as clinicians, as well as being the attitudes we hope to nurture in parents (and, by extension, children). Indeed, many techniques of mindfulness practice (e.g., focusing on the breath in the here and now, simple guided meditations) can be enormously helpful in encouraging parents to slow down, regulate, and become aware of their responses to threat (Kabat-Zinn, 1994). The first step is helping them pause enough to attend to their thoughts, feelings, and bodily sensations, to be present in the here and now. They may become aware that their thoughts are racing or that they are filled with intense feelings. They may begin to identify bodily symptoms such as headaches, muscle tension, or a racing heart. Once they have begun to identify these experiences and can accept them without defense and shame, they can begin to cultivate openness and curiosity about the experiences that trigger such dysregulation.

A clinician notes that a mother's response to her child's inconsolable crying is to stiffen her torso and fold her arms over her chest, trying—as it were—to push her feelings down. In response, the clinician asks the mother to describe how her body feels, helping the mother be present and compassionate about her own feelings of anxiety and frustration. The clinician can then wonder out loud how the baby interprets the tension in her arms as she holds him. Once the mother is able to take a few deep breaths, relax her body, and hold the baby more loosely, the baby calms. Only then, when the mother is more regulated, can she acknowledge that the baby's crying frightened and upset her and that it triggered her.

Other nonverbal and creative modes of self-expression can also be regulating and organizing. A pregnant woman who seems to the clinician somewhat frozen and inaccessible may be able to draw a picture for her unborn child or knit them a hat. She can begin a scrapbook of pictures and poems. Any of these activities help bring the child into focus for the parent in a nonthreatening way and free some of her fears as she creates images that are pleasant and calming (and that likely engage the pleasure centers of her brain). Of course, mothers may use drawing or poetry or even movement to convey their deepest fears; put in the language of art or movement, however, these fears can become less overwhelming and contained and thus regulated (Gray, 2018; Malchiodi, 2020). Sometimes putting our darkest worries into movement and imagery can make them less "hot" and dangerous. Artists have been doing this for millennia.

Openness to Relationship

Safety and regulation pave the way to relationships; in the absence of threat, social engagement and communication becomes possible. Once parents feel reasonably safe and somewhat regulated, they can begin to open themselves to the relationship with the clinician. Of course, as we noted earlier, these are all reciprocal processes; the clinician will be instrumental in helping the parent feel safe and regulated, but the softening of defenses that comes with safety and regulation are essential to the parents' allowing themselves to be reached by the clinician and changed by their relationship.

We have noted at several points that many of the families we see in health, mental health, and educational settings have had difficult if not overtly frightening and traumatic relationships with their own parents and other caregivers (e.g., extended family members, foster parents). These experiences are destructive to an individual's sense of themselves and to their basic willingness and ability to trust others. In the language of attachment theory, the parents' state of mind with respect to attachment is likely quite insecure; this is especially the case in the absence of BCEs, such as a loving grandparent, a mother who managed to keep her family together even though she was very depressed, and so forth (Lieberman et al., 2005a; Narayan et al., 2017). What this means concretely for any provider is that individuals who have never fully trusted the people meant to care for and protect them are not going to trust us at first and possibly not for quite a while, regardless of how open we may be to a relationship with them. What we are more likely to experience for quite a while are their attempts to push us away, test us, ignore us, overwhelm us, or reject us and our efforts outright. We may be subject, as they themselves have been, to swings in their affect, to negative projections, and to manipulation. These are manifestations of insecure internal working models of attachment; in other words, parents' negative representations of past relationships intrude in the present. This is a major stressor for practitioners and one of the reasons that supervision and self-care are so critical. Without these supports, we can easily feel endangered and dysregulated.

As we also discussed earlier, the relative lack of safety in their primary relationships may lead parents to assume that our intentions are malevolent (as were those of an abusing parent), to believe that if we are unable to make an appointment it means that we have given up on them, or to idealize us to the extent that we are doomed to failure (as, e.g., when a treatment we suggest is not particularly effective). That is, at the beginning of the work, we may not be real people to them but the embodiment of their worst fears and greatest hopes. It is only when we start to become real and they can begin to trust our motives, our suggestions, and *who we are* that reparative work and true relationship building can begin.

It is important to remember that the simple fact of our offering a relationship to a parent (or to their child) can itself be threatening, particularly if their past experiences have been negative and people they might have thought were going to protect and care for them did not. Why would we be any different? Why *should* they trust us? Why *would* they trust us? It is here that our patience, our consistency, our humanity and full presence, and our willingness to return, again and again, to trust that some part of them wants to connect and be heard will finally open the door to a deeper relationship. In Courtois's (2004) paper on treating complex trauma, she notes that, particularly with traumatized adults, the establishment of a safe relationship can take a very long time, even years. The more an individual has been wounded and hurt, the longer it will take them to feel safe and to trust.

A parent's expectations of us tell us so much about their own primary relationships. If a parent is pushing us away, it is likely because they are seeing us through the lens of their own experience. If the parent sees us as nosy and out to get them, we learn something, too. The parent's stance toward us tells us something important about their experience of seeking and receiving care. Ultimately, our knowledge of their experience will become more textured and clear with time and will help us find a way to relate to a particular parent in a way that helps them feel safe and understood. A parent's attachment organization also creates the lens through which they experience our feelings for them. If the parent is fundamentally suspicious, and we are, in fact, irritated and annoyed with them, then their convictions are confirmed. It is for that reason that it is so important for clinicians to monitor their feelings about a parent or child closely, because their anger, frustration, and fear can simply reinforce a parent's lack of trust in any helper. We are humans, and we are bound to feel some of these feelings, but we also have the opportunity and the requirement to process them.

The Child

In the following sections, we describe some of the ways to establish safety, regulation, and openness to relationship in the child.

Safety

Evolutionarily programmed threat detection is present from earliest infancy, at the hormonal and neural level (Gunnar et al., 1996), at the bodily level by shifts in heart rate and skin tone (Hofer, 2006), and at the behavioral level in the form of startles, apprehension, and shifts in the deployment of attention (Hoehl et al., 2008; Striano et al., 2007). Once the child's social communicative system has begun to mature, by about 2–3 months, responses to threat are much more tangible. As Porges (2011) points out, when they feel safe, infants can initiate social interaction by making eye contact, vocalizing with an appealing inflection and rhythm, displaying contingent facial expressions, and modulating the middle-ear muscles to distinguish the human voice from background sounds more efficiently. We would add to this the many bodily signs that the infant is open to communication: The chest is open, the torso engaged, limbs are mobile, and the head is held upright. When they feel threatened, however, "the eyelids droop, the voice loses inflection, positive facial expressions dwindle, awareness of the sound of the human voice becomes less acute, and sensitivity to others' social engagement behaviors decrease" (Porges, 2011, p. 15). They seem not to see, to hear, or to be interested in the world around them. By about 6 or 7 months old, infants begin to show fear reactions. Interestingly, however, studies of traumatized infants suggest that frightening experiences (such as physical abuse) can dramatically accelerate the development of the fear response (Gaensbauer, 1982).

Main and Solomon's (1986, 1990) descriptions of the behavior of infants who are "disorganized" in relation to attachment provide yet another way of detecting fear and threat in young children. Inherent in Main and Solomon's description of disorganized attachment is the notion of *conflict*: In a variety of ways, the child appears to be both seeking and turning away from the caregiver, "who is at once the source of and solution to its alarm" (Main & Hesse, 1990, p. 163). This leads to "a diverse array of inexplicable, odd, disorganized, disoriented, and overtly conflicted behaviors in the parent's presence" (Main, 2000, p. 1099), particularly when the child is seeking comfort from or proximity to the caregiver. Main and Solomon (1990) described seven key manifestations of fear and conflict in infantile behavior (pp. 136–140):

1. *Sequential displays of contradictory behavior patterns* (e.g., child suddenly becomes flat and quiet after displaying intense attachment behaviors).

2. *Simultaneous display of contradictory behavior patterns* (e.g., child expresses distress and wish for contact but at the same time avoids and turns away from parent).

3. *Undirected, misdirected, incomplete, and interrupted movements and expressions* (e.g., infant begins to approach parent but falls on the floor in an apparently "depressed" position; slow or limp movements in approaching a parent).

4. *Stereotypies, asymmetrical movements, mistimed movements, and anomalous postures* (e.g., rocking, ear pulling, hair twisting, or other rhythmical, repeated movements without visible function).

5. *Freezing, stilling, and slowed movements and expressions* (e.g., freezing and stilling suggestive of more than momentary interruption of activity).

6. *Direct indices of apprehension regarding the parent* (e.g., jerking back when mother enters the room, dashing away from parent with hunched or tucked head and shoulders).

7. *Direct indices of disorganization, disorientation, and confusion* (e.g., raising hands to mouth directly upon the return of the parent with a clearly confused or wary expression).

These signs can be very subtle (especially if an infant "seems" OK), although sometimes we can see the infant or young child's fear more easily than the parent's, as children are less skillful at disguise and defense. In any event, the child's fear is a critical signal and may well alert us to something we might not otherwise see or suspect. When we do see these signs, we think about gentle and nonthreatening ways we can bring them to the parent's attention.

As part of an assessment protocol, Jimmy was videotaped interacting with his mother, age 18, when he was about 4 months old. He is in an infant seat; Mom has been asked to play with him as she normally would. The tape is painful to watch: She "playfully" looms over him, pokes him, violates his physical boundaries, and ignores his signals. She mocks him when he protests and whimpers after hitting his finger. The child's fear responses are clear: He startles, seems almost to try to pull himself further back into the infant seat, and blinks repeatedly. Most telling are his mixed facial signals: He seems to be trying to smile, as if to signal to his mother that he is having fun. But his smile is more like a grimace; thus his communication of fun is laced with distress, a failed smile. His eyes betray no fun but are wary and fearful. His face is full of contradictions. And—contrary to the regular engagement–disengagement cycles so typical of infant–parent interactions (Beebe & Stern, 1977), in which children look away and then look back to the parent's face in cycles—he rarely breaks gaze with his mother, but instead keeps his eyes focused on her face.

> It's as if he wants to keep her in his sights so he can see danger as soon as it arises. The mother (likely driven by her own anxiety) sees none of this, but keeps up her steady stream of intrusions and frightening behavior.

This vignette captures vividly how fear escalates and penetrates the child's experience at multiple levels. Had this occurred during a home visit or during a session, the clinician would hopefully pick up quickly on how the child was responding to his mother's intrusions. She might gently ask, "What do think's going on with Jimmy right now?" Just a simple question might slow the mother down a bit. "Is he a little surprised . . . do you think?" These kinds of very simple nonjudgmental comments alert Mom to the fact that there is something to be noticed and may get her, albeit briefly, to attend. "And what's goin' on with you? What's this like for you?" Here, too, Mom might pause, and the child would be able to regain his equilibrium a little. Perhaps he'd calm and smile genuinely, giving the clinician an opportunity to say, "Wow. He likes that. What a sweet smile!" The clinician would *not* say, "Oh goodness! Look how scared he is!"—which the mother would unquestionably deny. Indeed, it has been our observation that parents often miss fear cues, mistaking them for interest or pleasurable excitement. Often, sadly, parents find the child's fear face funny.

In this instance, Jimmy's mother reviewed the tape with her clinician after 10 months of intensive intervention. She was very upset by what she saw. "It's so hard to watch this. He was trying to tell me he'd had enough. I remember that he hadn't had a good nap and hadn't even had lunch. He was trying to tell me what I didn't know. I had no idea what he wanted." The cues to his distress, his manifest fear, at first unseen, were now painfully apparent to her. Her impaired mentalizing had given way, and she could now "see" and "hear" him.

Physical Safety

It hardly needs saying that we need to ensure the child's physical safety. When there are overt threats to the child's safety, we must act immediately and remain with the child so their safety can be assured. Most clinicians working with high-risk young families will, at some point in their careers, find themselves in situations in which a child has been injured or is in immediate danger. But there are more subtle threats that can have just as powerful an effect on the child and their development as direct threats to their physical safety. Think of situations in which the infant's parents are always fighting. Voices rise to scary levels, and parents *look* scared and angry and become disorganized. Objects crash, doors slam. Threats multiply and build on each other; the world is uncertain, and it feels as if everything is falling apart. This affects the child at the level of the body. Although the child can and does habituate to everyday, normally occurring threats (a dog's barking, a loudly slamming door), the degree to which the fear system is chronically elevated by threats to their physical safety (even if the baby is not literally in harm's way) is the issue. We want both to watch for signs that this is happening and to do what we can to lessen the threat, as well as the activation of the child's autonomic nervous system.

A physical sense of safety also derives from physical health and the parent's capacity to care for the child's body. Minoritized women living below the poverty line, whose educations have been interrupted and who are without partners, tend to have the poorest outcomes and the most limited access to care (e.g., Basu et al., 2016). Such health disparities have typically persisted for generations, such that parents' own physical needs might well have been overlooked or ignored when they were children. As a result, they can have a hard time attending to their children's health. They can miss cues of hunger, of needing sleep, of being too cold or too hot, or of illness. They can forget to administer medications, wait until the last minute to take an ill child to the doctor, let a diaper rash get red and ugly. The sequelae of these unintentional oversights on the parents' part can be experienced by the children as mild to serious assaults on their sense of physical integrity. They feel hungry, tired, or just uncomfortable. Their rash itches, their diapers hurt, they feel sick. And they are without any means to rectify the situation. These circumstances, too, are threatening, in this instance to the child's sense of the body's trustworthiness and wholeness.

Internal Safety

Infants and toddlers let us know whether or not they are comfortable with their feelings in a variety of ways: Delight extends to the tips of their fingers and toes; sadness sinks their bodies, their eyes, and their mouths; fear leads them straight to Dad; a momentary lapse in confidence propels them up on Mom's lap for a huge hug. Over time, we see an increasing differentiation of the affect array (Pine, 1985), meaning that the child's affect repertoire grows over time to express more subtle and complex emotions: pride, shame, and so forth. And by the time they are around 2 years old, children can give voice to simple feelings: "I am mad; I am happy; I like that; I am sad" (Bretherton & Beeghly, 1982). But when feelings threaten a child's equilibrium or primary relationships, we can also see trepidation, constriction, hesitation, and extreme referencing of the other, all of which communicate: "Is this OK? Are you with me? Should I hold back?" These signs are subtle in infants but become more tangible and observable by the end of the first year (Sorce & Emde, 1981). And so we watch for the fullness of their feelings, for the freedom to express them, and note the subtle development of defenses against those that feel dangerous and disruptive.

We can also measure a child's sense of safety by the degree to which they feel free to explore the world and the confidence and competence with which they do so. We look for full, curious, engaged, and sustained exploration at all developmental stages. The 2-month-old infant looks at the mobile steadily, moving her head to see it from different angles. The 6-month-old infant grasps a rattle and bangs it on his high chair, varying the speed of his movements and chortling at the sound the rattle makes. The 1-year-old heads into the kitchen, pulls out all the plastic containers in the kitchen cabinet, and scatters them across the floor; she chews on a few to see how they taste, grinning at her mother's playful reproach. By contrast, the attachment strategies of avoidance and resistance, or the absence of strategy in disorganized attachment, help us make sense of children's approach to exploration. The avoidant infant's or young child's exploration of the world is thin because it is missing the gusto that comes from sharing it with trusted others. The resistant infant's explorations are limited and constricted because of their need to keep a close eye on the caregiver and maintain proximity at all costs. And, finally, the disorganized infant's explorations cannot help but be fragmented and incoherent, as the infant's primary concern is managing fear. Sometimes the disruptions in exploration are very subtle, manifest in the child's inability to maintain attention for more than a few seconds, as they move rapidly from object to object, or in the tendency to drift off and lose concentration, suspend movement, and so forth.

Relational Safety

Recall that in Chapter 2 we described insecure attachment as a response to threat, in particular the threat of losing vital ties to the caregiver. We also described the varying levels and types of threat that lead to particular insecure attachment organizations. The most pernicious kind of threat, so often linked to disorganized attachment in children, is *relational threat*: that in which the person meant to protect the child is also a "source of alarm" (Main & Hesse, 1990). This insoluble dilemma robs the child of the haven of safety that makes development possible and leads to various forms of psychological collapse.

As we've described, there are various forms of "hostile" relational threat: the father who becomes cold and hard in the face of his child's distress; the mother who frightens her child with her raging, causing him to try and placate her; the mother who violates her infant's physical boundaries and misses his signals out of her own anxiety. Remember that active threat can be as subtle as a snarl or bared teeth. At the other, "helpless" extreme, some parents fail to care for their children in the most basic ways, propping the baby's bottle up against his chest and returning to bed, dissociating in the face of the infant's distress, and so on. Researchers have proposed that these two types of environmental influence—active, hostile threat on the one hand and deprivation (parental helplessness or absence) on the other— have distinct neural correlates and stress the infant in quite different ways (McLaughlin et al., 2014). At the same time, it is often the case that we see both extremes clinically, with parents vacillating between the two, depending on the circumstances and the nature of the threat. In any event, it is very important for clinicians to be aware of such threats, which invariably leave the child feeling afraid and alone. Fraiberg and her colleagues (1975) made a similar point: that the caregiver's unmetabolized aggression (manifest in both abuse and neglect) derails the child's development and provides the mechanism for the intergenerational transmission of trauma. The experience of seeking care from a dangerous caregiver leaves the child without a coherent strategy, with collapse—in one form or another—the only option. Again, the bodily cues that alert us to the child's fear and apprehension are those we look for in assessing relational safety and in directing our interventions to repair disrupted interactions.

Regulation

We see the same extremes of arousal in infants and young children as we do in their parents. There are infants who cannot be soothed, or who cannot be aroused, or who vacillate between the two. In some instances, difficulties in regulation have underlying biological causes that must be addressed (e.g., gastrointestinal reflux, food allergies, fatigue and lethargy caused by a viral illness). Once these are ruled out, however, we are left to consider other reasons for their dysregulation. In infancy, and throughout much of early childhood, it is the caregiver who first helps the child regulate their physical and emotional states. A mother wraps her newborn son in a swaddle so that his hand and leg movements don't keep him from falling asleep. A dad holds his daughter's hands and arms tenderly as he feeds her a bottle, so that she can suckle most productively. She has the experience over and over that the bottle and the liquid it holds are associated with the disappearance of her hunger and the arrival of satisfaction. And that both are associated with Dad's tender care. A mother soothes her toddler with gentle coos when he is crying and reassures him that he's going to be all right. Ideally, these moments of regulation happen all the time, and the child gradually learns, through experience, that physical states, body movements, and emotions can be regulated, contained, and modulated. The parents' ministrations are slowly internalized over time, marked by the infant's and toddler's increasing capacities for self-regulation.

What we so often see clinically is that parents struggle—usually because of their own dysregulation and consequent difficulty attuning to the child's cues—with regulating their children in these basic ways. Often they are themselves in survival mode, in flight, fight, or freezing. None of these defensive postures are conducive to regulating their children. And so we begin by helping parents feel less threatened, less dysregulated, and more open to the child so that they can begin to respond to the cues that abound in everyday interactions.

> When Luca was first born, Vivian's handling of him was choppy and disconnected. She jiggled him too forcefully when she wanted him to calm down, and she missed his distress when she laid him down on his stomach so that he had to continually struggle to take a breath. The home visitor—who had from Vivian's second trimester onward been working to establish at least some trust between them and a feeling of safety during their visits—kept up a steady but slow (i.e., not overwhelming or annoying) stream of simple observations, sometimes speaking for the baby. "Oh, Mom, I love this, but I feel like I'm on a speedboat!" "How's that look for him?" "Oh, he likes that! Now he can find his hand. . . ." "You must feel much better after a good night's sleep. I'm glad, I know it's been hard." Slowly, as the child came more clearly into Vivian's view (in part because the clinician was able to see her), as she began to see and hear him, the home visitor saw that Vivian's movements were slower, more synchronous with Luca's. She saw that Vivian began to anticipate positions that would be comfortable for Luca. And she saw Vivian being more physically comforting and containing.

The clinician's sustained attention to the child's subtle and not-so-subtle struggles to manage his body and his needs made it possible for her to slowly and respectfully bring them to the mother's attention. She provided a "holding environment" (Winnicott, 1965) for the mother, so that the mother could provide the same for her son. The home visitor's observations allowed her to highlight, notice, and give voice to the infant's experiences in ways that the mother could make use of them. Her comments were gentle, simple, and digestible.

Although we would hardly expect the regulating strategies we mentioned previously—meditation, deep breathing and relaxation, expressive movement, and a range of creative activities—to be useful to babies, we can help parents develop their repertoire of baby-friendly regulatory activities by introducing them to infant massage (Field, 2018) and simple baby yoga stretches or by encouraging them to sing familiar and pleasing songs to the baby (Pixley, 2015). Simply massaging an infant's arms and legs or playfully moving their arms to the side can at first seem strange to parents, but once they see the baby relax and engage, they are hooked. Likewise, the idea of singing to the baby can feel odd and embarrassing; here again, however, the results can be immediate and tremendously reinforcing.

Openness to Relationship

A young depressed mother sought the help of a psychotherapist. She left her baby in the waiting room with her own mother. After her first session, she returned to the waiting room and picked up the baby, beaming. "I never knew I was the center of your universe!" she crowed, holding him to her tightly. Through the fog of her depression, she had lost sight of him and failed to realize that indeed nothing was more important to him than she was.

The psychotherapist's intervention had shifted her attention from her terror and sense of emptiness to the full relationship forming right before her. Although such dramatic transformations are, of course, rare, this story reminds us of the power of the relationship to transform both the parent's and child's experience.

As we discussed in Chapter 2, the child is born *ready* for relationships, able to signal with whatever capacities they have that they are ready for and open to connection. And, when things are going well, new parents realize within days of their infant's birth how very much these connections quiet, regulate, and please the baby. And how much they themselves are also quieted, regulated, and pleased by the baby. However, parents who are struggling with their own ghosts and demons or with the depleting and continuous stresses of chronic poverty and other forms of toxic stress can miss these signals. Their own social engagement system is derailed. But as they become less frightened, more regulated, and more comfortable trusting others themselves, they can create the same experience in their child. And so, just as we bring the young child's dysregulation to the parent's attention, so do we bring the child's bids for closeness, affection, reassurance, protection, and comfort to the parent's attention, as they themselves become more willing to both trust the child and trust that they can, in fact, let themselves be what they, in fact, are: the most important person in the child's universe!

Jimmy, whom we described earlier, had been startled and wary in the derailed interaction with his mother at 4 months. At 14 months, after 10 more months of intervention, mother and baby were seen in the Strange Situation. Jimmy was very distressed, particularly by the second separation. When Mom returned to the room, he rushed, crying and with outstretched hands, to his mother and climbed up into her arms. He leaned his head into her neck and wrapped his arms around her tightly. She murmured to him soothingly, "Everything's OK. I'm here. You're OK." She held him and rubbed his back and head for about a minute as he gradually calmed. She then slowly lowered him to the ground and picked up a book lying nearby. She sat beside him on the floor, opened it, and drew his attention to the pictures. His shaky breathing gradually calmed, and he looked at the pictures, all the while holding on to her leg for both physical and emotional support. Finally, he cracked a smile and slowly turned his body fully toward the book. He was calm and ready to read.

Jimmy's relationship with his mother had moved from one of fear and wariness to one in which he relied on her as a safe and secure base. He knew she would protect and comfort him, and she knew she could do that, too. In every way, he communicated that this was a relationship he could trust. He felt safe, regulated, and open to all the relationship had to offer.

Summary

The parents' sense of safety, their capacity to regulate themselves, and their openness to relationship are critical to their emerging capacity to see themselves and their children in new ways. They are also essential to the children's feeling safe, to their beginning to regulate their bodies and their feelings, and to their developing trust in their caregivers.

▲▲▲▲▲▲▲▲ QUESTIONS FOR CLINICIANS ▲▲▲▲▲▲▲▲

The following questions orient clinicians to locating parent and child on the RFR triangle. In a given clinical encounter:

▶ Does the parent seem threatened (wary, distrustful), or are they open to social communication (good eye contact, body open, speech communicative)?

▶ Does the parent tend to shut down or become overly aroused in clinical encounters?

▶ Are their descriptions of themselves or the child coherent?

▶ Do they represent themselves or the child in hostile or helpless ways?

▶ Is the parent able to talk about emotions?

▶ Does the parent seem open to a relationship, or are they inclined to see others (including the clinician) in light of their own projections?

▶ Does the child seem fearful or wary?

▶ Do we see odd, inexplicable, or contradictory behavior in the child?

▶ Does the child seem to feel comfortable in their body and moving in space?

▶ Does the child show signs of shutting down or being overaroused?

▶ Does the child seem open to a relationship with the parent or the clinician?

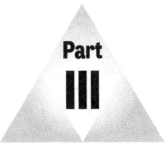

Part

III

Building Reflective Capacities

We now turn to the question that anchors this book: How can we, as practitioners, enhance parental mentalizing capacities or promote "reflective" parenting? It has taken us this long to come to this question because it is so important to understand the context and necessary preludes to the development and stability of reflective parenting. The parent feels reasonably safe, is fairly regulated, and has begun to trust the clinician. All of these may falter and require repair, and indeed it is important to see each as part of a dynamic process. But let us assume that the parent is ready to consider *what* their child is telling them and has set aside more negative interpretations, helplessness, hostility, and an urge to *do* something, to act, to fix. They are ready to wonder.

In the first chapter of Part III, Chapter 10, we begin with a set of general principles for enhancing reflective parenting. In Chapter 11, we discuss the application of these principles to nursing practice. In Chapter 12, we consider some of the challenges of working with parents who are struggling with mental health difficulties. Finally, in Chapter 13, we discuss the clinical applications of the Pregnancy and Parent Development Interviews.

Chapter

10

Enhancing Parental Reflective Functioning

GENERAL CONSIDERATIONS

Jaycee, 16 months old, is sitting in her high chair with her dinner in front of her. After a few minutes, during which she has been happily eating and looking quite content, she starts to pitch her food off her high chair and grabs her bowl, with the obvious intention of flinging it down. It is the well-known toddler game of "watching things fall," combined with the other well-known toddler game of colluding with the dog, who is patiently waiting for morsels to fly his way. Jaycee's mom—who has seen this trick before—intervenes and moves the bowl out of her reach. She asks, "You done? You had enough?" looking to Jaycee for an explanation and tentatively offering her a piece of food. Mom is wondering, not assuming. Jaycee takes the proffered piece of carrot and chews happily. But soon she is again lobbing food off her high chair; the dog, sitting close by, is thrilled. Mom looks at her inquisitively and waves her hands slightly, their sign for "all done." "You're done?" Jaycee waves her hands animatedly. She is done. Mom clears off the high chair, gives Jaycee's face and hands a quick wipe, and puts her down on the floor to play.

Throughout this typical exchange, Jaycee's mother is focused on her child's intentions. Contrast this with a mother who—when the first bit of food is thrown to the floor—quickly responds: "No! That's enough. Don't do that. You're being bad. You're done." She removes the food. Her daughter fusses, and Mom lifts her wordlessly out of the high chair. The difference between these two very common scenarios is that, in the first, Mom sees her daughter as *having* intentions, as having desires. This is a mentalizing

197

interaction. In the second, Mom is not curious and takes over. She tells the child what she (the child) wants, which is really what she (the mother) wants. She thus misses a small opportunity to wonder why her daughter has suddenly moved from eating happily to recreating a scene from the iconic movie *Animal House* and to communicate with her daughter about her intentions. This is a nonmentalizing interaction.

For many parents, curiosity is second nature; for others, becoming curious marks a profound shift from *assuming* they know what the child is feeling or wants or what the child needs to do (and likely trying to change or control it) to *wondering*: "What are they trying to tell me?" Although it is a profound shift, it is also a very simple one, noticeable in the tiniest moments.

The important clinical question is, of course, how we help a parent move from assuming (controlling, directing, overlooking, projecting, ignoring) to asking and being curious? How do we enhance a parent's capacity to reflect upon and make meaning of the child's experience and to appreciate that the child has thoughts, feelings, desires, and intentions that are different from the parent's own? How do we create a reflective space for the parent so that they can eventually begin to wonder about and make sense of the baby, first with the clinician's help and eventually on their own? And how do we help parents describe *their own* thoughts and feelings and soften the defenses that protect them from strong and unmanageable emotions?

Maintain a Reflective Stance

This work starts and ends with the clinician, whose capacity to maintain a mentalizing stance is central to the reflective parenting approach and the primary mechanism of therapeutic change (Suchman et al., 2012). As we described in Chapter 4, reflective parenting programs clearly help parents develop the basic tools necessary to mentalize and move out of prementalizing modes. The clinicians' steady mentalizing, their effort to *wonder* and not *assume,* gets parents moving in the right direction, not necessarily to full reflective functioning but perhaps to recognizing their child's basic thoughts and feelings. Recall Sally Provence's wise words: "Don't just *do* something. Stand there and pay attention. The *parent and the child* are trying to tell you something." *What* are they trying to tell us? We understand that behaviors *mean* something, that they communicate something, and that our job is to make sense of what that might be. Rather than taking behaviors at face value (or trying to change them), we approach behavior as indicative of underlying feelings and thoughts that we have to *discover.* And the discovery is a mutual process, with us always checking our understanding against that of the parent. Maintaining a mentalizing stance is not a "separate" part of our work; it provides an approach that frames all of what we do: drafting a labor plan, resolving a housing crisis, or responding to a parent's depression. It is a process we engage in as much as we can throughout the work.

In this chapter, we outline what we see as the stages of nurturing and supporting the parent's nascent mentalizing abilities: Engage the relationship, Observe/Listen, Mirror, Wonder, Hypothesize, and (when necessary) Repair. Whenever we initiate a clinical encounter, we begin at the beginning and engage the relationship with the parent. Then, we move sequentially, deciding when and whether the parent is ready for the next step. As the encounter proceeds, of course, we move back and forth across these various stances as is clinically appropriate. But we always begin with the relationship, and we repair whenever it is necessary. Once we have described each of these stages, we discuss some of the specific strategies for engaging the parent's reflective capacities and the means whereby the clinician can assess their success in staying reflective, even in the face of great challenges.

Throughout this chapter, we focus primarily on how we engage the parent, mirror their experience, and encourage them to wonder and hypothesize. But we never ignore the child. As should be evident in all of the following examples, we use the child's responses to guide us in our mirroring, affirming, wondering, and hypothesizing. And to return to a point we've made repeatedly in earlier chapters, we are trying to reach the child *through* the parent. Sometimes focusing on the parent may feel as if it is coming at the expense of the child's needs; one experienced clinician referred to this as the "MTB dilemma," the delicate balancing act of connecting with the parent while managing our concerns about the child. Doing so reflects our core belief that in order for the parent to attend to the child and become aware of and curious about the child's experience, the parent must themselves be held and nurtured by the relationship with the clinician. This may require the clinician to temporarily set aside concerns about the child while attending to the parent, with the ultimate intention of helping the caregiver quiet down enough to make room for the child.

This approach is quite different from a more child-centered approach, in which the primary clinical aim is to address the child's needs. One of our guiding principles is the belief that if clinicians skip the step of keeping the parents in mind and turn directly to the child (albeit for legitimate reasons), they will not have nurtured the parents' capacities to keep the baby in mind but have taken over their role for them. Naturally, there are instances in which the baby's needs are primary and imperative, notably when the child is in danger. That is, when the parent cannot fulfill their biological caregiving role to protect the child, we must step in. However, what we are ultimately trying to do is to create enough safety for the parent so that they can listen to the baby (Close, 2002). When parents can pay attention and listen, the child will flourish.

Engage the Relationship

As we emphasized throughout Part II, a trusting relationship with the parent is what supports reflection, exploration, and learning. As such, we—in any encounter—convey empathy, warmth, and support for the parent's strengths and capacities. We always highlight what they are doing well. Our care and the trust that develops between us and a parent not only gives the parent the secure base from which to mentalize but also gives us the foundation from which to address conflicts and challenges. We also always highlight the parent–baby connection. In this way, we are always underscoring not only the importance of their emotional bonds and connections but pointing to the specific ways in which these are maintained.

STRATEGIES FOR ENGAGING THE RELATIONSHIP

- Be emotionally present.
- Be supportive and empathic.
- Highlight and praise competencies in reflection and other areas.
- Validate the parent's experience.
- Highlight the parent–child connection.

Observe/Listen

We then try to join the parent *wherever they are*. To do this, we must first see and hear where that is. If we start anywhere else, we will lose them. And so we begin by observing and listening. Our goal in doing so is to have a sense of both the parent's experience *and* the baby's experience. What is it like to be *them* in that moment? How do they see and feel others in their lives? As Allen and his colleagues (2008) have noted, "patients' mentalizing capacities vary considerably within and across sessions; hence as a mentalizing therapist, you will be monitoring the patient's state of mind continually and intervening accordingly. A basic principle: the more fragile the patient's ability to mentalize, the simpler your interventions must be. This simple principle can be difficult for therapists to follow because most of us tend to become more complicated in our interventions as we understand less" (p. 185). Thus observing and listening as a means of monitoring *where the parent is at* is crucial.

As we described in Chapter 4, the capacity to reflect upon mental states can be conveyed *implicitly* in the way a person interacts with others or *explicitly* in language, namely, in the way an individual talks about themselves and others. In populations where verbal expression or vocabulary may be limited as a function of trauma, educational opportunities, the way language is used in the family, or developmental/cognitive capacity, watching for *implicit* forms of mentalizing is particularly important. Thus, when we *observe* a parent and child, we are—among other things—looking for signs that the parent is implicitly mentalizing, namely, reading the baby's bodily cues and responding contingently. When we *listen* to a parent or child, we are listening for signs of a willingness to consider and imagine what is in the other's mind. In the Jaycee example earlier, the mother is both implicitly mentalizing (paying close attention to the baby's bodily cues and behaving in kind) and explicitly mentalizing (asking, with curiosity, "You done? You had enough?").

Observe

We observe the parent, the child, and their interaction, focusing on the physical body, the feeling tone of the interaction, and the quality of arousal.

The Body

What is the parent's body posture? What is their facial expression? How are they holding themselves? Is their stance open? Relaxed? Are there signs of contentment, pleasure? Are they crumpled, disengaged, not making eye contact? Are their movements sharp? Sluggish? Do they seem tense, angry, anxious, distracted? Do they seem frightening or frightened? What about the sound of their voice: Is it melodic? Flat? Pressured?

And what about the child? How do they hold themselves? What is the quality of their movement? Are they open and engaged? Or shut down and flat? Is the child physically relaxed or tense and edgy? Passive and floppy? Are their body movements calm and assured or timid? Is the child cooing or chatting, or is their voice flat? Are the child's eyes open and responsive, or do they avoid the parent's gaze? Does the child appear to feel safe with the parent, or are there subtle signs of threat and dysregulation? Does the child—as described by Main and Solomon (1990) and reviewed in Chapters 3 and 9—display contradictory behavior patterns, incomplete or interrupted movements, stereotypies, freezing, apprehension, disorientation, or confusion? These are all signs of fear and conflict.

And the parent and child together: How does the parent hold and handle the child? Do they seem comfortable being face to face? Can they establish a comfortable closeness, not too distant, not too close (gluey, sticky) but "just right"? Do we see signs of the capacity for "serve and return" (National Scientific Council on the Developing Child, 2012, 2020), for maintaining reciprocal, mutually regulating interactions? Is the child an interactive *partner*? How does the child seek proximity and maintain contact? Is the parent interested in and reading the child's cues (following the infant's gaze, following the child's lead in play) with reasonable accuracy or overriding these in subtle or not-so-subtle ways? Is the parent making sense of the child's nonverbal signals?

OBSERVING PARENT AND CHILD

- Body posture
- Facial expression
- Physical stance
- Vocal tone
- Quality of eye contact
- Quality of the interaction
  - Ease of proximity seeking and contact maintenance
  - Reciprocity and mutual engagement
  - Parent's capacity to pick up on the child's lead and follow it
- Level of arousal in parent and child

Arousal Level

Returning to the arousal curve (see Figure 10.1), we observe the level of arousal in the parent and in the child. Where do they fall on the curve? What state are they in? Is the parent activated and highly aroused or shut down and remote? Or are they open and ready to engage? And what about the child? Are they excited, overexcited, or passive and withdrawn? Or are they engaged, focused, and regulated? As we described in Chapter 2, the arousal curve provides another way of describing an individual's state of consciousness. When a person is open and regulated, they are in a state to receive what we have to give; when they are shut down or overaroused, they cannot process their experiences and open themselves to change. To return to some of the material we reviewed in Chapter 9, when the parent is in a regulated state, the prefrontal cortex, or reasoning part of the brain, can be engaged to organize and make sense of emotional experience and thus allow for transformation. Note that parent and child can be in different states of arousal, a mismatch that can in and of itself be problematic. For instance, a child might respond to the parent's agitation by shutting down and withdrawing. Thus, as in the example of Sandy in Chapter 9, the mother is very distressed, yelling, pacing, and the child is wandering around looking apologetic. One clinical aim would be to help them get back in sync with each other. The home visitor attempted to do this by asking Sandy to take

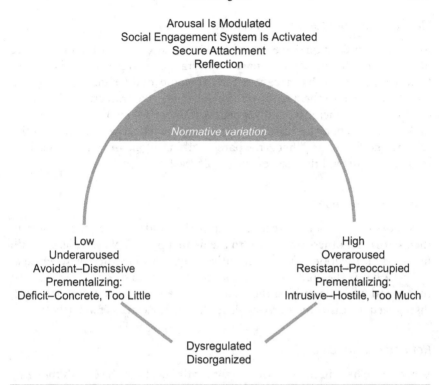

Arousal Is Modulated
Social Engagement System Is Activated
Secure Attachment
Reflection

Normative variation

Low
Underaroused
Avoidant–Dismissive
Prementalizing:
Deficit–Concrete, Too Little

High
Overaroused
Resistant–Preoccupied
Prementalizing:
Intrusive–Hostile, Too Much

Dysregulated
Disorganized

FIGURE 10.1 Arousal in the clinical situation.

note of her daughter, which might have calmed her down. Unfortunately, she was too agitated to pay attention to the home visitor's suggestion.

Listen

Anne Gearity, a social worker, infant mental health supervisor, and reflective practitioner in Minneapolis, Minnesota, regularly hands out cards to her supervisees that have only two words printed on them: "STOP TALKING." You can't listen with your mouth open. Making any sense of what is going on with a parent and/or child requires that we listen to what they are telling us. Silence is an open invitation to the parent to think and talk. This may seem like a simple and obvious point, but in fact it can be the hardest thing to do. We so often feel an urgency to do something, to solve a problem, to fill in the blanks, fill the silences, to get to *the work*. It may be uncomfortable, but this *is* the work. If we are going to join them, we have to know where they are.

Quality and Coherence of Narrative

Recall that in Chapter 2 we described Main's discovery of the importance of evaluating the quality of a parent's narrative, as this reveals the degree to which the parent has access to their thoughts and feelings (Main et al., 1985). We listen to the narrative for incoherence, contradictions, blocking, oscillations, incoherence, and vagueness. Can we follow the story? Does it make sense? When there are disruptions in the narrative, can we identify what triggered them? What is the parent talking about and why might there be a need to defend themselves, to get off track?

Quality of Representations

How does the parent represent or describe the child? How do they represent themselves and others important to them? In a positive way, inflected with humor and affection? Or in a negative way, with hostility or disengagement? What is the content of their stories? What kinds of things come to their mind when describing the child? Are their representations balanced, disengaged, or distorted (Vreeswijk et al., 2012; Zeanah et al., 1994).

Reflective Capacities

What do we hear in the way the parent is talking about the child's thoughts and feelings, and about their own? Where are they, more or less, along the continuum of reflective functioning?

Reflective Functioning Scale (RFS)

Prementalizing

- –1 Bizarre, hostile, or negative RF
- 1 Disavowed or absent mental states

The Foundations of Reflective Functioning

- 3 Identifying thoughts and feelings

Reflective Functioning

- 5 Average RF; reflecting on the nature and impact of thoughts and feelings
- 7 Complex or sophisticated RF
- 9 Exceptional RF

At the most basic level, is there evidence of the parent's mentalizing abilities? Are they, at any level, aware of their thoughts and feelings? Of others' thoughts and feelings (Level 3)? Or are they primarily stuck in pre-mentalizing modes, either having little interest in or sense of what is going on in the child, or projecting onto and distorting the child's experience (Level 1)? Do they think about mental states when trying to understand their own or others' behavior (Level 5)? Are they curious or do they make assumptions about others' mental states? Do they try to understand behavior in light of mental states? Can they be flexible and open in the way they think about internal experience? As we discuss more fully in Chapter 13, we do not expect clinicians to be expert coders or able to make precise assessments of the level of PRF, but we do hope that they can listen to the parent's speech with these distinctions in mind, as they will guide what the clinician says and does in working with the family.

LISTENING

- To the way language is used (to create closeness or distance)
- To the coherence of the parent's narrative
- To the ways the parent represents the child and others
- Does the parent assume they know what others are thinking or feeling?
- Is there evidence of projections or misattributions or an absence of interest in the child's mind?
- Can the parent acknowledge feelings?
- Can the parent be curious?
- Can the parent infer feelings and thoughts from behavior?
- Can the parent be flexible in imagining possibilities?

Mirror

Once we have a sense—by observing and listening—of where the parent is "at," we often begin by mirroring what the parent or child is saying. Recall Allen and his colleagues' (2008) reminder to start simple, especially when a parent is struggling to mentalize. Mirroring is a simple and powerful way to communicate interest in another's experience, to indicate that we are present and engaged. We saw this in the example of Sandy and Joni in Chapter 9. The clinician first says, *"You're mad, furious, in fact"*; Sandy agrees with and expands upon this. The clinician then mirrors, *"You are so mad you want to hurt her,"* which is also right on target. However, when the clinician then asks Mom to think about her behavior or, later, to think about other ways to understand the situation or reactions, Sandy feels threatened, gets defensive, and slips into prementalizing. The clinician has asked her to do too much, and there is little working with her in those moments; the clinician has to move back to curiosity and mirroring.

Mother–infant researchers noted long ago that the simple act of mirroring validates the child's affective experience, makes it more real, marks it, and acknowledges it (Stern, 1985). Mirroring a parent's stated experience can have the same effect. And it is always a good place to start, even when things are settled and calm. It can take many forms, in all of which the clinician stays *close to the feelings*. The first is simply repeating back what the parent has said, using the same words. The second, which is what the home visitor did in the example of Sandy, is to offer words to describe the parent's diffuse state or behavior. Another strategy is to clarify: "*So you're angry, and not scared?*"; "*Did I get that right?*"; and the like. In doing this, the clinician communicates in a variety of ways that they are open to and interested in understanding and knowing what the parent (or child) is feeling, rather than telling the parent or assuming that the parent knows. The clinician makes it clear that they hope to be accurate and in tune.

MIRRORING

- Stay in the moment and close to the parent's experience.
- Reflect the parent's feelings back to them, sometimes simply repeating what they said, at other times using other words, but staying close to the feelings. This can be regulating and containing.
  Example: "You are really mad. Furious, in fact."
- Ask a parent to clarify what they mean, so that you're sure you understand.
  Example: "You thought she was going around spreading stories about you? Is that it?"
- Ask the parent to tell you more, to elaborate on what they are saying.
  Example: "Can you say more about what you were feeling?"

Wonder

Here we come to the question of understanding the parent's state of mind. *What is going on* internally? Although we may well note denial, prementalizing, distortion, or projection, we take a stance of wondering, of trying to imagine what the child (or the parent's partner, family member, or the parent themselves) might be thinking or feeling. To discover this (and it *is* a process of discovery), the clinician wonders and doesn't assume. They take a stance of *not-knowing*, of wanting to understand, tolerating uncertainty. The clinician acts—as it were—"like an alien" (Allen et al., 2008), trying to learn about a new culture. *"What's this like for you?"*; *"I want to know you. I want to understand."* The clinician tries to remember, even when things get very hot (the parent is very upset), or very cool (the parent is shut down), that helping the parent cool down or warm up depends upon keeping the parent's thoughts, feelings, and mind in mind.

> The mentalizing, or not-knowing stance is not synonymous with having no knowledge. Not-knowing captures a sense that mental states are opaque and that you can have no *more* idea of what is in the patient's mind than the patient has and, in fact, you will probably have a lot less of an idea. Mentalizing, you demonstrate a willingness to find out about patients, what makes them tick, how they feel, and the reasons for their underlying problems. The mentalizing stance is respectful and devoid of assumptions. (Allen et al., 2008, p. 183)

Wondering can take many forms and can be conveyed nonverbally (a curious look, an open, interested look) or verbally: *"So, tell me what's going on. . . . "* *"What's that been like for you?"* *"How's that feeling?"* *"What do you think about his not wanting to let you go at school?"* *"What do you think made that feel so bad?"* *"Why do you think he had such a bad night?"* These statements not only convey curiosity, but they also convey that there are meanings, motivations, and causes to be discovered and understood.

Fearon and his colleagues (2006a) refer to mentalizing as an *attitude* rather than a skill. The word *attitude* conveys nicely that mentalizing is not something we are always doing *explicitly*, as in wondering out loud or asking a parent about their experience. It is an *internal* process, a way of approaching another human being. Oftentimes clinicians can interpret the word *wonder* rather concretely and begin statements that are veiled directives with it: *"I wonder why you didn't do such and such."* Rather than being curious, the clinician is in this instance scolding the parent, which can easily be humiliating. Clinicians can ask too many questions, leaving the parent feeling badgered and—if they have no answer—shamed. For these reasons, we try to remain open-minded, interested, and engaged; we try to keep mentalizing, but not necessarily out loud. Parents (and older children) need time to process, to listen to and observe their own thoughts and feelings. This is how we hope they will approach their own children. And when we do wonder explicitly, we do so judiciously, respecting their tempo and level of engagement. To return, once again, to the question of threat, the mentalizing or reflective stance is inherently nonthreatening, in that we invite the parent to share their experience in whatever way they are able; the clinician and parents are partners on a journey.

In the videotaped session described below, the clinician, Lisa, uses a variety of wondering approaches to help Belinda, age 17, become more curious about her 8-week-old baby, Carlos. We can well imagine, reading this passage, that the clinician wanted, first, to tell Belinda to pick up the baby and, second, to pick up the baby herself. But she is patient, and it pays off.

In the background is the sound of a television crime show, as well as rhythmic music. Infant and mother are seated on a double bed; the mother's younger sister is in the room, although not on camera. Belinda is holding Carlos loosely on her lap, facing away from her; she has a kind of half-smile on her face. She puts a pacifier in his mouth. He looks disoriented, floppy, kind of lost, fusses slightly, pushes back against her, refuses pacifier. She jiggles him and laughs nervously as he fusses. She continues to jiggle him and tries to get pacifier in his mouth. He continues to fuss.

She then picks him up and puts him face down on the bed (which is actually in line with pediatric guidelines for "tummy time" but implemented without apparent intention). He naturally tries to take a crawling position but does not have the muscle strength in his arms to do so; he fusses, moves his face from side to side to breathe. Belinda's sister notes twice that he is trying to get up, and Belinda remarks, "he's frustrated." He is obviously very uncomfortable and struggling. She is kind of laughing, not meanly, but anxiously. She pats his bottom, but otherwise there is no contact—she is observing impassively.

LISA: What do you think he wants? (*Lisa is inquiring.*)

BELINDA: He gets frustrated when he can't do what he wants to do. . . .

LISA: What do you think he wants to do? (*Her inquiries follow what Belinda has said.*)

BELINDA: Tryin' to crawl. . . . (*She rubs his bottom in a vigorous way while he fusses.*) You need help? (*She is speaking to the baby. She does not move, continues to passively observe.*)

We can well imagine that the clinician is likely itching to tell the mother to pick up the baby and hold him. But that would rob the mother of discovering the baby's needs on her own, albeit with the clinician's support. And it runs the risk of making the mother feel ever so slightly shamed for not recognizing the baby's needs on her own. And so the clinician proceeds slowly.

LISA: What do you think? Does he need help? (*Inviting Mom to explore her observation.*)

BELINDA: I don't know. . . . (*Shrugs.*)

LISA: How do you think he's feeling? (*Hoping Mom will pick up on what is apparent to the home visitor as well as Belinda's sister.*)

BELINDA: He feels frustrated. . . .

LISA: At?

BELINDA: Cuz he can't crawl?

LISA: You think he wants to crawl? (*She is affirming Mom's observation and encouraging her to keep observing.*)

BELINDA: I don't know. . . .

LISA: (*speaking for the baby*) Hey, Mom, it's kind of hard to hold my head up. . . . My arms aren't that strong yet. . . . (*Here she is imparting developmental information in hopes of getting Mom to imagine what it is like to be the baby.*)

BELINDA: (*Gazes at the baby with a little bit of curiosity.*)

LISA: (*to the baby*) You tryin' to find your mamma? You lookin' for her? (*Here, using a series of questions, she is highlighting the activation of the baby's attachment system as he signals that he needs help.*)

(*As if slightly roused, Belinda reaches over and pulls the baby into her lap. Gradually, she puts her arms around him and pats him vigorously, rocking him side to side. It's a little rough, but at the same time he calms and settles against her. She smiles slightly.*)

LISA: There, he likes that. . . . (*She is mirroring and thus marking baby's pleasure for Mom, thus reinforcing Mom's success.*)

In her next session, Belinda seemed much more attuned to the baby and was able to describe the infant's obvious pleasure in their feeding interaction. And when a loud noise in the room startled the baby, she readily and naturally moved in to protect and comfort him.

WONDERING

- Model and encourage curiosity and wondering ("not-knowing") about feelings and thoughts.
- Ask questions to promote exploration and clarity, rather than taking answers at face value or assuming you know the answer.
- Avoid certainty (you are not an expert on *them*).
- Ask parent to think about the feelings of all those involved (i.e., the parent, the baby, the grandmother).
- Work to identify and label hidden feeling states.

- Speak for the parent—sometimes parents have limited feeling vocabulary or little practice putting their own feelings into words.
- Speak for the baby—verbalize the baby's perspective, talk to the baby, describe the baby's world and experience to the dyad.
- Use humor judiciously when it feels right.

Hypothesize

Many of the parents we see really struggle to make sense of their own or their child's experience. Their parents, their friends, and their partners may all be quite mysterious to them; mentalizing is hard. And that is why we often need not only to wonder but also to *hypothesize* about what is going on in a way that offers the parent new ways of thinking and of being. Hypotheses are just that, *hypotheses*, and not certainties. They are not assumptions but a guide to considering alternatives and to developing a broader sense of why people do the things they do. Most important, they demonstrate that the clinician, too, is open to possibilities and to various ways of seeing a situation.

As clinicians, we know something about feelings, about people, about causes of trouble in relationships, and about what makes people unhappy and happy; we understand the role of unconscious dynamic processes in human relationships. And we know something about child development, about adult development, about learning. We don't have the answers, but we know something about the possibilities. And we can use this knowledge to speculate, to wonder "what if it's . . . ?" In training clinicians, we have noted many times that they can be reluctant to hypothesize and fall back on mirroring and wondering. At times, actively mentalizing for the parent or child is crucial, because this offers a new way of understanding a situation that is painful and confusing. We are knowledgeable about the impact of the past on the present, about relationships, and about development. And we can use this knowledge to inform the hypotheses we offer.

Note that we use the word *offer*; the parent can accept or reject them. It is so important that hypotheses not be presented as certainties. Nor are they "lessons" that a practitioner needs to teach the parent. We do not know for sure what the parent or child means to communicate, nor why they are doing one thing or the other. It is also important that we offer hypotheses in a way a parent can understand and make sense of. Language should be simple and clear; sentences should be short and coherent. And the "level" of the hypothesis should be close to the parent's level of understanding. Thus, for example, if a parent who had herself been abused as a child was describing a wish to hurt her son, we would not begin by linking this to her childhood experience. We would first ask her to think about why she was so provoked and angry, what she imagined the child was feeling, and how she understood her own feelings. We might then hypothesize that she felt disrespected and helpless. Only once she was fully grounded in the present experience might we ask her to think about some of her own childhood experiences and how they might be triggered in the present.

In the following example, the clinician hypothesizes in a way that communicates developmental information. Marta, age 13 months, loves to hang on to the TV's remote control and to wave it around and press all the buttons. As a result, of course, the TV comes on and off randomly, and the volume fluctuates dramatically.

> Marta's mother, Lucia, is upset and frustrated. When the clinician asks her why she thinks Marta won't let go of the remote, Lucia resorts to relatively benign prementalizing: "Oh, she just wants to do whatever she wants!" The clinician might say, "Well, you're right that toddlers love to feel in charge . . . they love to press things and see what happens. Toddlers also like to copy their mommies, and . . . ? What if she's kind of enjoying being just like Mommy?"

What the clinician is doing here is first affirming Mom's efforts to understand her child and her observation about toddlers and their need for control. She then offers a couple of alternative explanations that are based on what she knows about toddlers and their development, and that also highlight the mother–child relationship. She is, in effect, saying, "Well, there might be some other ways to understand this. . . . How about this?" She is not saying, "*This* is what your child is doing," but rather, "Well, there could be all sorts of ways to think about Marta's behavior. . . . Can we think about them?" These subtle reframings, particularly the suggestion that Marta wants to be like her mommy, place the behavior in a positive light and hopefully will soften Mom's frustration. It may also help her find other, quieter ways for Marta to be like her mother.

The clinician's understanding of the parent's history can also often inform their understanding of what is going on with the child.

> A mother had recently separated from her abusive partner. Her son witnessed numerous fights between her and his father, and he has since been very aggressive toward his mother. When the clinician arrives, the mother is distraught and very upset with her child. "I can't take this anymore. He's hitting and biting me and I just want to smack him!" The clinician wonders to herself what this upsurge of aggression in the child is about. Does he miss his dad? Is he mad at his dad for leaving and taking it out on Mom? Is he copying his dad? And she wonders about the mom's wish to fight or flee. Is she frightened by the child? Is her rage at her partner being directed at the child? Is she feeling

that she wants to retaliate? Likely both the child and she are feeling a range of things, all understandable within the context of what's been happening in the family. The clinician offers some hypotheses. "Wow, you've been dealing with your partner's anger for so long. . . . This must not be what you expected. This sounds a little scary. . . ." Mom replies, "That is for sure. What if he turns out just like his dad, who is such a lowlife?" The clinician replies, "I can sure understand why you'd feel this way . . . but you know, maybe he's confused about why his dad left? And about why his dad was hitting you? Sometimes that's how kids act when they're feeling confused and lost."

The clinician is providing the parent with various ways to potentially understand what is going on with both her and her son; she is also trying to gently dislodge the negative attribution that the boy is going to grow up to be a loser like his dad. She is doing this using a relational and developmental framework, gently offering a range of possibilities that will hopefully allow the mother to see herself and her child in a different way. Such hypotheses will often be rejected by a parent who is still closed to reflection, usually because they are too shut down or agitated, as we saw in the case of Sandy. But even if the parent doesn't accept our hypotheses, our thinking about them may be helpful in the long run. And when there is a team of clinicians working with the family, the parent can hear different (though hopefully not contradictory) points of view from different clinicians. This directly conveys the idea that there are often multiple ways to view most situations.

In the following exchange between Leticia and the social worker she has been working with for more than 2 years, the clinician uses mirroring and wondering to support hypothesizing. Leticia is a full-time caregiver for her 4-year-old nephew, Marco, whose mother is unable to care for him. In this session, Leticia is able to use the clinician's hypotheses to expand her thinking about Marco and to understand some of the links between her own childhood experiences with her mother and her feelings about her nephew. It's important to note that—throughout the exchange—the clinician's efforts are working, in the sense that the mother doesn't become defensive, pull back, or resist. This allows the clinician to deepen her inquiries and gently push the mother toward more compassion toward her nephew and for herself.

Marco just returned from a trip to Disney World with his father, with whom he had little prior contact. The session took place outside, where Julia (Leticia's 18-month-old daughter) and Marco were playing. Julia got frustrated and grabbed a toy out of Marco's hand. Marco let out a woeful cry.

LETICIA: (*to Marco*) Why are you crying so bad? You're a big boy. Big boys don't cry! (*Marco cries even harder and goes over and tries to sit on Leticia's lap.*)

Go on, you don't need to sit here, go play with Julia, she wants to play with you, that's why she grabbed the toy. (*Marco puts his head down and cries harder.*)

LETICIA: (*to the clinician*) I don't understand. He just got back from this great vacation but he's been crying and clingy and whiney.

CLINICIAN: Seems like you knew from Julia's grabbing the toy that she wasn't "just being mean" or anything but just wanted to play. What do you think might be going on for Marco? (*Here the clinician is praising Leticia's accurate reading of her daughter's intention and inviting her to think about Marco's.*)

LETICIA: I have no idea, but it's really getting on my nerves.

CLINICIAN: It seems like it's hard for you to see him upset, especially when you think he should be "relaxed" from vacation. (*Here the clinician is offering a hypothesis [note: not with certainty!] about why Marco is getting on her nerves.*)

LETICIA: Yeah, I would love for someone to take me on vacation!

CLINICIAN: No doubt! It'd be nice for you or me. (*Here she empathizes with the mother.*) But I wonder, do you think it might feel the same for a 4-year-old? I was thinking it might feel a little different. He was traveling with a dad he doesn't know well and was away from all the family he does know well. (*Here she offers another way of thinking about Marco's behavior, an alternative perspective.*)

LETICIA: Yeah, I guess maybe he might feel kinda insecure or something. (*She softens and offers the possibility that Marco might not be feeling so great.*)

CLINICIAN: Yeah, that would make sense to me. Maybe being close to you, crying, wanting a hug or to sit on your lap is his way of saying, "I missed you and I feel kind of stressed. I want to be close to you because being close to you helps me feel better." (*The clinician praises Mom's recognition of the child's distress and then proceeds both to offer a possible explanation of Marco's need for Leticia and to speak for Marco directly.*)

LETICIA: Ugh! But sometimes I feel like, ugh, like just saying, "Get away! I need my space!"

CLINICIAN: Yeah, I can understand that. Sometimes he wants to be close to you and you don't like that. It makes you feel . . . "ugh." (*The clinician echoes the mother's feelings and supports them.*) It might be a silly question, but what is that feeling, "ugh"? . . . Can you describe it? (*Here she invites Mom to think more deeply about this feeling. This kind of inquiry will only work if the parent is open and receptive.*)

LETICIA: Stressed—like too much pressure. It just feels like too much to be with him, AND Julia, AND work, and everything I'm trying to juggle on my own.

And it's not like my sister ever even asked if I could take care of Marco, she just left him here one day. (*Mom's feelings come pouring out, clearly and coherently.*)

CLINICIAN: Yeah, it's very hard. You didn't sign up for this job taking care of him . . . and you already do so much on your own. (*The clinician empathizes with Mom and acknowledges the pain she is feeling.*)

LETICIA: And my mom—she was really my aunt, but I called her "Mom"—always encouraged that. She told me not to depend on anyone, that I didn't need a man or anything to get by. She really wanted me to be an independent strong woman. Needing someone or something wasn't something to be proud of! (*Here the mother has herself taken the conversation to a new level, spurred by the clinician's empathy and her invitation to deeper reflection.*)

CLINICIAN: Hmmm, I wonder if maybe that makes it hard for you to know what to do when Marco needs something from you. Do you remember what that was like for you—when you needed something from your mom or felt stressed and wanted to be close to her? (*Here the clinician is able to use what the mother has told her to begin to make links to the mother's own history and experience of feeling needy. Such moments are possible when the parent is not defensive or threatened and when she fully trusts the clinician. In this case, mother and clinician have known each other for 2 years.*)

LETICIA: Oh yeah, my mom usually pushed us away—if we cried she'd send us to our room and tell us not to come back until we could act like a big girl . . . or else she would really give us something to cry about—she never really wanted to hear why we were crying. (*The clinician notes but does not mention that Leticia has just described her interaction with Marco to a "T."*)

CLINICIAN: What do you remember about what that was like for you? (*The clinician is following the mother's lead, once again inviting Leticia to tell her more.*)

LETICIA: Well, on the one hand, when I could pull it together and stop crying, I felt proud. I believed her when she said that not crying meant I was acting like a big girl. On the other hand, I hated being pushed away. I always felt like I was being pushed out from under my mom's feet, like I was in the way and needed to learn how to be on my own faster so I wouldn't be a burden to her. (*Here Leticia describes her ambivalence clearly and coherently and makes clear why she is activated by Marco's neediness.*)

CLINICIAN: It makes me feel sad thinking about how that might have felt for you then—sad about you as a little girl wanting her mom and being pushed away. Do you think any of that ever influences any of the decisions you make about taking care of Marco? (*As we discuss below, here the clinician is using her own experience to imagine Marco's experience. She is also invicing her to reflect on how her past feelings influence her behavior with Marco.*)

LETICIA: Well, I guess sometimes, especially when I'm stressed, I'm doing the same thing my mom did—I'm pushing him away when he needs something from me. (*Here she makes the link explicitly.*)

CLINICIAN: Sometimes it helps me to think about Marco's behaviors as his own kind of language, like he's saying, "I'm anxious, and it was hard for me to be away from you. I need to be close to you to feel better AND, Mommy, it will be hard for me to act better until I feel better." I think his being "clingy or whiney" might mean he needs to get close to you to feel more settled or safe. I wonder what it would be like when you are stressed and have those feelings, the ones that make you want to push him away, to do the opposite—to pull him close instead, stop and give him some attention, a hug or space on your lap for a few minutes? (*Now that Mom is open and reflective, and making complex connections across time, and between feelings, thoughts, and behaviors, she can take in the clinician's mentalizing for the child and potentially try out the clinician's suggestion.*)

LETICIA: It would probably feel awkward!

CLINICIAN: Awkward. Yup, I bet it would. Lots of times when we try something new it feels pretty awkward at first. (*The clinician is empathizing with and supporting Leticia.*)

LETICIA: I guess I could try. You mean if I try, it might help him feel better so he'll do what I want? (*Leticia uses humor, a good sign that she is feeling softer and more playful and considers alternatives.*)

CLINICIAN: Well, I do think it will help him feel better, but I wouldn't promise you it will always get him to do what you want in that moment! (*Clinician responds with humor and offers a little developmental guidance.*)

LETICIA: (*with laughter*) No, sometimes there is nothing that I can do to get him to do what I want. (*Continued humor and an apparent appreciation of Marco's complexity.*)

CLINICIAN: (*laughing, too*) That's true! Well, after all, he is his own little person with a mind of his own—and as hard as that can be on you sometimes, I think you do want him to keep using that mind! (*The clinician praises Leticia for her reflectiveness.*)

LETICIA: Yes, and I'd really like to figure out a way to keep letting him know that he can come to me when he's happy or stressed, trust me, and trust that I love him and won't push him away. (*Mom appears to have come to a new understanding and appreciation of Marco and her circumstances.*)

CLINICIAN: I think he'd really like that, too. (*The clinician again reinforces Mom's reflectiveness.*)

HYPOTHESIZING

- Think of this as expanding the parent's mentalizing capacities.
- Do so in moments when the parent seems receptive and open to reflecting.
- Elaborate possible alternatives when you have their attention.
- Validate the parent's experience before offering alternative perspectives or reframing.
- Use a "what if?" stance; encourage family members to play with new ideas.
- Generate multiple perspectives: "What else could be going on?"
- Use your knowledge and understanding of the parent, their history and way of regulating to reframe their perceptions of the child, themselves, or others.
- Gently challenge parent's beliefs about themselves or others.
- Use humor judiciously; be playful when it feels right.

Ideally, with mirroring, wondering, and hypothesizing, parents can begin to move out of prementalizing, nonreflective modes, name feelings, wonder about their own reactions and try to understand them, wonder about their child's reactions, focus less on behavior, respond more sensitively to the child, and have fewer disrupted interactions.

Repair Ruptures

Ruptures between interactive partners occur all the time (Tronick & Gold, 2020), including between parents and clinicians. We have noted throughout the book that cycles of rupture and repair are at the heart of all relationships. Thus clinicians should acknowledge mistakes when they arise, pay attention to ruptures in the relationship, and do what they can to repair them. The repairs can be subtle and swift, or—when there has been a painful rupture—they can take a long time and be very hard work. But they are so necessary. For this reason, clinicians must be very attuned to ruptures and not let them get too far along. Sometimes the repair can be made in the moment: *"Oh, I see, it works to keep her in bed with you until she falls asleep. I got that wrong. Sorry."* In the Sandy transcript, the clinician's attempts to regroup and rewind are unsuccessful, but she tries. At the end of the session, she acknowledges the rupture. Mom has retreated to being defensive and shut down. This rupture will have to await another visit to be repaired. The clinician can begin the next session by acknowledging the rupture directly: *"You know, I think that somehow I really wasn't hearing you the other day when you were telling me about the woman who said you had crabs. . . . I've been thinking about that, and about you, and I realize just how hard that must have been. You try so hard to do what's right for your daughter and best for you. You must have been upset that I couldn't quite hear you.*" Or the clinician might send the mother a text in a few days to see how she's doing, implicitly trying to mend fences. Whether or not the mother responds is less important than that the clinician conveys to the mother that she's been thinking about her, that she (the mother) matters to the clinician, and that her voice is valued.

Use Your Own Experience

Throughout this book, we have discussed how important it is for practitioners to attend to their own reactions in clinical encounters. The way we feel in a situation, our gut reactions, our triggers, our impulses, our fantasies all tell us something about what the parent is experiencing. This can help us think about how to frame things, what hypotheses make sense, and when to back off and wait. Take, for example, the vignette described in Chapter 9, when the mother, Sandy, is in a rage at a woman who has insulted her. When the clinician could not move Sandy out of her angry state, she tried to elicit Mom's protectiveness by sharing her worries about Joni. Sandy could not hear the clinician, however, and eventually the clinician stepped back, acknowledged her uncertainty, and tried to step to the surface, pause, and rewind.

USING YOUR OWN EXPERIENCE

- Know yourself—pay attention to your own reactions and feelings.
- Make use of yourself as a clinician, your own feelings, and your experience.
- Share your feelings when therapeutically useful.
- Acknowledge when, as clinician, you do not know what to say or do.
- If overwhelmed with affect or content, step to the surface, pause, and rewind.
- Put your feelings and thoughts into words.

The Challenges of Working in a Reflective Way

We have found again and again that clinicians who adopt this approach, often after decades of working in a more behavioral, problem-focused way, are quickly persuaded that the changes they see in families are deep and long-lasting. A nurse described it as "the gift of time" (Birgitte Bjerg, personal communication, April 2019). What this gift does, very simply, is greatly reduce the risk of the parent's feeling threatened, shamed, and disrespected. This allows them to discover the child and discover themselves. But such developments can be very hard won. Parents often come to intervention prone to being reactive, impulsive, and out of touch with their emotional lives. These defenses have been essential to their emotional survival. Such survival mechanisms are not going to yield quickly or easily, and, in fact, clinical progress often means that they shift just a little. We often remind clinicians to "cherish small shifts" because, although parents may, even after a course of treatment, be only fleetingly able to name feelings and contain their behavior, these are enormous steps forward for their own and their babies' development. Recall from Chapter 4 that simply being able to identify and recognize mental states can be quite therapeutic and an antidote to a position of threat, shame, and defense.

The main challenges in this way of working revolve around the clinician's very real struggle to balance reflecting on the one hand and taking a more active, directive stance on the other, to navigate what we call the "dance of reflecting and directing." There are, in fact, many times when parents need advice, guidance, and concrete resources. Typically, practitioners are able and willing to do this. They know a lot about how children develop and thrive; they have useful information and knowledge about parent and child health; they can link the parent to a range of resources. The key is doing this in a reflective and not directive way: *would,* not *should.* So, for example, a parent may ask: *"What's the best position to encourage her to nurse?" "Do you think my son is ready for day care?" "I just got an eviction notice—what do I do now?" "Can you show me how to meditate?"* In these situations, parents are *inviting* us to share our expertise, our thoughts. They are open, asking, curious. We offer advice within the framework of a mentalizing stance: *"What positions have you tried to encourage her nursing? Let me watch you . . . have you tried supporting her head?" "Well, what options are you considering for day care? How would you feel about sending him to the Park Lane Day Care? Shall we call them together and see whether they have openings?"* Our relationship with the parent makes us a trusted source of knowledge; as such, our expertise can be valued and not threatening. We try in every way not to threaten the parent or make them feel (consciously or unconsciously) that we are saying we know better than they do. That is—in any form—an invitation to resistance and defense. We never know for sure what is in another's mind, so it behooves us to find out!

It can be very difficult to keep listening and wondering. Even when concrete support or guidance is needed, it's important to maintain a slow pace and try to help the parent(s) discover what they feel and/or what the child feels. The absorption of knowledge and the ability to make use of concrete advice and to modify behavior depends upon *experiential* understanding, and particularly the experience of getting to know oneself and one's child. By letting the parents come to a solution on their own, clinicians promote autonomy and sharpen the parents' awareness of their or the child's inner experience. And for many parents, the discovery that they *have* thoughts and feelings and that the baby also has thoughts and feelings can be utterly transforming.

Threat is often at the heart of therapeutic breakdowns, or what Fearon and his colleagues (2006a) have described as "nonmentalizing cycles of interaction." By this they mean interactions in which neither interactive partner is considering the thoughts and feelings of the other; as a result, both members—because they are unable to make any sense of the other—become more controlling and coercive, and reciprocity or attunement is impossible. These are forms of rupture that are perpetuated over time. In nonmentalizing interactions, the clinician has abandoned wondering and is imposing their assumptions and beliefs upon those of the parent. This is the essence of prementalizing; the clinician is *certain* of what is right. Let us return again to Sandy, first mentioned in Chapter 9. The clinician is able, at first, to remain curious about what it is that has so offended Sandy, staying close to Sandy's experience with her inquiries. But as her anxiety grows about the intensity of Sandy's rage and her repeated threats to go out and beat up her accuser, the home visitor moves too fast, and in effect tries to get Sandy to see how unreasonable she's being. This just sets Sandy off again. This is a nonmentalizing cycle of interaction, with both Sandy and the home visitor triggering more nonmentalizing in the other. Of course, there might well be moments when stopping Sandy might be the only possible course for the clinician (e.g., if she were storming out the door). In the moment, however, the home visitor might have had more success had she been able to fight her impulse to try to get Sandy to be reasonable, because it just led Sandy to be more unreasonable and allowed nonmentalizing cycles to continue.

Practitioners working with young families are almost always from the "helping" professions. Often their professional disciplines (social work, nursing, education) emphasize taking action to fix problems and restore health. As a result, the pace and subtlety of a reflective approach may leave them feeling that they are not "doing enough" and that not much is happening. Add to this that the "gift of time" may make clinicians very anxious. They've got to *do* something. Sometimes practitioners respond to this by *pushing* parents to reflect, peppering them with questions they cannot answer. Sometimes practitioners label, diagnose, or "other" the parent (Shapiro, 2008). "That's his ADD; I read about it in his chart." "She is such a borderline, getting everyone all worked up and sowing chaos." They find themselves judging and critical: "Why would she see her boyfriend again after all we've talked about?" "Why didn't he give his son his medicine?" "He didn't show up at work *again*?" "*Why* would she leave the baby with her friend?" "Why couldn't he get himself to school?" Although these seem like questions, they're actually judgments, rather than attempts to imagine the parent or child's experiences. Practitioners can also resort to assuming, which is, in essence, disrespectful: "I know what you are *really* thinking." "I know what you want for your child/family." "I know the best way for you to behave." "I know what your behavior means." "I can see what is important in this situation." Once a clinician says, implicitly or explicitly, "I know what you feel. I know what you should do," they have created a power dynamic that—especially for young, disenfranchised, or marginalized parents—provokes defensiveness born of shame and threat. This dynamic is likely magnified when the clinician is White and inherently privileged.

Many early-intervention models offer guidance, education, and support without engaging the parent's reflective capacities. But knowledge that is offered without an opportunity to learn it *from the inside out* (Suchman et al., 2017) cannot be internalized in a meaningful way or used to support their agency and autonomy. To return to the central message of Part II, by attending to threat and dysregulation, by building on the relationship we have developed with parents, by being willing to repair when we've gotten it wrong or have threatened the parent, we create the foundation for increasingly complex reflection and the development of a sense of competency and confidence as a parent.

Self-Assessment: Maintaining a Mentalizing Stance

In an attempt to help clinicians keep track of how they're doing in maintaining a mentalizing stance, we recommend regular "self-assessment" checks. Adapted from Allen et al. (2008), these gentle self-correctives remind the clinician to step back and try to understand and listen. They can also help identify areas for improvement and potentially inform supervision. It is easy to step into a directing, educating, advice-giving mode or to make assumptions about the parent's internal experience, and these inquiries help reorient the clinician. Of course, to reiterate what we have said before and what we describe in more detail in subsequent chapters, there are times when giving advice and guidance, or directly intervening to curtail a behavior, is crucial.

CLINICIAN MENTALIZING SELF-ASSESSMENT

- I take a stance of not knowing what the parent's or the baby's experience is, and I am interested in finding out.

  Example: "Tell me more. I'd like to understand what that was like for you and what you were thinking."

- I ask questions to promote exploration and clarity, rather than taking answers at face value or not following up or assuming I understand.

  Example: "How do you understand it when she cries and falls to the floor? What do you make of that behavior?"

- I encourage curiosity.

  Example: "What do you think he made of that big crash?"

- I validate the parent's experience before I offer alternative perspectives or reframing.

  Example: "Wow! It sounds like reading her comments on Facebook made you furious."

- I always try to keep the baby in mind, even if they never enter our conversation in a given session. When I can, I try to bring the baby into the conversation. When I can't, I respect the fact that, for the moment, the parent needs my undivided attention.

- I highlight and praise competencies in reflection and other areas.

  Example: "You really figured out what she needed, and now she's smiling and relaxed!"

- I help the parent to imagine, "What if?"

  Example: "What if he's copying you, wanting to be more like you?"

- I ask the parent how they understand the motivations of the child or of family members.

  Example: "Why do you think Elsie did that? What do you think she's feeling when she does that?"

- When I can, I try to speak for the parent, putting a complicated experience into words.

  Example: "So when your mom said the baby was crying because he was hungry, and your aunt went to buy formula, it sounds like you were worried about your milk supply and the baby not eating, and things were happening so fast it was hard to think about what the baby really needed right then."

- I try to speak for the baby if the parent makes misattributions or isn't engaged.

  Example: "Oh, Mommy, I'm crying so hard because you left the room and I didn't know where you went!"

- I try to elaborate in moments when the parent can consider alternative perspectives.

  Example: "Ah . . . It seems as though you were wondering if his cry meant he really was hungry or if it meant that he was trying to tell you something else. What else did you think the crying meant right then?"

- I reflect the parent's feelings back to them in a modified form, that is, in a regulated, contained, and organized way.

  Example: "A toddler's crying can be so hard to handle! That cry just gets to you and you get worried, frustrated, and upset all at the same time. It's hard to know what to do when you have so many feelings at one time."

- I frequently highlight parent–child bond.

  Example: "Look! He is really looking into your eyes. When you look back at him he seems so loving and peaceful!"

- I use humor judiciously and I try to be playful when it feels right.

When parents are resistant or negative:

- When a parent can only see things in one way or in a negative way, I try to generate multiple perspectives.

  Example: "Can you think of other reasons why she's tantrumming?"

- I try to reframe the parent's perceptions of the baby or of herself.

  Example: "Do you suppose we can think about that in a different way? I wonder, when he makes that face and he looks like he is mad, I wonder if he might actually feeling sad."

- I gently challenge a parent's beliefs about me or herself or others.

  Example: "In your experience with other social workers, it seemed they just wanted to be in your business. Are you wondering if I will be the same way?"

- I stay in the moment and with the parent's current thoughts and feelings.

  Example: "You seem really angry"; "That sounds like it feels really scary to you."

- I stay away from complex explanations for her and her child's feelings. I tend not to bring up her past history as an explanation for her current reaction.

  Example: I avoid saying things like "Oh, the reason you are feeling so mad at your child is because your mom used to feel mad at you."

- When a parent is seeing things in black or white and with absolute certainty, I do not confront her but use techniques like exploration, considering alternatives together, and attending to current emotions.

  Example: Parent says, "My sister is a brat. She always gets what she wants and I hate her." I reply, "How does that happen? How does your sister get what she wants?"

- During an emotional outburst, I maintain our dialogue, and I don't comment on the reasons behind the outburst. I try to clarify what the parent is feeling without interpretation.

- I only consider underlying causes when the parent is no longer acutely upset.

- I try to identify triggers in recent interpersonal experience, including interactions with me.

- When things get too "hot," I try to stop, look, listen, rewind, and explore.

  Example: "You just got so upset. . . . Can we stop a minute and think about what happened there?"

In supporting myself as a clinician, I pay attention to my own experience:

- I pay attention to my own reactions and feelings and bring them to supervision, especially when I am upset during a home visit.

- I pay attention to ruptures in my interaction with the parent and try to sort out, from both of our sides, what led to the rupture.

  Example: "Perhaps you were trying to tell me that you didn't want to talk about that issue anymore, and I wasn't understanding what you were telling me."

- I use my own experience in the home visit to help me imagine what the parent or baby might be feeling.

- I share my feelings when it is therapeutically useful.

  Example: "I'm worried about you. If you decide to go beat up that girl who made you so angry, you could get hurt, or arrested, or even go to jail."

- I acknowledge when I do not know what to say or do.

- When I feel overwhelmed by affect or content, I put my feelings and thoughts into words.

  Example: "This is really hard to talk about. It brings up so many feelings. Let's take a breath and talk about what would help you feel supported."

Summary

Enhancing a parent's reflective capacities is best conceived of as a stepwise process, where we begin by engaging the relationship, observing and listening, gauging the parent's openness and capacity to be curious and open to the child's experience. This can be a painstaking, tentative process. As Allen and his colleagues (2008) suggest: "First, go slowly; second, when in doubt, be more supportive and less challenging of the patient's perspective" (p. 185). We use the relationship we have established with the parent to first support simply mirroring their experiences and then moving on to wondering and hypothesizing or offering new and different frames for their experiences. We always keep an eye out for ruptures and the need for repair.

▲▲▲▲▲▲▲ QUESTIONS FOR CLINICIANS ▲▲▲▲▲▲▲

▶ Does the parent appear open and ready to reflect?

▶ Are you and the parent open to the relationship?

▶ Observe both parent and child behavior.

▶ Listen to the content, structure, and manner of the parent's speech.

▶ Note what happens when you simply mirror the parent's observations. Does this lead to their opening up and becoming more regulated?

▶ How do they respond to wondering, to your asking them to consider their experience, to describe it to you?

▶ Is the parent open to hypotheses offered in a respectful and curious way? Does this expand their understanding? Are they able to consider alternate perspectives?

▶ Have there been ruptures that need repair?

▶ Are you able to slow down and appreciate the gift of time?

Chapter

11

Reflective Nursing

U p to this point, we have written about reflective practice with parents and young children from a transdisciplinary perspective, in hopes of "speaking" to a range of clinicians: social workers, psychologists, counselors, and health care providers. In this chapter, we focus specifically on what we call reflective *nursing*. We do this for several reasons. The first is that nurses—public health nurses, hospital-based nurses, nurse midwives, and nurse practitioners—provide the lion's share of care to pregnant women, young children, and their parents around the globe. They do so as home visitors (in North America), health visitors (in a number of countries worldwide), nurse midwives, lactation consultants, and clinic or office-based practitioners. The second is that it is has been our experience that the basic principles of MTB-P can expand and enrich nursing practice, particularly within the framework of home visiting. In the following sections, we (1) describe the primary tasks of nurses working with young families; (2) define reflective nursing and describe its particular relevance for stressed families; (3) describe a range of strategies for reflective nursing, using case examples as illustrations of key points; (4) outline some of the particular challenges of this way of working; and (5) consider the application of reflective nursing to more traditional forms of nursing practice.[1] It is important to note that, despite our specific focus on nursing in this chapter,

---

[1] In preparation for writing this chapter, we interviewed a number of MTB-HV nurses— Birgitte Bjerg, Kendra Davis, Kim Davis, Kelly Mosher, Rosie Price, Debra Samuel, and Melissa Smith—about their experiences of working in the program. We are grateful for their input; their voices expanded our understanding in so many ways.

we believe that most of everything we have to say here is relevant to reflective practice and reflective practitioners generally.

Nursing Practice

Nursing is an enormously diverse discipline, and nurses enter the profession with different levels of education and experience. Registered nurses (RNs), whether practicing in hospitals, health care settings, or the community, usually have an associate's or undergraduate degree, whereas advanced practice nurses have either master's or doctor of nursing practice degrees. A PhD or other related doctoral degree (e.g., EdD) prepares an individual for a career in teaching and research. Whatever their level of training and area of expertise, nurses aim to promote health and well-being and/ or prevent or treat illness or disability (Henderson & Nite, 1978). And, depending on their professional role(s), nurses may also work in advocacy, research, health policy and systems management, and education (International Council of Nurses, 2002).

Nurses have been central to MTB from its inception. Expecting and new parents welcome and need the information and guidance about their own and the baby's health and development that nurses provide. Nurses are usually seen as trustworthy and helpful and free from the stigma that families associate with mental health providers. And they are well equipped to address the particular ways that trauma and toxic stress live on in the body. Over the years, MTB nurse home visitors have included RNs, nurse midwives, and nurse practitioners, most with some background in maternal and child health care. Despite this broad similarity, they have had different levels of experience, different backgrounds, and different areas of specialization. Some worked previously in hospital settings and some worked in clinic-based practices and thus came to MTB having practiced in more "typical" nursing settings, where patient care was fast-paced, acute, and very targeted and outpatient clinical encounters were widely spaced. Other MTB home visitors were educated and had worked as health visitors[2] in the United Kingdom and Denmark.

The orientation and tasks of the MTB nurse home visitor are somewhat different from those in other forms of nursing practice. Meetings are frequent and ideally take place over a long period of time. The "dyad" (and often the "triad") is the unit of care. The scope of care is quite diverse. The

---

[2]The practice of health visiting is widespread in many countries; typically, health visitors are specially educated nurses who work with families over the course of the baby's first year of life, providing infant health assessment and health care, supplementing primary care practice, and providing support and developmental guidance as needed.

nurse attends to the child's and parent's health, to child and parent development, and to the promotion of maternal and infant mental health, the relational health of the dyad, secure attachment, and supportive, sensitive parenting. They facilitate triage, referrals to team members, and outside referrals. And they do so while maintaining a reflective stance, supported by ongoing supervision and self-reflection. This wide scope of practice obviously requires a range of competencies and knowledge across many domains. Nevertheless, we find—almost without exception—that our model is a good fit for nurses; MTB-HV nurses consistently describe it as deepening their work and allowing them to care for parents and children in ways that feel very meaningful. And while MTB approaches may seem, in and of themselves, new to some nurses, they are in fact consistent with many of the core goals of holistic nursing practice. As one MTB nurse home visitor noted, "Reflective nursing *is* nursing!"

What Is Reflective Nursing?

The simplest way to describe reflective nursing is that nurses[3] approach their clinical goals *through the lens of reflective practice.* Nurses enter most clinical situations with the aim of assessment, education/guidance, prevention, and (in many cases) treatment. In community-based nursing, their role is to assess, educate, problem-solve, and intervene, especially when health or safety issues are present. These goals don't change when nurses are working reflectively; rather, their *way of achieving* them does. That is, while they continue to make critical assessments and think about potential solutions as they interact with parent and child, they work to cultivate a stance of "not-knowing" *at the same time*, to assess and remain curious while continuing to apply their clinical knowledge to the situation before them. In this, they balance a reflective and a directive stance. There are times, of course, when health or safety are endangered, that the nurse must step in and address a situation immediately, albeit in a respectful and collaborative way. But in nonurgent situations, "*I see the problem/understand the issue and here's what can be done to solve it*" can be replaced by "*Let's try and understand what might be going on and how I can help.*" The nurse is, in effect, adding yet another layer to their work, addressing health and wellness while at the same time remaining open to the family's perspectives, curious about their thoughts and feelings and the multiple cultural and contextual issues informing their thinking and behavior. For some nurses, this perspective is consistent with their education in holistic

---

[3] Although we focus solely on nurses in this chapter, these approaches are relevant for any health care practitioner (a doctor, physician's assistant, respiratory therapist, etc.).

health care. For others, the MTB approach feels very new and, at times, like a kind of "culture shock." Their education and practice may have been geared solely toward identifying and solving problems. Often, nurses work in settings where there is great pressure to work quickly and efficiently, to chart extensively, to follow guidelines, checklists, or curricula, and to produce outcomes. As an MTB nurse put it, "We would educate all patients the same way. We never thought 'Did she understand me?'" To tolerate *not* providing immediate solutions, to pause and investigate, to listen rather than teach or give advice immediately require a shift in technique that can seem unfamiliar. As such, it requires a great deal of patience and self-compassion. Yet the value of slowing down, of listening, of remaining open and curious, becomes clear very quickly.

The following example provides a look at some of the complexities of this way of working.

> The nurse arrives to find Malcolm cooking for his 6-month-old son, Henry, who is happily banging an empty cup on his high chair. Malcolm is frying up some sausage and scrambled eggs, and it seems—from the small plate sitting on the counter—that he is planning to share these with Henry. The nurse thinks about several things at once. The child has only recently begun eating small portions of soft, solid food such as baby cereal and pureed fruit. Small pieces of scrambled eggs might be OK. However, fried sausage is a choking hazard for a 6-month-old; it is also difficult to chew and digest, and Henry has no teeth yet. So at one level she knows she has to provide guidance about nutrition and food safety before either food is placed in front of Henry. At the same time, she immediately recognizes that something special is happening between father and child. This is a father who has had a great deal of difficulty allowing himself to engage with his infant son and who has kept a distance between them, leaving all the child care to the baby's mother. He is almost never home when the nurse visits, and yet today she is welcomed. This marks a shift, on many levels. Malcolm and the baby are interacting in a sweet, playful way, and Malcolm is obviously pleased with his efforts at cooking and sharing time with his son. He seems comfortable having the nurse in the room.
>
> This leaves the nurse facing a dilemma: how to have a conversation about safe foods and what's healthy for a 6-month-old while at the same time supporting this very special and absolutely critical shift in the father–child relationship. How can she realize her goals (the immediate one being to make sure Henry isn't offered a chunk of sausage) without pushing the father away? She doesn't want to create a rupture with the father, to make him feel threatened and shut down. Were that to happen, he would be quite unlikely to change his behavior with respect to feeding his son. She needs to find a way to leverage the father's pleasure and pride in nurturing his son as a means to gently providing guidance that he can hear and follow. Trust must be nurtured first,

as this is the foundation for the parent's capacity to be curious and open to new information.

The nurse might begin by turning to the father and noting the great pleasure between them. "Oh, I can see you two are having a wonderful time! It's so great that Henry can hang out with you while you're cooking. I can see how much he loves being with you" (her observation). "You are a lot of fun to watch, Dad! I like being with you!" (speaking for the baby). "It smells great in here! Looks like you are the breakfast cook for the grown-ups, Dad!" She might turn to the baby and say, "Daddy's cooking today . . . and one day when you are bigger and can chew and swallow better you'll get some of this yummy food, too, Henry!" (The nurse says this in this way so Dad can ask a question about swallowing and perhaps save face.) Ideally, Dad might then ask, "Oh! I was just gonna give him some of both . . . you think that's OK?" The nurse can then do some directing, providing the health and safety education around signs that the baby is ready for some solids and foods to avoid because of safety and choking hazards. "Maybe a little bit of scrambled egg? Let's see what he thinks of that. . . ." She might then turn to a more reflective stance: "How does Henry tell you what he thinks of a new food? How can you tell?" All of these comments are geared toward getting the father, now in a more relaxed, open state, to observe the baby. The nurse has highlighted for the dad the importance of observing, of noting the baby's response. This helps him be curious about it.

The nurse might then inquire about his own family. "Do you like to cook? Did your dad cook? With you?" "What were your favorite foods that he cooked?" This conversation might well lead to the nurse realizing that sausage was a staple in Malcolm's family, and indeed in the wider culture in which he grew up, or it might lead to his describing how deprived he felt in relationship to his own father or to traumatic ruptures in his childhood relationships. The nurse is building her relationship with the dad and helping him observe the baby at multiple different levels. She is also listening to him and to his story. She is communicating knowledge to him after having made sure not to threaten him or provoke his defenses; then he is able to listen, be curious, and learn.

The nurse has, in this instance, achieved her goal of developmental guidance. She has also greatly increased the likelihood that Malcolm has heard the information she provided and may actually make use of it going forward. But she has not done this by following a simple or direct route. Rather, she has had to think actively and quickly about how she is going to reach her goal while preserving her relationship with the parent. She has done this by first taking a stance of not-knowing—I don't know why he wants to feed the baby sausage and I don't know the backstory—and tolerating this as she comes to understand and connect with the father. She is both an expert and not an expert at the same time, tolerating her uncertainty as she gains understanding. Then there will be a place for her expertise and a willingness to hear it.

The harder scenario would be if the sausage was already on Henry's plate or Dad challenged the nurse when she said the baby wasn't ready to chew and swallow the sausage. In this instance, the nurse would have to be a lot more directive faster. "Oops—that sausage is just the right size to get stuck in his throat so he couldn't breathe. I love that you want to share breakfast with Henry. In a few more months it will be easier for him to sit up straighter, chew and eat tiny bits of sausage safely. I can give you some ideas of other foods you can share right now, OK? Maybe a little piece of the scrambled egg? Let's see how he does with that."

Why Reflective Nursing?

There are many ways to answer this question. The first has to do with how families experience "expert" advice and guidance. Even the most savvy of us ignore excellent advice; we know we should exercise, eat healthy foods, and get plenty of sleep, and yet we often don't. Advice, knowledge, or guidance do not necessarily change behavior. This reality is amplified when we work with stressed families, where there is often a built-in power differential and, in many instances, a distrust of the "system" and of outsiders. The lived experience of many marginalized families coping with a range of other health and social inequities often makes it difficult for them to trust health professionals and the organizations in which they work. This is quite understandable. They have often been told by medical professionals what to do and then rebuked (implicitly or explicitly) for their failure to comply; this can leave families feeling shamed, criticized, and disrespected and their cultural values diminished. For instance, Malcolm might respond from the "gut": "Who is this woman telling me what to do?" Or he may have an arrest record and fear the interference of any outsiders, particularly those associated with local health authorities. Or he may be so worried about his capacity to father that he feels shamed and disrespected when he's told (implicitly) that he put his son in danger. His fear that he is going to do as lousy a job as his own dad rises to the surface in an instant. As we have discussed throughout the book, this is likely to make him feel quite threatened and defensive, and any opportunity for either a relationship or for learning and reflection will be lost.

Nurses—particularly those who work reflectively—are in a prime position to alter these negative expectations, to ease families' distrust, and to build bridges between patients and health care systems. In the preceding example, Malcolm's sensitivity to criticism was softened by the nurse's appreciation of his spending sweet and fun time with his son, by her interest in his own experiences with food, and by her curiosity about his hopes for his son. He felt understood and thus was able to accept the nurse's guidance about how to best feed his child.

Another value of the "help me understand" approach to nursing care is that it allows the nurse to consider the ways the parent's history has affected their capacity to hear and metabolize health information or developmental guidance. Many parents who have histories of abuse and neglect find it difficult to listen to and understand their bodies, which—as the "scene of the crime" (van der Kolk, 2014)—can be experienced as foreign, and even dangerous, and as such must be dissociated. Add to this that a variety of unhealthy coping strategies (drugs, alcohol, poor diet, lack of exercise) are the manifest sequelae of decades and generations of ACEs and toxic stress (Felitti et al., 1998). And, just as they may have lacked the support and holding to come to know their own bodies, parents may have little experience in understanding the physical and emotional needs of infants. Often they may have been asked to care for younger siblings and cousins from a very young age. They do the best they can. Some become intuitive and loving caregivers themselves; others approach child care from an entirely utilitarian perspective. Whatever the circumstances, the nurse helps them better understand and care for their own and their children's physical health.

Key Elements of Reflective Nursing

The fundamentals of reflective practice in nursing are quite like those we have discussed throughout the book. We ensure safety and regulation and slowly build a trusting and open relationship. We maintain a reflective stance, observing, listening, soliciting parents' perspectives and observations, mirroring, wondering, and sharing our observations and (when a parent is engaged) our hypotheses. At the same time, there are particular issues that arise in applying these principles to nursing practice. We address these next.

Establish Safety, Regulation, and the Relationship

As we have described throughout the book, until they feel safe and engaged, parents may struggle with taking advice and adhering to guidance. Learning and synthesis, like mentalizing, requires trust (Allen, 2022; Fonagy & Allison, 2014). Thus one of the goals of reflective practice is to create the space that allows parents to trust what nurses have to offer. This begins with building the clinician–parent relationship, one of the cornerstones of nursing practice. This relationship develops within the framework of safety and regulation. So nurses work to provide relational safety, to minimize defensiveness, and to slowly build trust. They watch for threat and dysregulation (Theede, 2018). They listen carefully, observe carefully, wait, remaining respectful and genuinely interested in what the parent has to say. They are caring and concerned and create a space for the parents to share their thoughts, questions, and beliefs, where the parent's expertise and experience is valued and heard. Creating this atmosphere, which may need to be reestablished many times over, will make it more likely that parents will feel safe, relax their defenses, and ultimately respond openly and accurately. It also allows them to fully consider advice and information. This is particularly the case with home visiting, in that the parent has *allowed* the clinician into their home. Home visitors are on their turf, which may be particularly stressful for some parents. Home visitors have the privilege of entering the family's private world, and—as such—have much to learn.

Maintain a Reflective Stance

Taking a stance of curiosity and wonder may, for the reasons we've described here, seem to run counter to some of the nurse's primary goals, specifically health education, problem solving, and treatment. And yet this stance facilitates and promotes learning, autonomy, and treatment adherence. The nurse's willingness to reflect conveys interest in the parents and their perspective: *"Let me understand that"*; *"How do you see it?"*; *"What's important to you?"* Nurses communicate, implicitly and explicitly, that they want to know how the parent sees things, what the parent cares about and wants for themselves and the child. Thus the parent becomes the nurse's partner, a respected voice in their shared dialogue. The parent shares their observations of the child, and the nurse shares theirs; parent and nurse learn from each other. The nurse is not *teaching* the parent how to be a good parent; the nurse is *exploring* with the parent how to be the kind of parent *they want* to be, which is almost universally a good parent, and often a better parent than their own parents were.

One of the core elements of a reflective stance is the effort to understand the other's intentions. Thus, for example, the nurse saw Malcolm's intention as wanting to have a good time with his son and feed him the things he, Malcolm, dearly loved. This thread runs throughout the examples in this chapter: The nurse waits and watches, trying to make sense of the parent's (usually benevolent and loving) intention. Then the nurse can frame the parent's intentions in a way that allows the parent to hear what the nurse has to offer without threatening them. Another core element of a reflective stance is reframing. Often parents (and indeed all human beings) see things the way they see them: *"My daughter keeps taking the pots and pans out of the cabinet to defy me." "My partner works all day long just to stay away from us. He doesn't care.*" A reflective practitioner implicitly and explicitly conveys to the parent that there are usually many ways to understand another's behavior. "*Maybe she sees you cooking and wants to be like you.*" "*Maybe he's so worried about making sure you keep your apartment and have plenty of food that he feels he has to work extra hard to provide for you.*" Such reframings can help the parent relax and refocus on the benevolent intentions underlying her child's or partner's behavior.

When working in a reflective way, nurses also help parents observe their own bodily experiences and sensations, as well as those of their child. In doing so, nurses are communicating that "*your body and your feelings are important, your child's body is important, and you can learn a lot by attending to them.*" That is, the nurse's attention and observations provide a form of experiential learning for the parent. Experiences a parent had ignored or found confusing become information that helps them understand themselves, their child or their partner more deeply.

Taking a reflective stance often means making a change in the way the nurse asks questions, even when making basic assessments. For instance, rather than asking a "yes" or "no" question, such as "*You're putting the baby on her back to sleep, right?*," the nurse might ask, "*How are you putting her to sleep? Tell me what those times are like. . . .*" Open-ended, clarifying questions are much less likely to provoke defensiveness and shut the parent down, as they invite the parent's participation and engagement by asking the parent to tell their story, in this case the story of bedtime.

Validate, Validate, Validate

In earlier chapters, we described the many critical ways that pleasure (delight, laughter, moments of shared intimacy) mitigates against stress and dysregulation. Part of the nurse's job is to reinforce and underscore these moments of pleasure and success. This happens first by highlighting pleasurable moments whenever possible ("*Oh, you two are having such fun!*"), by noting and validating progress ("*She's so steady on her feet now!*"), and by validating moments when the parent is reflective ("*You saw that he wanted to share and wasn't just being greedy—that's great.*"). Thus, as difficult as things can get with a family, it is important to validate, to look for the "one good thing" and shine a light on it. These are moments we want to grow.

Start Where the Parent Is "At"

The nurse begins, as we emphasized in Chapter 10, wherever the parent is "at," and not with their own agenda. This can be very difficult when the nurse is expected to follow an explicit curriculum and accomplish specific tasks in each session. If the nurse begins with this agenda before allowing the parent to set the stage, it will almost inevitably set up the cycle of threat and dysregulation described throughout this book. At some level, the parent will quickly register that they are not being heard, and this will lead to subtle or overt defensiveness and resistance or to passive, but ultimately thin, compliance. Let's imagine a very common scenario.

> Maria, the nurse, plans to talk about safe sleep in her upcoming visit with Elva and her infant daughter. She arrives to find the mother in a state of collapse; her boyfriend had punched her in the face during a fight the night before. Terrified for her child and her own safety, Elva had called the police, and her boyfriend had been arrested. Maria realizes immediately that her job on that particular day is to support Elva and help her sort out what she can do to protect herself and provide for herself and her child. Both mother and child have been up half the night, and the mother may need medical attention; if her boyfriend is released, she may not be safe in the home. That is where the nurse begins, assessing for safety and harm, while taking a reflective stance. She will listen, she will comfort, she will be there for Elva. "What happened? Tell me about it. How are you now? I see that you have a bruise. Do you have others? Does anything else hurt? Can I take a look? Did you fall at any point? What about the baby? What did she see? Was she hurt at all? Is it OK if I check her out a little? Where did she sleep? How did she sleep? You must have felt so scared. How are you feeling now? We'll sort this out. What's worrying you the most?"

This approach—which is informed by the nurse's wide knowledge base and various competencies—makes possible a number of assessments, for safety, for harm, for the need for treatment. Over the course of the visit, the approach gives way to a series of plans, for Elva's and her daughter's safety, for shelter, and for food assistance. The nurse may even get to discuss safe sleep as part of it, but the day's "plan" has gone out the window. As it had to. That is the essence of sensitive and reflective care.[4]

Slow Down, Listen, and Observe

One of the great benefits of home visiting is the "gift of time." Except in emergencies, there is time to slow down, to listen, to observe, and to learn. There is time to come back to issues that were left unresolved, there is

---

[4] Very few but the most inexperienced practitioners would push forward with a curriculum in a situation like this. What often causes tension is the expectation from program managers and supervisors that specific goals be met within each session.

time for repair, and there is time to come back to information until it is fully understood. This can seem quite different from a more typical nursing practice pace, and yet MTB nurses regularly report that once they can adjust their pace, "park" their worries for a bit, and "be with" the parent's concerns (as opposed to feeling that they must immediately "do" something about them), the work really flourishes. They "wait, watch, and wonder" (Cohen et al., 2003), gathering the story. As one nurse noted, "You need grace, space, and time" to connect and bring about change. Slowing down builds trust and communicates to the parent that the nurse is really interested in them and their story. "Parking" does not mean that nurses ignore their concerns; rather, they appreciate that they need to know a lot more and engage the parent fully before they can address the issues at hand. As one nurse put it, "If you can help the parent with a small change, it's a good day."

Repeat as Necessary

For most of us, learning takes place over time. For new parents, trying to absorb an extraordinary amount of knowledge against the backdrop of pregnancy and early infancy, certainly among the most stressful (and wonderful) times in a new parent's life, really takes time. It takes language that is simple and clear. It takes repetition. The beauty of home visiting is that knowledge and information can be repeated again and again. At times information is offered before it is directly relevant (anticipatory guidance and foreshadowing) and then is repeated as needed. This is also the reason that videos and written handouts that complement clinical conversations can be so helpful; they allow parents to review materials, to let them sink in and make sense over time. When nurses understand the challenges of learning so much, so fast, particularly when a parent may lack support, guidance, and relevant life experience, they can be more patient, less frustrated, and more willing to start from the top all over again.

A nurse home visitor gives a teenage mother instructions on administering medication to her infant for his painful, itchy eczema. A week later she finds that the mother has apparently "ignored" her advice, leaving the medicine unopened. The nurse fights the impulse to lecture the mother, as she is alarmed by the fact that the baby is not getting the medicine. The eczema is worse, and he is miserable. But she takes a deep breath, and (she hopes) gently inquires about what might have happened. She learns that the young mom couldn't remember the nurse's instructions, nor could she read the instructions on the label, as she was primarily Spanish-speaking and the instructions were in English. She was too embarrassed to text the nurse and ask for help. Hearing this, the nurse gives the mom clear and specific instructions and then backs them up with a text message that the mom can refer back to as needed. The child immediately starts to improve.

The Dance of Reflecting and Directing

We have, at many times throughout this book, talked about the complexity of balancing reflecting and directing. This issue is particularly relevant for nurses. Most nurses are good at solving problems. They like to solve problems, as it brings a sense of accomplishment and closure. They are very good "doers." But parents want and need to have a sense of accomplishment, autonomy, and closure themselves. If the nurse solves problems for them, they are not doing it for themselves. This can be very infantilizing and disempowering. At the same time, parents, especially young, stressed parents, need scaffolding and support; this is not enabling, it is facilitating. Reflective practitioners slow their pace, break down the problem, invite parents to share their view of the problem, and support their taking action and arriving at their own solutions. Balancing "doing" and "being" can be very challenging and requires great patience. Sometimes nurses have no choice but to direct; but, ideally, that is not the initial approach. A seasoned MTB nurse put it this way: "I realized it was important not to make the mistake of feeling I needed to *do* something. That would be more traditional nursing: Assess the problem, make the diagnosis, and decide on a treatment. Or see a need and educate the patient. Now, it's listen, reflect, and decide together: Does something need to be done? What? What if nothing can be done? Will listening in a caring way, witnessing the family's challenge, be enough to help them make decisions or think differently?" Another MTB-HV nurse spoke about the ways MTB changed the way she taught: "Now when I teach, I add reflecting. Like asking, 'Why do you imagine someone might shake their baby? Why might you get stressed?' Then I talk with them about their bodies and ask how they might calm themselves down. Or I might say, 'Have you heard about safe sleep?' Then I give them some information and then I stop and invite them to reflect."

Tolerate Difficult Material

When they feel heard and see that their stories are valued, parents will often disclose or discuss painful material: their own histories of sexual abuse, current domestic violence, severe depression, and the like. In our experience, this can be challenging at first, as nurses may feel that they are not "equipped" to manage these situations. It is hard to hear these stories; without training and support from one's colleagues and from supervisors, it can be triggering or retraumatizing. Depending upon a nurse's education, this may feel more like the job of social workers. Many of the nurses we worked with spoke to this point. They had not necessarily learned about trauma and toxic stress in their own nursing education and may have had limited exposure to these concepts in the course of their daily work. When they had, they had not necessarily been educated to work with trauma: "We knew about women's sexual abuse but were never given any continuing education in it when we worked on Labor and Delivery units. Now, thinking about it, I think about how retraumatizing [labor] was for those patients." "We would do a screening, but we didn't learn how to *do* the screening or what to read in the body language to see how the mom was affected by her history." But being willing to listen and "sit with" a parent helps a nurse manage painful, emotionally complex situations: "Now I am slower and read body language and am less afraid to 'go there.' I used to think that whatever had happened to the mom didn't matter. It was like 'Don't ask about it and you won't feel bad if you can't help them.' But meeting them where they are at is so helpful, even if you can't make big changes." The disclosure of painful life events is an indication that a trusting relationship has developed between nurse and parent and, as such, it becomes part of the context and care.

These concepts ultimately help nurses understand their patients more deeply—"I used to just say, 'She's a difficult patient,' but now I have a very different perspective." But this kind of work may often feel alien at first. "Am I supposed to be doing this?" "Am I doing anything? Am I really working? Am I still working as a nurse and not a social worker?" "It was definitely a challenge. I would say, 'That's a social worker thing.' But no, anyone can do it. It's a learning curve." In fact, in many cases, there are social workers or other mental health clinicians working with the families. But this does not obviate the importance of the nurse being willing to tolerate difficult feelings, to hear them and really listen. This is one of the most healing and therapeutic things a nurse can do. As one nurse put it, "I'm not a social worker, but I can listen, and I can be empathic."

The shift to more reflective nursing can also alter a practitioner's technique in quite specific ways. For example, an awareness of the impact of trauma can change the way the nurse prepares a mother for labor and delivery. Worry about giving birth is universal, but for women with PTSD or complex trauma related to sexual abuse, the anticipation of labor or labor itself can be overwhelming and shattering (Simkin, 1992). Women who have suffered other traumas related to poverty and violence can likewise feel powerless and violated while in labor. In MTB-HV, we adapted a labor planning method developed by Simkin and Klaus (2004) to help mothers cope with these fears as they plan for their birth experience (see also Chapter 15). Well before delivery, the mother is invited to talk through the specifics of labor with the nurse and to make choices about those aspects of labor that can be individualized, such as how pain is managed, who she would like with her, what she can expect, and so on. Developing a labor plan, which can often take several visits, gives the nurse an opportunity to explore a pregnant woman's feelings and concerns and to provide concrete information about the hospital and birth experience. And it gives women a sense of control during a time when many aspects of life feel out of control. It can also be shared with her support partner and with the birth attendant (midwife, obstetrician) during the actual labor and delivery.

Maintain Cultural Responsiveness and Cultural Humility

As we have emphasized throughout this book, cultures vary in their unique values, traditions, beliefs, and behaviors; such differences are often particularly evident when it comes to parenting and child care. As such, cultural complexities are an important aspect of home visiting (Kitzman et al., 1997). Aspects of a family's background may be unfamiliar or alien to the nurse. Similarly, parents may find the home visitor's vocabulary strange and suggestions inconsistent with how they understand their world. The possibility of misunderstanding or misinterpreting behavior or advice can be very real. As we have noted in previous chapters, a reflective stance is inherently curious about and respectful of differences; "cultural humility" (Parisa et al., 2016; Tervalon & Murray-Garcia, 1998), the willingness to examine one's own assumptions and beliefs, is at its core. The clinician remains open to multiple perspectives and understands that there is no one "right" way to parent. A reflective practitioner *wants to know* what matters to the parent; often what matters is based in their family's culture and the broader culture in which they were raised. Aiming for "cultural responsiveness" rather than "cultural competence," the nurse remains responsive to and curious about differences and works in a way that takes these differences into account (Hart, 2017).

Critically, the nurse's willingness to examine their own assumptions and beliefs about family structures, childrearing, cultural contexts, and parenting of infants and young children allows them to distinguish global and essential areas of advice for families (e.g., that infants will be harmed if shaken) versus more arbitrary or culturally based beliefs (e.g., that children should be eating independently by age 2). It also helps the nurse differentiate between cultural or familial beliefs (e.g., a grandmother advising a mother to drink only warm liquids after a Cesarean section) from those actions or traditions that could cause harm (e.g., using home remedies containing mercury). When a parent is adhering to practices that are harmful, then the nurse does, in fact, need to act; when they are not, the nurse need only understand and not interfere. The MTB-P approach also helps nurses put what they have learned about cultural sensitivity into practice:

"I always thought about my work in a context of the family's culture, but I didn't know how to work with their stories. I only knew the facts." As we saw with Malcolm and Henry, and as is shown in many of the following examples, this is part of the parent's "story." Culture deeply informs areas that are obvious foci of nursing practice: an individual's relationship to food, to the body, to discipline, to family planning, to child development, and to illness.

Who's the Patient?

As we've discussed in earlier chapters, practitioners, be they nurses, mental health providers, or other family care professionals, often see themselves as working with an "identified" patient; thus, in this case, the child *or* the parent. This is a core assumption of many disciplines. As anyone who bills for their services knows, this assumption is also built into the billing codes that allow for insurance reimbursement. In MTB-P, the identified "patient" is the dyad (parent–child) or the triad (mother–child–other parent/caregiver). Working through the parent is often the best (and only) way to reach the child. For nurses, this can be a real shift: "I hadn't heard of dyadic work—I was trained to care for *either* the mother *or* the infant." Opening up the space to include parent *and* child, or parent, child, and grandparent, or mother, child, and father can seem overwhelming. But as we have seen again and again, once the nurse has the tools to see the bigger picture, to reflect, to engage, and to listen, her practice expands exponentially.

Case Vignettes

In the following sections, we present a series of case vignettes as a means of bringing these approaches to life.

"My Daughter's Too Angry to Breastfeed": Family Lore and Breastfeeding

The nurse is working with a very young mother and her mother, the grandmother-to-be. The grandmother and the nurse have a very different take on one of the most important aspects of newborn child care: feeding the baby. In this instance, the nurse is hoping that Laura will consider breastfeeding her baby (which many adolescent parents find to be difficult for many reasons; SmithBattle et al., 2020). The nurse is promoting a behavior that is known to be beneficial to the child's health. The grandmother, on the other hand, thinks that Laura will endanger her baby if she breastfeeds. The techniques the nurse is using are indicated in parentheses.

The nurse meets 14-year-old Laura, accompanied by her mother, for the first time, and explains that she hopes to support Laura as her pregnancy progresses by providing information about her pregnancy and the changes that come with being a mother. When she touches on the possibility of Laura breast-feeding, Laura nods and listens. Her mother, however, laughs derisively.

GRANDMA: She'll never be able to breastfeed! She's too angry all the time.

The nurse wonders internally what the grandmother might mean. Is she afraid her daughter will become angry with the baby and harm him? The laughter seems derisive but hard to understand in this context. The nurse thinks, "Where do I start? I want to have a relationship with this family." She knows that if she just forges ahead with advice, there will be some pushback from Grandma. So she pauses, and engages the grandmother, trying to understand what she might have on her mind.

NURSE: Sounds like you are concerned. Can you tell me more about what worries you about Laura breastfeeding?
GRANDMA: My mother told me a story about my great aunt, who was breast-feeding. Then something happened between her and her husband and she got really mad. After that, the baby died because her breast milk became poisoned with her anger.

The nurse nods and thinks to herself that Grandma is the important support Laura needs. She provides shelter, food, and clothing and will be the person to teach and support Laura as she learns about infants. "How do I respond respectfully but still give accurate information to Laura? How can I work with Grandma and earn her trust?" The nurse shares her feelings with Grandma.

NURSE: That must have been so sad and hard when her baby died. I can see why you'd want to be sure nothing like that were to happen with your grandchild. [*Not agreeing or disagreeing regarding the poisoned breast milk but validating Grandma's intention of making sure her grandchild is safe.*]

Grandma leans forward, listening. Laura is listening intently. The nurse thinks, "I wonder if Grandma can be curious? Or open to another possibility? Can I build trust by not being the expert here and have her help me understand what might have happened?"

NURSE: I haven't heard of that happening before—the breast milk changing when someone is angry. Can you tell me more? When did this happen? I wonder if anything else might have caused the baby's death?

Grandma says that she heard this story many years ago when she lived in Cuba. She then mentions that she visited her old home last year and found so much had changed on the island even from when she was young. The nurse picks up on Grandma's words, "so much has changed."

NURSE: Yes, I know. So much has changed since my daughter was a baby. We were told that it was good for babies to sleep on their stomachs, and now we know from research that it's much safer for them to sleep on their backs. It can be hard to know what to believe. Nurses have to keep up with all the newest information. I'm happy to share it with you.

The nurse feels the feeling in the room shift. The grandmother sits back and seems more relaxed and open. The nurse returns to the subject of the baby who died.

NURSE: I wonder if something else could have caused the baby's death back then, like an infection or something. We may never really know what happened. You know, many mothers breastfeed, and all mothers have hard and difficult feelings at times, and their babies do well. Breast milk can be protective for babies when they are new and growing.

Several months later, Laura's baby was born. He was healthy but had a high bilirubin count and significant jaundice. He needed to stay in the hospital for a few days after Laura was discharged. The nurses at the hospital asked if Laura would consider feeding her infant breast milk, as it was one of the best ways to reduce jaundice. Laura successfully breastfed her son in the hospital, and continued for several months after discharge. Grandma supported this fully.

This example vividly demonstrates the value of slowing down, taking time, and inviting the grandmother to share her observations and tell the nurse a story that has haunted her since her childhood. The nurse is modeling curiosity for both Laura and her mother and is respectful and interested in the grandmother's point of view. Hearing that the grandmother thought her daughter would poison the baby with breast milk could so easily have led to a quick "correction" (e.g., "Breast milk is the best thing for babies and certainly not dangerous"). The grandmother might have been very annoyed and clung to her position more strongly, having felt that her fears weren't being heard. But because the nurse recognized the grandmother's intention, regulated herself, did not threaten or challenge the grandmother, and expressed genuine interest in the grandmother's point of view, the grandmother relaxed and began to open herself up to new information. This allowed Laura to take in the nurse's guidance and do what was indeed best for her baby. An atmosphere of trust was slowly being established, with both grandmother and Laura coming to trust the nurse's guidance.

This example also raises an important issue about the treatment "unit." With adolescent and even young adult parents, grandmothers (or other female caretaking figures, such as aunts or older siblings) often play a very major role in supporting them through the transition to parenthood (Sadler et al., 2001; Sadler & Clemmens, 2004). Although this support is critical, it can also be very complicated for both the young parent and the care provider. Nevertheless, the grandparent often becomes a de facto part of the treatment unit, and engaging her in the treatment process becomes essential to positive outcomes. Without the grandmother's buy-in, the young mother will inevitably feel torn and conflicted at a very challenging and complex time. Bringing the grandmother into the work often requires managing her feelings of being wounded, left out, or needing to compete with the clinician. In the preceding vignette, what the nurse managed to do was align herself with the grandmother *in the service of* helping Laura feel more comfortable with breastfeeding.

"I Miss Having a Little Baby": Family Planning

In the following vignette, the mother of an 8-month-old baby muses about getting pregnant and having another baby soon. The nurse is faced with the delicate task of hearing out the mother and father while managing her concerns about adequate spacing between pregnancies, a factor tied to a range of positive developmental and parental outcomes (Nerlander et al., 2015; Regan et al., 2019).

> Eighteen-year-old Moira lives with her boyfriend, Joseph, and his family. Baby Mirabel is a busy 8-month-old who has learned to crawl and is starting to pull up to stand.
>
> When she arrives, the nurse notices the baby happily exploring a basket of toys. Hearing a new voice, Mirabel turns to look and quickly crawls over to her father's lap while watching her mother give the nurse a warm greeting. Mirabel then crawls over and brings the nurse a toy.
>
> NURSE: Hello, my little friend. What have you there? A little red car! (To Moira) Look at her crawl!
>
> MOIRA: I know! She's gotten so fast and she's into everything.
>
> NURSE: What a change over the past few months. It wasn't long ago that she was just learning to sit up. What's it like for you now that she's on the move? (*Wondering*)

MOIRA: I like watching her grow and learn things. She's so smart. But it's like she doesn't need me anymore.

NURSE: Oh? (*Using mirroring, the nurse notes the importance of the mother's feelings of rejection/loss.*)

MOIRA: I miss that feeling of having a baby. You know? Like just holding her and feeding her and all.

NURSE: (*Nods her head.*) (*Using silence*)

MOIRA: And now look at her—she is full speed ahead away from me. She wants to hold her spoon and feed herself. And she doesn't want to be held and be still and cuddle. It's hard. I just want to scoop her up and hug her, but if I do she gets mad at me and pushes me away.

NURSE: She doesn't want to stop moving and exploring? (*Clarifying; reframing baby's intention*)

MOIRA: Yeah, I guess. But it makes me sad. We've been talking about having another baby. (*Moira looks at Joseph, who shrugs and makes a "maybe" gesture.*)

The nurse, looking at both parents, considers her thoughts before speaking (self-reflection). The parents have done a lovely job raising Mirabel. She isn't sure what is behind their thoughts about having a second child sooner than their original goal of seeking better jobs and renting their own home. She hears that Moira feels saddened by what she imagines is her daughter rejecting her but also wonders whether Joseph may have mixed feelings about a second child in the near future. On the one hand, she would like to support them without telling them what to do. On the other hand, she is concerned that a second pregnancy at this time might derail the young couple's plans for an independent life and affect their capacity to be attentive parents. She takes a breath (self-regulation).

NURSE: I remember when you were pregnant you had mentioned wanting more than one child.

MOIRA: I've always wanted children. I know I probably could have waited 'til I finished high school, but I'm almost finished now. And my birth control appointment is in a couple of weeks, so I could just not get it and then I could get pregnant.

NURSE: I remember finishing school was one of your goals before having more children. (*The nurse is holding the mother's prior intentions, voiced during the Pregnancy Interview, in mind and offering them for both parents to contemplate.*) You are almost done with your GED? (*Clarifying*)

MOIRA: Yes! I want to get a better job. Joseph wants a good job, too. He's finishing his apprenticeship next year. We want to have enough money to pay for our own place so Mirabel can have her own room.

JOSEPH: Yeah, that's what we want—our own apartment. We've looked but we don't have enough saved yet. We want Mirabel to have a nice home. We want her to grow up and feel like we've been good parents and really gave her everything she needed.

NURSE: You've both been working really hard towards those goals. It's impressive! (*Validating*) I also remember some other wishes you had. One was for your daughter to be able to trust she could come to you when she was worried or something happened to her. For her to know you were always available for her.

PARENTS: (*Nod*)

NURSE: I can see Mirabel certainly knows her parents care for her. When I came in the door, did you notice how she crawled to you, Joseph? She wasn't sure who had walked in and she knew you'd keep her safe. And then she watched to see Moira's reaction. When she saw her mother smile, she realized everything was OK and she could go back to playing. (*Sharing observations*)

JOSEPH: That's pretty cool! I didn't think about how she comes to us to feel OK.

NURSE: You've both really made her feel secure and that allows her to go out and learn about her world. Look how confident she is—she's even trying to pull herself up to stand.

Mirabel teeters trying to stand and holds onto the couch.

MOIRA: See—she's going to be walking soon and then she really won't need me.

NURSE: Are you wondering whether Mirabel will need you, as she gets older? (*Clarifying*)

MOIRA: It's so different from when she was little.

NURSE: That's true. What she needs has changed a bit as she becomes more independent. (*Validating their observations*) Your roles as parents have changed, too. You are helping her learn to feed herself and keeping her safe as she learns to walk. You are helping her feel safe and secure as she tries out new skills. I wonder what it would be like for you to have another baby in 9 months when Mirabel is one and a half years old? A newborn and a walking baby? (*Wondering*)

JOSEPH: I remember those first months with Mirabel. I don't think we ever slept. We were exhausted.

MOIRA: Yeah. That was hard. We were lucky Joseph's parents helped us out. It would be pretty tight having all of us in one room, too.

NURSE: It is exhausting caring for a newborn! And pretty tiring watching out for a toddler. *(The nurse pauses as the parents silently process/visualize having two babies.)* I wonder what it would be like for Mirabel to have a baby sister or brother at that age.

Mirabel lets go of the couch, falls, and startles herself. She looks around quickly and finds her mother and crawls into her lap. (The nurse seizes this opportunity as a port of entry/teachable moment.)

MOIRA: *(rocking her gently)* You're OK, baby! You are OK.
NURSE: "That surprised me, Mom! I'm glad you are here to tell me it's OK." *(Speaking for the baby, using baby as her partner in the visit)*
MOIRA: *(looking at Mirabel and giving her a kiss)* Yep, I'm here.
NURSE: She still needs you to comfort her when she is surprised or scared. Let's talk more about your thoughts about having another baby before your appointment. We can think about what your goals are for yourselves and for Mirabel before you have another baby. And when you are ready we can discuss how to plan a healthy pregnancy. How does that sound?
JOSEPH AND MOIRA: *(nodding)* Sounds good!

In this example, the nurse uses a variety of strategies to help Moira and Joseph think about family planning and to offer developmental guidance. She hears the mother's longing for her snuggly infant and the sense of loss she is struggling with. She reminds Moira that she is still so important to Mirabel. She also reminds the parents that they had hoped to get better jobs, to create their own home, and to give Mirabel her own room. The nurse gives voice to two sets of conflicting feelings, gently holding the need for family planning in mind. At the same time, she reminds Moira and Joseph that Mirabel needs her parents as much as ever, just in a different way. She hopes that this will soothe Moira's sense of loss and longing and help her delay a second pregnancy until things are a little more stable. By reframing and taking a step back, the nurse helps Moira and Joseph make decisions based on a bigger picture and on their larger hopes and dreams.

Conflict, Abandonment, and Maternal Depression

Sixteen-year-old Cece and her 6-month-old baby are just resuming home visits after a 5-month period during which the nurse was unable to find them. They had moved unexpectedly, and Cece did not have a phone. She had called the nurse as soon as she could, and the nurse finds them living in an apartment with Cece's sister and mother (who is largely absent). Cece's boyfriend is living in another city, and they can only meet infrequently. Cece (understandably) seems depressed and shut down; the baby looks flat and disengaged. All of these things are in the nurse's mind as she works slowly to bring the mom and baby to the point of lively and satisfying connection.

When the nurse enters the small bedroom, she finds Cece sitting quietly on her neatly made single bed, hands in her lap. The lights are off and the only illumination comes through the curtained window. Carl is lying silently in his crib, looking up at a colorful mobile about 6 inches from his face. The nurse notes that the crib mattress is still at the height appropriate for a much younger baby and that the mobile looks like a strangling hazard. In the past the young mother had good intentions and wanted to be attentive to her child and keep him safe, and the nurse is startled to now find Carl at risk for injury. She finds herself wanting to address the safety issues immediately and reminds herself to slow down (paying attention to pacing of information; self-regulation) and imagine what might be happening for the mother (wondering).

The mother appears to have little energy, her affect is flat, and she seems vulnerable. The nurse wonders why Cece is keeping him in the crib during the visit, but she "parks" her question, feeling it's important to first reestablish the congenial relationship they had been building before the break in treatment. What might be going on? Could there be a misunderstanding about the baby's needs and abilities at his age? Might Cece have a postpartum mood disorder? Did something happen during the months Cece was out of touch? Did the mother's past history of neglect as a child influence the situation (hypothesizing)? The nurse wants to give a benevolent interpretation of the situation and decides to be curious and explore the mother's thoughts.

NURSE: (*sitting in the desk chair near the bed*) It's so nice to see you and Carl! It's been a while, and he has really grown.

CECE: (*smiling but not moving off the bed*) Yeah—he's bigger. I'm sorry I couldn't call you when we moved. I didn't have a phone for a while. I share one with my sister now.

NURSE: I'm really glad you called. I missed you. Tell me about the past couple of months.

CECE: (*Shrugs*) Not much happened. Mom said we had to move someplace bigger.

NURSE: This is a nice room! How have you been?

CECE: Tired. Carl still doesn't sleep through the night. And I have to keep him quiet so my sister can sleep 'cos she goes to school and 'cos mom gets annoyed.

NURSE: That is hard to get up at night and keep an awake baby quiet! (*Validation*) Tell me more about the night waking.

CECE: He cries and then I feed him and then he just wants to talk and move around. I put him back on his back and put on his music. Then I get in bed so he doesn't see I'm awake. Eventually he stops talking, and I guess he goes to sleep.

NURSE: What's that like for you?

CECE: It's hard. I mean, he's a baby and he can't help it, but I get so tired and I don't want to be annoyed with him. Or have my mom annoyed with me.

NURSE: That's lovely that you have soothing music for him, but I can imagine being tired and not having as much patience in the middle of the night. (*Normalizing her feelings*)

Turning to the little boy in the crib, the nurse sees he is dressed nicely and looks well nourished, but he also looks somewhat flat, like his mother.

NURSE: I wonder what keeps you up at night, little one? (*To Cece*) May I say hi to Carl?

CECE: (*still not standing up*) Sure.

NURSE: Could you pick him up and bring him over? I don't want to startle him, and I don't know that he'd remember me.

Cece picks Carl up gently and lays him on the bed without speaking.

NURSE: Let's see how you are growing! He is so tall! Can you put him on his tummy? Let's see what he does. (*Modeling curiosity and observing*)

Carl lifts his head and looks around, then reaches out his hand to touch the bedspread.

NURSE: "This is pretty, Mommy." (*Speaking for the baby*)

The nurse continues to coach the mother to move the baby into different positions and notes his interest in what he sees. When Carl is able to sit with support, Cece smiles.

CECE: I didn't know he could do those things!

NURSE: I have some toys you can show him.

Cece offers her son a toy key ring.

NURSE: "Look, Mom! I can shake it and make sounds." (*Speaking for the baby*)

CARL: (*Smiles for the first time*) (*Teachable moment, baby as nurse's partner*)

CECE: He likes it!

NURSE: He really does! Let's see what else he likes to do.

Nurse offers other toys for mother to show to Carl and helps her scaffold his beginning motor skills, encouraging her to be more active. After 10 minutes, Carl begins to yawn and rub his eyes.

NURSE: Is it his naptime? I bet all that play has tired him a bit.

CECE: I wish that would happen at night!

NURSE: Sometimes babies at this age need to move around and get a little exercise. Sometimes that helps them sleep better at night, too.

CECE: I didn't know that. I feel kinda bad now.

NURSE: Babies keep changing! Sometimes it's hard to know what comes next in a baby this age; they grow so fast. You made sure he was safe as an infant sleeping on his back, you've kept him well fed, and you've given him some nice soothing music for sleep. (*Highlighting what she has done well*) Now he's learning new things. We can talk about other ways for him to move and learn about his world. And help him sleep better!

CECE: (*more animated and relaxed*) That sounds good!

NURSE: I also want you to feel better. You are important, too. Sometimes it can be lonely being a mother. (*Offering a feeling word in nonthreatening way, speaking for the mother*) I'm wondering what your day is like and how you are feeling being a mom of a growing baby.

At this point the nurse feels that the atmosphere between her and the mother has changed. Cece is leaning forward to listen to the nurse and opening up about her experience of the past months. The nurse judges that Cece is now likely to be open to hearing some information on the safety, sleep, and feeding needs of a 6-month-old. She offers to help change the height of the crib mattress and moves the mobile to a safe distance. Cece and the nurse agree to meet again in 2 weeks to continue their discussion of the baby's development. The nurse hopes she might also address the mother's mood in the next visits and assess for changes in the child's affect.

"Failures" and What They Teach Us

As we've described in earlier chapters, there are plenty of times when our efforts fail. Usually there are a number of reasons for this: The parent is too upset to hear the clinician, the parent has been triggered and cannot take a broader perspective, or the clinician has somehow triggered and upset the parent. As we described in Chapter 8, the clinician is not immune to being activated, particularly when a parent or child is in danger. The fact that we are triggered or vulnerable to our own "core sensitivities" (Powell et al., 2013) does not mean that we have failed. It means that we are human. The effort to be self-aware never ends but is always an inherent part of any professional practice. Without it, we may cross boundaries, get careless, zone out, and/or (unintentionally) cause harm. With it, we grow and flourish, as do those for whom we care.

In the following example, the nurse unwittingly offends Mom and leaves her feeling like a bad mother.

The nurse visits and finds Annya frustrated by her 9-month-old son's grabbing her hair and earrings while she is feeding him. The nurse makes a suggestion, which doesn't go well.

NURSE: Do you think there are other things he can practice holding onto during meals? Have you tried any foods like small bits of banana mashed up or little pieces of scrambled egg? I wonder if he would be interested in using those muscles to pick up food and try to put it into his mouth? (*Wondering*) Noting the mother's scowl, she adds: He might still try to touch your hair or help feed himself! (*Trying some humor*) Soon he'll have more control of his muscles. Feeding himself foods that are safe at this age would give him some practice.

ANNYA: (*Seeming pleased that Ahmed is developing*) OK, little man. Let's give that a try next time I have some banana to mash up and give you!

At the next home visit the nurse finds Annya out of sorts. The baby is asleep, and it doesn't take long for Annya to tell the nurse she was all wrong about giving Ahmed mashed bananas.

ANNYA: That did not work at all! I don't know what you were thinking telling me he could try mashed banana. . . . There was banana on his hands and then it was in his hair and all over the high chair and his clothes. I mean sometimes he gets a little messy and all when I feed him, but this was just too much! It looked like he'd got a whole banana and taken a bath in it. It took me forever to clean up. I had to give him another bath, and we were out of clothes, too.

The nurse could feel the mother's anger but was confused. The anger seemed more than the situation called for. The nurse wondered if normalizing the baby's behavior and clarifying that his intention wasn't to make a mess would be helpful.

NURSE: That's pretty common. Those first times a baby tries to feed himself might be really messy while he's learning to use those hand muscles. I'm sorry it was so much cleanup for you.

ANNYA: (*Still very upset*) Well, that was just bad advice, and I don't think that makes sense for any baby to feed himself something so messy.

NURSE: I'm really sorry, Annya. It really made a mess of your mealtime with Ahmed and caused you extra work. (*Trying to repair the rupture with apology*)

ANNYA: It did. And I was all out of clothes. I can't just let him go around being messy like that, and I couldn't get to the laundromat, so I looked like a bad mother.

The nurse was beginning to understand what Annya was saying. It wasn't only the mess; it was also the importance of demonstrating that she is a thoughtful and good mother by showing her baby is clean and cared for. The nurse hypothesizes that Annya's early history may have made her very sensitive to being judged by how the baby looks. The nurse realizes she has not taken into account the family's situation in terms of resources or what a messy baby might mean to Annya. She sees that it has triggered Annya's fear that she will be seen as a bad mother.

NURSE: On top of it all you needed to get laundry done for him, and you didn't have time. And you were concerned about how people might think about you having a baby with dirty clothes. (*Restating to show Annya has been heard*)

ANNYA: Yes. That advice is all wrong, and I don't think you should tell anyone that ever again.

NURSE: OK. I can see that. I should have thought about how Ahmed learning to feed himself a banana might cause messy problems for you. I am truly sorry. (*Still trying to repair*)

Annya feels heard and her body relaxes somewhat.

ANNYA: Just don't tell anyone that again.

The Challenges of Reflective Nursing

As we've noted throughout this chapter, reflective nursing may appear to run counter to the way nurses have worked in the past—in hospitals, in busy office practices, or even as home or health visitors—where they were expected to follow prescribed topics or curricula. Despite the fact that holistic practice is the goal of nursing education, this goal is not always foremost when nurses are working in fast-paced, real-world settings. One MTB nurse observed, "I think nurses are naturally empathic and use open-ended questions, but often there aren't enough chances to use these skills." As a result, it can be hard to shift to this "new" way of working; MTB nurses can feel deskilled and unsure of what to do, setting aside "doing" for "reflecting." One nurse put it this way: "I felt like I wasn't a nurse. Am I doing anything? I would come with a plan and then the mother would talk for an hour about her boyfriend." Another noted: "It was hard to *do silence* and give Mom space to reflect on her own. I used to do all the talking and coaching: 'I show you, and now you do this,' as opposed to 'What do you want to learn?'" Some nurses spoke about the sense that they were failing: "It's hard not to think, 'Maybe I'm not a good nurse,' if patients don't do what I educated them in." "Sometimes I would ask myself: Do you even need a nurse?" "I wanted them to parent the 'right way,' and I felt like a failure when they didn't."

MTB nurses also described how—even after they had become comfortable with the reflective approach—they would have to work not to slip into a more "directing" stance: "I keep catching myself, saying I need to slow down and let the mom ask questions." "I ask myself: 'Am I being reflective?'" "I still ask myself, 'Did I just tell that mom what to do?'" It can be hard to think about multiple viewpoints rather than the one "right" way to do something. It can be hard to slow down and listen, as this can feel quite inefficient. Sometimes, of course, frustration wins out. One nurse ruefully described finally just throwing up her hands in frustration, saying to the mother: "It is time for you to go back on birth control! You told me you want to space your children, but you are having unprotected sex!" For many nurses, coming around to reflective nursing is a process. It takes time to trust that this approach can be more fruitful than those they are used to or that this new approach gives them an opportunity to work in the way they had wanted to from the beginning.

Supervision is essential to reflective practice. For nurses, who may find this "new" way of working particularly challenging, a blend of reflective and clinical supervision (see Chapter 8) is particularly important. The availability of a safe space with a trusted supervisor who listens in a nonjudgmental way, who can create the "gift of time" with the supervisee, is essential to developing the multiple skills at the heart of reflective nursing.

Summary

The reflective approach to nursing has a great deal to offer nurses in practice in a range of settings. It also has an important place in primary care and may well—as we have discussed earlier—enhance the likelihood that nurses can achieve their clinical goals (Ordway et al., 2015). This point was brought home to us clearly when two nurses who worked in the Labor and Delivery unit of a community hospital joined MTB-HV as part-time home visitors. What they found was that their experience in MTB-HV changed the way they worked with women giving birth in the hospital. One nurse described her "old" stance as a Labor and Delivery nurse: "In the hospital, we did our job and cared deeply for the mothers and did the best we knew how. But we never wondered what went on after they got home. For example, when a baby died during delivery, we brought in hospice, and we knew about grieving, but we didn't know how to bring it up to parents. It made us uncomfortable. We didn't want to upset the parent by talking about it." She described another situation in which a mother planned to give her baby up for adoption; the adoptive mother was there to help deliver the baby. But the biological maternal grandmother was also there and—at the sight of the baby—lost control and began screaming and crying. She had to be removed by the staff. The nurse reflected: "After working in MTB-HV, I was better prepared to just be with the mom afterward and ask her how she was doing. 'What was that like for you?' I was able to meet her where she was *at*." There are many barriers to such practices in large, overloaded health systems. Yet the simplest forms of reflection, offered in moments of distress and dysregulation, can be enormously helpful and meaningful.

QUESTIONS FOR CLINICIANS

Here are a set of key questions a nurse aiming to work in a reflective way might ask themselves:

▶ How do I think the parent(s) felt during our meeting: Open and comfortable? Anxious? Judged? Confused? Informed?

▶ Did I listen more often than I spoke? Did I use open-ended questions?

▶ Did I understand the parents' agenda? Let them take the lead?

▶ Was I able to use a reflective stance while offering health and safety information?

▶ Did I balance teaching the parents and reflecting with them about their experience?

▶ Did I bring the baby's experience into the conversation?

▶ How well did I pace the visit? Did it feel rushed?

▶ Was I able to link parents' hopes and dreams for their child with the way they are parenting?

▶ Was I able to acknowledge mistakes and repair ruptures?

▶ Was I too corrective? Too focused on problem solving and fixing?

▶ What set me off?

▶ Did I rush in and get "teachy" or solve the problem for the mother?

▶ What made *me* anxious?

Chapter

12

Parental Mental Health

In this chapter, we focus specifically on the challenges of working with parental mental health difficulties.[1] Mental health disturbances are common in the general population,[2] but they increase with high levels of adversity and trauma (Felitti et al., 1998; Hogg et al., 2022; Putnam et al., 2013). Indeed, adult mental health difficulties are among the most tangible effects of early trauma, adversity, and toxic stress. Given the fact that nearly all of our implementations (in the United States, Western Europe, and South America) were carried out with families living in high-need, high-stress neighborhoods and municipalities, it was not surprising that many of the parents we saw were struggling emotionally, be it from depression, anxiety, or—more significantly—PTSD, complex trauma disorders (see also Chapters 5 and 16), severe personality problems (many, if not all, of which were also trauma-related), substance use disorders, and, on occasion, psychotic disorders. Many also came to MTB-HV carrying prior mental health histories and diagnoses, and many were living with impaired family members. We anticipated much of this when we developed an interdisciplinary service model that combined health and mental health approaches to working with

---

[1] We thank Heather Bonitz-Moore for her contributions to this chapter.

[2] In the United States alone, 1 in 5 adults experience some form of mental illness in their lifetimes, and 1 in 20 live with a serious mental illness. Likewise, 1 in 6 children between 6 and 17 years old experience some form of mental illness. Suicide is the second leading cause of death in individuals between 10 and 14 years of age. Depression and anxiety disorders cost the global economy $1 trillion in lost productivity each year, and depression is the leading cause of disability worldwide (National Alliance on Mental Illness, *nami.org/About-Mental-Illness*, January, 2023).

young families. However, we consistently found that practitioners (working in MTB, as well as other intervention programs) often needed a good deal of help managing the many complexities of parents' mental health difficulties.

This was particularly the case with beginning practitioners, as well as those who had little prior experience working clinically with adults. It became increasingly clear that we needed to develop ways of thinking about and working with adult mental health issues within the framework of our parent–child intervention.

The roots of the relative neglect of adult mental health difficulties in infant mental health practice are tangled and complex. There is a general neglect of mental health across all levels of health care; these inequities are more pronounced among high-stress families living in underresourced and marginalized communities. There are the stigmas surrounding mental illness that affect parents and clinicians alike. There is the failure to realize that *by definition* being trauma-informed means being mental health–informed, that trauma-related pathology and mental health pathology are one and the same. This would seem to dictate that practitioners working with young, stressed families should have at least some training in adult mental health, and yet many do not. Many do not have training in child mental health, either. Add to this the broad tendency—at least in the United States—to assume that more generic, low-touch, psychoeducational approaches are suitable for all families, regardless of their experiences of adversity and toxic stress (Condon, 2019). This despite the fact that parents in significant psychological distress often drop out of or disappear from prevention or intervention programs, and are deemed intervention "failures." In point of fact, it is the families who have been failed. Unfortunately, given that systems of care tend to be underresourced and isolated, many of these difficulties show no sign of abating soon.

Our goal in this chapter is to create a road map for bringing adult mental health issues into clearer focus for practitioners working with parents and young children. Ideally, of course, practitioners working with stressed and traumatized families would have advanced training in adult and child mental health, as well as in psychodynamics, clinical formulation, and psychotherapeutic foundations. But in light of the fact that this is often not the case, we describe here what we see as the essentials, many of which are well within the reach of a broad array of practitioners. We begin by discussing how important it is that infant mental health work focus on both the parent's and the child's mental health. We then discuss how difficult this balance can be for practitioners, who must integrate work with parents— many of whom are struggling mightily—into their work with young children. In the last sections, we describe potential "levels" of adult mental health competence in clinicians.

Psychotherapy in the Kitchen

Selma Fraiberg's classic and deeply influential paper "Ghosts in the Nursery" (Fraiberg et al., 1975) beautifully described the devastating impact of two mothers' psychological struggles on the emotional lives of their infants. When Fraiberg and her team, who were all experienced psychotherapists, initially met their first patient, Mrs. March, they immediately recognized the severity of her depression and the extent of her trauma. They also saw clearly the devastating effect these struggles were having on her baby, Mary. They began by following what was then the "usual" treatment protocol of referring Mrs. March for psychotherapy with a psychiatrist, while Edna Adelson met with the mother and baby for developmental guidance. But the young male psychiatrist triggered Mrs. March's decades of trauma at the hands of men, and the treatment stalled completely. And Mrs. Adelson's attempts at developmental guidance foundered; despite Mary's obvious failure to thrive, Mrs. March seemed oblivious to the baby's clear signs of distress and despair.

It was at this point that Fraiberg and her team tried a different tack, one that was to change the field of psychotherapy forever. Adelson worked with the mother and baby *together*. Mary became the guide to the mother's inner life and to her early terrors; exploration of these in the presence of her baby and with the "holding" of a skilled practitioner helped Mrs. March heal the scars of abuse and neglect and *discover* her baby. The outcome was nothing short of miraculous; over months of painful, cautious work, mother and baby began to thrive. "Finding" the baby became a way for the mother to find herself and recover from deep, deep wounds. Fraiberg likened this process, with the baby providing the entrée into the mother's pain, to having "God on your side" (Fraiberg, 1980, p. 53).

We retell this familiar story to make the point that *in order to ensure the child's emotional and physical survival*, Fraiberg and her team had to recognize and address Mrs. March's severe depression and complex attachment trauma therapeutically. "When [the] mother's own cries are heard, she will hear her child's cries" (Fraiberg et al., 1975, p. 396). Without this, Mrs. March could not see her child and her needs.

> What emerged, then, was a form of "psychotherapy in the kitchen," so to speak, which will strike you as both familiar in its methods and unfamiliar in its setting. The method, a variant of psychoanalytic psychotherapy, makes use of transference, the repetition of the past in the present, and interpretation. Equally important, the method included continuous developmental observations of the baby and a tactful, nondidactic education of the mother in the recognition of her baby's needs and her signals. (Fraiberg et al., 1975, p. 394)

Though they approached Mrs. March through her baby, Fraiberg and her team *identified* her significant mental health difficulties, and focused on these to ensure the mental health of the infant.

It is worth thinking about the circumstances that allowed them to create a model that was to have such a remarkable and sustained impact on children and families. First, they were very experienced psychotherapists who had been working with adults and children for decades. They knew how to diagnose and work with severe psychopathology. This allowed them to trust their own instincts in trying something new when they realized that referring parents out for a mental health evaluation was *not working*. Mrs. March brought to the consulting room decades of shame and pain at the hands of men and "helpful" social services. Being sent to a psychiatrist likely confirmed for her that she was "crazy" and "unfit" to mother her baby. In addition, separate psychotherapy was *not what she needed at that moment*. She needed to get beyond the demons that were *evoked by mothering a small, helpless infant* so that she could care for her. Her pain and profound trauma could not be disentangled from the act of mothering, and, in fact, treating complex trauma and caring for the baby as *one* was essential. How did Fraiberg and her colleagues have the prescience to understand this? In addition to having the confidence and faith that come from years of growing from success and learning from failure, the founding team of clinical social workers—Fraiberg, Adelson, and Shapiro—was steeped in the psychoanalytic tradition, in which infantile and adult experiences are inextricably linked. As such, they were willing to take some very big risks to save Mrs. and Mr. March and their baby.

Adult Mental Health Concerns and the Clinician's Experience

Despite the broad impact of Fraiberg and her colleagues' remarkable work, working with adult mental illness continues to be a challenge for many infant mental health practitioners. This is so even though knowledge of adult mental illness is an expected competency for endorsed infant mental health specialists and mentors (Michigan Association for Infant Mental Health, 2017; Weatherston et al., 2009), as well as advanced practice nurses. Knowledge does not necessarily translate to confidence and competence, however, and across the board providers need more support in this area. The infant mental health workforce is extremely heterogeneous in terms of discipline, education, and training, and many have little, if any, clinical experience working with adults. That is why, as we describe in this chapter, multiple layers of training and clinical supervision (see also Chapter 8) are necessary.

Obviously, increased attention to adult mental health issues will benefit families (Ammerman et al., 2013). But having the training and support necessary to develop more sophisticated mental health awareness is also *good for practitioners*. When confronted with, for example, severe depression or signs of complex trauma, clinicians may quite *reasonably* feel that they don't know what to do and find themselves overwhelmed, shut down, frustrated, angry, or unable to empathize and remain present with parents' distress. They may (in essence) throw up their hands (*"I don't work with psychosis!"*) or minimize the severity of a situation (*"The dad's just having a few strange thoughts"*), essentially wearing rose-colored glasses when high-strength bifocals are needed. Practitioners can also close their eyes to expectable vulnerabilities in the parents' earliest interactions with the baby. Evidence of the intergenerational transmission of trauma can emerge within the earliest weeks of life.

When aspects of the work are experienced as frightening and alien, practitioners can so easily avoid asking questions or taking steps that make them uncomfortable and for which they do not feel prepared. What you don't know can scare you and often does. Anxiety and dread quickly take hold. *"What should I do??? How can I fix this? I don't know how to handle this!!!"* Sitting with emotional pain can be very difficult. It is natural to feel helpless, frightened, or deeply uncomfortable, to want to shut out the pain, or to rush to remedy feelings that are not, as such, "remediable." It is natural to search for concrete solutions or to become so distressed that it is nearly impossible to hear the parent. Without skills in this area, clinicians can also become very frustrated and end up, in effect, "blaming" the victims for not doing what they're "supposed" to do. We see this particularly when clinicians have very large caseloads and little supervision. But with more specific training in adult mental health, as well as the availability of mental health consultation and supervision, practitioners can feel more confident approaching, rather than avoiding, these situations. Of course, not even experienced mental health professionals are immune to avoidance and dread in certain cases, and, indeed, we found that practitioners at all levels needed ongoing training and supervisory support to feel prepared and competent to integrate developmentally informed mental health approaches into their work. The more challenging families that practitioners have in their caseloads, the more difficult it will be to remain open and available and to move toward rather than away from the problems that are often hidden in plain sight.

Today, referring parents out for ancillary evaluation and treatment remains one of the most common approaches to addressing parental mental health challenges within the framework of infant–parent or child–parent work (Ammerman et al., 2006). As we mentioned earlier, it was the failure of this approach that led Fraiberg and her colleagues to try something else. We, too, found that referring parents out was rarely effective, for a variety of reasons. Generations of less-than-optimal care and historical trauma leave many parents extremely distrustful of the mental health care system. There is also considerable stigma attached to mental health treatment; this is especially the case in marginalized populations who are already fighting stigma on many levels. The suggestion that parents need "help" can be insulting and threatening, and often they simply do not follow through. In addition, when there *are* mental health services available, the interventions being offered (usually short-term behavioral treatments) have rarely been developed or tested in high-need, under-resourced communities. And rarely are there developmentally appropriate, trauma-informed, culturally relevant mental health services focused specifically on *parents and parenting*[3,4] Thus we often found that we were the first and—for quite a long time— only line of "defense" in helping parents navigate the transition to parenthood, in all its complexity. Ultimately, however, once parents experienced a *different* kind of health care and mental health care (see Chapter 11 on reflective nursing), they were much more open to different kinds of therapeutic experiences and began to trust themselves to navigate care systems and find the additional help they needed.

Cultivating Mental Health Awareness

We have come to think of the development of clinicians' adult mental health awareness as dependent upon a graded set of competencies. We describe these in some detail below. The first is the basic capacity to create a therapeutic space. The next level is the development of the capacity to think clinically and critically about assessment and diagnosis. The most advanced level is the development of clinical skills that allow practitioners to deepen their therapeutic work with parents and to intervene in more effective and expert ways.

---

[3]This is less the case in a number of Western European countries (e.g., Denmark), where a range of services is available for struggling parents and young children, including short- and long-term residential facilities offering intensive family-based interventions. By contrast, mental health systems in the United States, particularly in underserved urban and rural areas, are often overwhelmed and grossly inadequate.

[4]An exception to this is the Family and Parent Development Program at the Yale Child Study Center, which is devoted to providing mental health care specifically geared toward parents and parenting.

Creating a Therapeutic Space

We begin with a fundamental skill that many practitioners have in abundance: the capacity to remain present, open, genuinely curious, willing to listen, and—most important—to *hear*. These are the capacities that create safety and regulation in the other person and that make healing relationships possible. As we have emphasized throughout this book, our humanity and willingness to care, connect, and listen can be the most therapeutic aspects of what we have to offer. It can be so transforming for parents and children to be seen and heard. Yet it can be easy for clinicians to forget—particularly when they are feeling overwhelmed and anxious—how helpful simply listening and creating a therapeutic space and a therapeutic alliance can be. No matter how distressed they are, parents (and their children) benefit from our simple willingness to observe, listen, and hear. Each of us, regardless of our discipline, has the capacity to be inherently therapeutic. Our "skill in being human" (Allen, 2013), to listen, to hear, to witness, and to join, is the first step in helping another feel less alone and less frightened. It is one of the most important skills we have in leveraging change. As Allen (2012) puts it, "plain old therapy" is often the best medicine we have to offer. Some readers may immediately protest that they are not trained psychotherapists, that they are not trained in evidence-based treatments for depression/anxiety/trauma (take your pick). Indeed. But it does not take an advanced degree to listen and to hear: "*That sounds so hard*"; "*You must be just overwhelmed and worried*"; "*That sounds really sad, and it'd be hard for you not to feel kind of depressed.*" It means accepting the parents *where they are* and hearing their turmoil, often saying it out loud. We may not know precisely what we are seeing, but that doesn't mean we can't be present for it. We show up and we bear witness. Nearly all parents will be helped and sustained by our willingness to accompany and hear them and ensure their safety in the face of the most paralyzing distress.

Often, the first layer of what we see or hear is a defense, a strategy for managing unbearable pain. That is, as we discussed throughout Part II, both adults and children *regulate* and contain their emotional experiences in a variety of ways. Fight, flight, or freezing, in their multiple manifestations, are survival mechanisms, extreme efforts to manage extraordinary stress. For example, the *absence* of distress (flight) is often the sign of a vigorous effort to suppress unbearable feelings. A teenage mother said of her father's raping her at age 4: "Oh, I don't even remember it. It didn't bother me." This was, plain and simple, a defense, a survival strategy aimed at managing the unimaginable and the unbearable. Recognizing it as such does not mean we rush in to confront or challenge it or that we take her denial at face value; rather, it alerts us to pain that must be approached very slowly and over time. Similarly, a young mother became enraged in remembering her own mother's abandonment, spitting out the words, "She's a pig!" with great venom (fight). She was using anger to defend against great sadness and longing. Were the clinician to back away and label her an "angry woman," they would not be incorrect, but they would be missing the boat. This mother was so hurt. To fail to see this and other survival mechanisms *as such* dramatically affects the clinician's capacity to recognize psychological distress in the parent.

Recognizing and Assessing Parental Mental Health Disturbances

We now turn to the next level of competence in recognizing and assessing parental mental health disturbances.

Assessment

There are many times when therapeutic listening and the capacity to maintain a reflective stance, though extremely valuable, are simply not enough. In order for the parent and child to thrive, the parent's mental health difficulties—which may or not meet criteria for a mental health disorder—must be *recognized* and *addressed*. A parent who does not respond to the infant's cries when the clinician visits seems dissociated. A father cannot get out of bed and cannot rouse himself to smile at the child. A mother cannot stop obsessively checking her infant, who she is sure is about to die. Another does not answer the door or repeated text messages. Or, as the clinician comes to know the parent, they may see evidence of entrenched character pathology, usually manifest in chronic relationship difficulties or in the parent's repetitively getting into self-destructive and self-defeating situations. In such situations, the clinician is also extremely likely to see signs of "trouble" in the child. What are the clinician's next steps?

The first is, quite simply, to approach *rather than avoid* the issue and to listen to one's own growing sense of concern. Otherwise, there is a very good chance that the parent's mental health difficulties—for example, postpartum depression, a manic episode, blossoming obsessive–compulsive disorder—will become the elephant in the room, unnamed and unrecognized but demoralizing and defeating for all involved. The failure to address them can scuttle even the most effective intervention: "*This isn't getting better. What else is going on? It looks to me like she's depressed, and I can see it's getting worse.*" Ideally, the practitioner asks the parent more about the symptoms and their course to get a better sense of what is going on. How severe are the symptoms and how long has the parent been aware of them? *"How bad are you feeling?"* *"Do you feel like hurting yourself?"* *"How long has this been going on? When did it start?"* These simple inquiries can be so helpful.

The next step would be to consider whether the parent's difficulties meet diagnostic criteria for a mental health disorder. For some practitioners, this is within their scope of practice; they are trained to diagnose mental health difficulties. They can consider the options: Is it debilitating anxiety? Is it the activation of an attachment trauma? For many others, however, diagnosing is not within their scope of practice. In this case, mental health consultation or support from clinical partners and supervisors becomes essential. In any event, it is so very important not to overlook signs of an impending mental health crisis. A case in point is the fact that, much to our surprise, 3 of the first 19 mothers in our entirely volunteer community sample had psychotic breaks around the birth of their children. The clinicians, a licensed clinical social worker and an advanced practice nurse, readily recognized the signs of the mothers' decompensation and were thus able to provide additional sessions and other forms of intensive support. As was so often the case with the parents we saw, all three declined referrals for psychiatric care, but they were greatly helped by the other levels of support we were able to offer.

Trish: A Brief Psychotic Episode

Trish was 18 years old and expecting her first child. She had an uneventful pregnancy and seemed prepared for labor and the early days of motherhood. She was living with her mother and two younger siblings. When Trish's water broke and she moved into labor, she became more and more disorganized, to the point that she was actively psychotic and had to be restrained by the time her baby boy was delivered. The staff at the hospital reached out to the MTB-HV social worker. What had happened made clinical sense to the social worker. As a child, Trish had been in a serious car accident, requiring her to have a series of surgeries and then wear a full body brace for nearly a year. Likely it was these experiences that had been triggered by the helplessness and pain of labor. The social worker made a plan to meet Trish the next day, who, though still quite fragile, was a little more oriented. They talked about what had happened, and the social worker offered her thoughts as to what might have triggered it. And together they marveled at Adam, her new baby. As Trish began to relax, she began to smile and "converse" with her infant son. Over the next month, the social worker met with Trish two times a week, intensifying support for the mom. She included Trish's mother in the effort to minimize stress on Trish and alerted them to warning signs that Trish might again be decompensating. Slowly, the remnants of Trish's panic and terror began to abate, and she began to connect with Adam. Because she was nursing and seemed slowly to be getting better, she declined medication but agreed that if she felt worse she would see a psychiatrist.

Magnolia: A Manic Episode

Magnolia was 19 years old and 3 months away from having her first child when she joined MTB-HV. She was working and living with her mother and siblings in a fairly chaotic household where emotions ran high. Her mother greeted her pregnancy with a plea to God for "help" and told her she wasn't fit to be a parent. Her sister reacted with contempt. The relationship with her baby's father ended shortly after she found out she was pregnant. In her Pregnancy Interview, Magnolia was clearly trying to make the best of things, but her loneliness and sense of isolation was unmistakable, as was her fear. When she was asked, "Are there things that you're afraid you'll do as a parent?" she responded, "I'm just . . . I'm just scared all the way 'round," and then spoke in an increasingly incoherent way about all of her fears, particularly of neglecting, spoiling, or abusing her child. But there were few signs of the mania that emerged after the baby was born. Within weeks of the birth, she was agitated and irritated and could not sleep. When she spoke, one idea flew into another. She was confused and overwhelmed by the sheer number of things she had to keep track of and felt completely unsupported by her family. The baby was lost in the shuffle. The social worker and the nurse both increased their visits and tried to create as much order as they could for Magnolia, who struggled to attend and not talk *at* the clinicians. They listened and reassured her, working to slowly bring the baby into the mother's "field of vision," so that she could begin to anchor herself as a mother. With their steady presence, their willingness to sit with her agitation, and their helping her establish concrete routines, she began to calm down. The team learned that, in fact, there was bipolar disorder in the family. Magnolia was highly affronted when a psychiatric consultation was suggested. She would not have been able to nurse while on neuroleptics, and nursing was one thing she *could* do. So the clinicians managed her therapeutically, trying in a variety of ways to help her feel safer and heard. She slowly calmed down, although she always tended to be somewhat hypomanic and would likely have been diagnosed as Bipolar II.

Nadine: A First Break?

Nadine lived with her mother and father. Her mother had major mental health challenges and had been in and out of hospitals throughout Nadine's childhood. The father of the baby had recently been sent to jail for an extended sentence. Nevertheless, Nadine spent a great deal of time imagining a joyful reconciliation with him after the baby's birth. Once she delivered her infant daughter and returned home to life with her often delusional and frightening mother, she became more and more paranoid in her own thinking. She would not allow the child to play on the floor, as she feared contamination, and she developed fixed and psychotic ideas about the baby's father and imagined that he was soon going to return and marry her. She seemed oblivious to the baby's cues and needs, and the baby began to look more and more neglected. Like so many mothers who fear and feel stigmatized by mental health intervention, Nadine also declined a psychiatric consultation. Nevertheless, sustained work with the social worker—who was a highly skilled diagnostician and clinician—led slowly to a remission of psychotic symptoms. Sadly, a severe depression emerged in its place, but this, too, softened as the intervention continued, and the baby began to thrive.

All three of these mothers completed the MTB intervention successfully, and in each case the acute symptoms of mental illness receded. Nevertheless, both clinicians' alertness to the problem and willingness to work with the mothers and provide extra support was essential.

Evaluating Prior Mental Health Diagnoses

It is often the case that parents come to services with one or more previous psychiatric diagnoses. Many are well known to child protective services (often because of their own involvement as children) or to other community educational, medical, and social service systems. As a result, they may enroll in parenting programs with lengthy case records and often a raft of "diagnoses," such as ADHD, bipolar disorder, and so forth. We put diagnoses in quotes here because such labels are often assigned without thorough and comprehensive evaluation and may reflect a range of biases and stereotypes and/or a lack of attention to development (e.g., any boy who misbehaves in school has a behavior disorder or ADHD; a teenager with dysregulated mood is bipolar). Or, as we discussed in Chapter 5, the signs of complex trauma disorder are missed in favor of the symptoms that reflect adaptation to trauma. Thus a mother's "depression" may in fact be a symptom of attachment trauma and not reflective of an underlying depressive illness. Sadly, these diagnoses often say much more about systems of care than about parents themselves.

Whatever diagnoses accompany a parent to a given prevention or intervention program, the practitioner needs to be able to think critically about them and what they mean—"*Does this diagnosis make sense to me, and how will it/should it affect my work?*" Here again, either some working knowledge of diagnosis or the availability of mental health consultation and supervision is essential. Consider a 24-year-old mother-to-be who received a diagnosis of bipolar disorder[5] as an adolescent after being seen once by a psychiatrist in her local hospital's emergency department (ED) following a suicide attempt. Let us imagine three different scenarios. In the first, the young woman was seen in follow-up for a complete evaluation. Medication and therapy were prescribed, and she complied and continued to be on medication and to see a therapist regularly. Under these circumstances, we would not necessarily expect her psychiatric diagnosis to interfere with her ability to participate in a parenting program, nor would it necessarily interfere with her capacity to parent, as long as she was followed and treated. It might, however, have implications for her children's later developmental trajectories (as it can be heritable), and informing her about the genetic risks of bipolar disorder for subsequent generations might be important at some point.

In a second hypothetical scenario, the young woman was not seen for follow-up after her trip to the ED, nor was medication prescribed. Nevertheless, despite the absence of crucial follow-ups and "tests" of the physician's hypothesis (e.g., full evaluation of her psychosocial and psychiatric history, ongoing psychotherapy, and a trial on a mood-stabilizing medication), this diagnosis became part of her case record, and she was routinely described as "bipolar." Let us assume that this diagnosis was, in fact, correct but that she had essentially been untreated (i.e., she was not on medication, nor had she received any ongoing therapy). In this case, the presence of a serious mood disorder (which could manifest in depression or mania or both) would likely have a number of effects on her ability to participate in whatever parenting program was offered to her. It would also have a great impact on her capacity to parent. And, of course, there are biological risks to her children as well. Clearly, managing these complexities necessarily falls to the practitioner, regardless of their training.

Conversely, let us imagine that the diagnosis is actually *not* correct but that a tired, overworked psychiatrist mistook teenage angst and misery for bipolar disorder. These symptoms, of course, lessened over time. The implications of this error are enormous for the child or adult, but unless the clinician thinks critically about the aptness of the diagnosis, they cannot begin to right the wrong. Do common descriptions of the symptoms of a particular disorder (which are clearly described in *DSM-5-TR* [American Psychiatric Association, 2022] or *ICD-11* [World Health Organization, 2019]) align with what the clinician sees in a parent? For example, does the mother described as bipolar show signs of significant depression, mania, or both? Or is there evidence of ongoing mood dysregulation? Does the diagnosis *make sense* to the practitioner or the mental health expert on her team?

---

[5] We use this particular disorder as it is one of a number of "garbage-can" diagnoses assigned to patients after incomplete evaluations.

What we sometimes see in our consultative work is that current practitioners accept these prior diagnoses at face value and continue to describe
the parent as "bipolar" or "having ADHD" without really considering
what these labels mean and whether or not they are actually correct. To
not evaluate prior mental health diagnoses for their accuracy is to place too
much stock in a system of care that—like all systems—can be vulnerable
to bias, overburdened, and sometimes just plain old wrong. If the diagnoses no longer make sense in light of the current clinical picture, then the
clinician should note this in the parent's clinical record and correct what
they can. By contrast, if the diagnosis (or diagnoses) seems accurate, then
it becomes very important to think about how such difficulties may affect
parenting. For instance, a father with a history of substance abuse is likely
to find the stresses of parenting a newborn quite overwhelming and will
need special support to anticipate and manage potential crises. Likewise,
a mother diagnosed with borderline personality disorder (BPD), which is
almost always tied to a history of relational trauma, is likely to find many
aspects of pregnancy and early parenthood quite dysregulating. A mother
diagnosed with an autistic spectrum disorder as a child may well find her
infant's need for emotional connection utterly incomprehensible. Whatever
mental health difficulties the parent brings to an intervention, the clinician
needs to keep them and their potential implications in mind throughout
their work with a family. This is what makes it possible to interfere with
intergenerational cycles of disrupted relationships.

Junie: The Utility of a Diagnosis

Junie joined our program at 17 years old and shortly after gave birth to a son.
She was living with her aging grandmother, who expected her to take care of
the house and prepare all the meals. Junie had no other sources of support;
her own mother had disappeared years earlier, and she had never known her
father. The case records indicated that her pediatric care provider diagnosed
her with ADHD at age 5; she had been prescribed Ritalin, but she had stopped
taking the medicine within a matter of months, as there had been no effort to
help her grandmother understand the diagnosis or the treatment. Now 17 and
enrolled in MTB-HV, Junie could not keep her appointments straight, was often
away from home when the clinician arrived for scheduled visits, dropped her
child off at day care late every morning, and hadn't made it to the pharmacy
to fill her child's prescription for medication to treat an ear infection. Nor had
she made an appointment to begin birth control. And she was often distracted
and randomly chatty during home visits.

The clinician was frustrated and at her wits' end. None of the strategies
she offered the mother were working, and she found herself becoming more
judgmental, impatient, and critical. She and her supervisor went back to her

original notes; there it was, hidden in plain sight: ADHD. This told the practitioner something vital about this mom and her mental health and cognitive challenges. Organizing anything was really difficult for her. Her disorganization was not a sign of laziness, intransigence, or willful resistance but a sign that she was overwhelmed, in part because organization was such a struggle for her and because she had more to organize than just about anyone, let alone a 17-year-old, would be able to handle. The simple realization that she wasn't being a pain on purpose immediately activated the clinician's empathy and willingness to understand. Junie wasn't lazy or uncaring. She had a disability and needed help managing it. And her current life circumstances likely overwhelmed any prior capacities she might have had to organize and regulate herself. The problem then shifted from "How can I get her to do x, y, and z?" (which is often an inherently adversarial stance) to "This must be so frustrating for her, and so hard. I wonder what will help her be more organized?" The clinician was then able to work with Junie to develop simple ways of organizing herself (using her phone for reminders, getting a calendar, making lists, etc.), and to connect her with community resources as necessary. She also gently suggested that Junie consult with her primary care physician for a reevaluation and potential resumption of stimulant medication.

Mental Health Screens Are Not Enough

In many programs, sadly, the only manifestation of adult mental health awareness is the administration of behavioral health screens at prescribed points in an intervention cycle; thus, for example, a program might administer the Edinburgh Prenatal Depression Scale (Cox et al., 1987), the PTSD Symptom Checklist (Blevins et al., 2015), or the ACE Questionnaire (Felitti et al., 1998) at regular intervals. Often these are administered without attention to the basic psychometric properties of the instrument; for instance, many measures are invalid if repeated too frequently, whereas others are not meant to be repeated at all (e.g., repeating a measure of childhood trauma exposure makes little sense because the events themselves would not be expected to change). More important, however, such screens are often administered without any effort made to use them *clinically*—to learn more about a particular parent and *their* feelings of despair or hopelessness, *their* fear and sense of danger, *their* anger and frustration, and whether they are, in fact, at mental health risk (but see Stob et al., 2019). Although administering a screening instrument may give a practitioner or program administrator the *sense* that they are addressing adult mental health issues, if these screens are not used to deepen assessments and to inform the practitioner's work in a meaningful way, they are clinically of no use (although they may be of use in research). The best example of this is the current infatuation with the ACE Questionnaire, which is often administered without an effort to help the clinician think about the particular ways an individual's history may be profoundly affecting their capacity to parent and without the effort to link the parent to services as necessary, if such services even exist (Finkelhor, 2018).

Add to this the fact that it is not uncommon for diagnostic screens and questionnaires to be quite inaccurate and/or culturally irrelevant. When filling out checklists, parents can, and often do, deny symptoms and minimize trauma histories. Many people routinely underreport their symptoms and struggles. And, depending on the cultural context, issues of literacy, or language, they may not have a framework for understanding the questions being asked.

> A teenage mother was having a very difficult time in high school. Velma was socially awkward, could relate only to the other "odd ducks" in her grade, and felt like a terrible misfit. She was miserable. At school, she would blow up in anger and then collapse in tears, often first threatening to hurt herself. When her therapist visited the school for a meeting, she stated the obvious, which was that the young girl was depressed. She also explained that this was one of the reasons Velma was in psychotherapy. The school psychologist, who had administered a depression screen, quickly retorted, "But no! I gave her a depression screen and she denies depression!"

The willingness to accept a false negative was a perfect example of ignoring the *obvious* data in favor of an "objective" measure of distress.

Treating Parental Mental Health Disturbances

The question of treatment brings us to yet another level of complexity in infant mental health work and of practitioner competence in adult mental health. We begin by returning to the point we made at the beginning of this chapter. Parents who are struggling emotionally will often take their first steps toward deeper self-understanding and psychological health within the context of parent–infant intervention. Using the relationship with a safe and trusted practitioner as ballast, they come to see their babies more fully and to uncover and take stock of long-buried ghosts and deep emotional scars. These transformations—which often seem nothing short of miraculous—are dependent not only upon the practitioner's capacity to observe the infant but upon their capacity to see and hold the parent's distress and pain, as well. To repeat, it does not take advanced training to listen and to hear. Clinicians' humanity and trustworthiness are often what parents need most.

The more training a practitioner has, however, the more they will be able to draw parents out, to recognize and thus soften defenses, and to consider the multiple factors that might be leading to the activation of critical but debilitating survival strategies. The more they know, the more their hypotheses are likely to be helpful and generative, the more they can bring to the act of listening, and the more expertise they can provide. The more the practitioner is able, for example, to recognize the signs of depression and anxiety or of psychosis or to think critically about prior diagnoses, the more they will bring to listening and the more frameworks they will have to understand and make meaning of the parent's difficulties. In addition, the more treatment skills the practitioner brings to the work, the more resources they will have available. We do not mean to suggest that clinicians should have the ability to provide a range of specific evidence-based treatments. But sitting with a practitioner who is at least versed in basic therapeutic approaches, who understands attachment and relationship dynamics, and who is relatively unafraid of a parent's pain and distress will help them make use of an intervention and potentially ease the way toward eventually getting the help they need for their own mental health difficulties.

As we discuss more fully in considering the case of Genevieve in Chapter 16, for parents who struggle with attachment trauma, the stage of relationship building and establishing safety can often take a very long time (Courtois, 2004). But without it, there is no true possibility of trauma processing. With Genevieve, the practitioners' capacity to respond to the multiple signs of complex trauma allowed them to provide the level of support that she needed to take care of both her child and herself. *Treating her complex trauma by creating safety in relationships and addressing her needs for physiological regulation and organization was essential to her baby's development on multiple fronts.*

It has been our experience that, although it is often the case that parents would, in fact, benefit from a referral to a psychiatrist or to an outside therapist, they often don't follow through with these referrals (although some, like Brenda, described in Chapter 14, did). While they were in MTB-HV, they saw *us as their treaters, and us as the ones they trusted.* Many parents also had their own (often justified) distrust of the medical system and/or felt keenly the stigma around mental health treatment. Sadly, even when parents are willing to seek outside help, they may have difficulty finding it. These factors once again put the onus back on the practitioners themselves.

Severe Mental Illness

When parents present with significant mental illness or behavioral problems (a psychotic disorder, substance use disorder, or dangerous or criminal behavior), they may well require a specialized parent–child program (those that are targeted toward severely mentally ill parents, toward substance using parents, etc.), or they may need to have their mental health disorders treated *before* they can meaningfully engage in infant mental health work. We found that there were a small number of parents in MTB-HV who were simply too impaired and too traumatized to benefit from even the intensive services we offered. We also found that we were less effective when young mothers and fathers were living with their seriously mentally ill parents. The grandparents' own difficulties created a level of chaos that was very difficult to penetrate. For example, as we describe in Chapter 15, Yolanda's mother's interference made it impossible for the clinicians to intervene in the way they saw fit.

Summary

A range of mental health concerns—from depression and anxiety to the more severe adaptations of complex trauma—are common sequelae of living in circumstances of extreme stress, high socioeconomic risk, and chronic relational disruption. These are not incidental to the work of infant mental health practitioners and home visitors; rather, they are central to it. Workforce education, training, and supervision should reflect these realities.

▲▲▲▲▲▲▲▲   QUESTIONS FOR CLINICIANS   ▲▲▲▲▲▲▲▲

▶ In thinking about your practice and caseload, do you see signs of significant emotional distress and/or psychopathology in the parents you're working with?

▶ To what extent are parents' mental health challenges affecting your work?

▶ Are you able to create a therapeutic space?

▶ Are you comfortable making assessments and evaluating prior diagnoses?

▶ Do you have the supervisory support you need to do so?

▶ Are there ways you can address the parents' difficulties within the framework of your work with them?

▶ Do you have mental health consultation available to you?

▶ Are there mental health providers within your community whom you can reliably collaborate with if outside referrals are necessary?

Chapter

13

Clinical Applications of the Pregnancy and Parent Development Interviews

As we described in Chapter 3, the Pregnancy Interview (PI) and Parent Development Interview (PDI) were developed to help us better understand parents' experience of pregnancy and early parenthood. Most published work focuses on the use of these instruments in research,[1] and indeed we used these interviews to assess PRF at the beginning and end of the MTB-HV intervention (Sadler et al., 2013; Slade et al., 2019). Aside from their utility in research and evaluation, many practitioners find them of great use in clinical practice. Part of the interviews' power is their sustained focus on both the parent's and child's emotional experience: Parents are asked again and again about the parent–child relationship, as well as a range of affects across a range of situations. The process of responding triggers both episodic memories and semantic generalizations (Main et al., 1985), activating both the attachment and the caregiving systems. The result is that strong affects and/or the defenses that are used to manage them are revealed. As such, we can hear in parents' responses their strengths, areas of fragility, potential ports of entry, and openness to change.

We begin this chapter[2] with a description of the interviews and a discussion of their integration into clinical practice. We then focus on (1) markers

[1] For information on how to obtain training in coding PRF on the PI or PDI for research, go to *www.pditraininginstitute.com*.

[2] We thank Jeppe Budde, Anne Corlin, and the "B5 group"—Jessie Borelli, Danielle Farrell, Marjo Flykt, Sanna Isosävi, Ruth Paris, Michelle Sleed, Ann Stacks, and Kristyn Wong—for their thoughtful and incisive comments on an earlier version of this chapter.

of mentalizing in parent narratives, (2) markers that parents are struggling to mentalize, and (3) markers of the quality of parental representations: affect quality, view of the child, and view of the self as parent. Finally, we consider the clinician's (or coder's) response to the parent. As we make clear, these domains are not mutually exclusive but rather provide a series of overlapping frames for thinking about clinical material. As such, they are meant as a guide for clinical listening and formulation, pointing the clinician to areas that need particular attention and that can be built upon, strengthened, and leveraged for change. In Chapters 14–16, we include discussion of material from both the PI and PDI in our case studies of Brenda, Yolanda, and Genevieve.

The Pregnancy Interview

The PI (see Appendix A) was developed in 1987 (Slade et al., 1987) and later adapted and revised in 2003 (Slade, 2003). The current version has 24 questions, many of which have follow-up probes. The primary areas explored in the interview are (1) the emotional experience of pregnancy, (2) preparedness for the baby, (3) feelings of connection to the child, and (4) imagining the future with the child. In developing the interview, we wanted to learn about how parents' capacity to manage the complex emotions of pregnancy and the transition to parenthood. As such, it provides a means to evaluating parents' capacity to reflect on their own and others' mental states, to imagine the baby's experience, to develop a relationship with the unborn child, and to envision the baby after birth. The interview has been adapted for use with fathers (FaPI; Slade, 2017).

The Parent Development Interview

The PDI was initially developed in 1985 (Aber et al., 1985). Twenty years later it was adapted and revised (PDI-R; Slade et al., 2004a). There are currently two versions in use: PDI–Full, which has 39 questions, and PDI–Short, which has 29 questions (see Appendix II). The primary areas explored in the interview are the (1) parent's representations of the relationship, (2) parent's representation of the child, (3) parent's representation of the self-as-parent, (4) child's response to separations and parental unavailability, and (5) intergenerational factors. In 2018, Sleed and her colleagues conducted a large-scale validation study of the psychometric properties of PDI-RF ratings across a large sample ($N = 323$) that included mothers from a normative community sample, a clinical sample, and a sample of mothers residing in prison with their babies (Sleed et al., 2018). The PDI has been adapted for use with a range of populations over the years: parents of adopted children (Steele et al., 2009), children with learning disabilities (Ilardi, 2010), children with autistic spectrum disorder (Enav, 2020), and children with physical disabilities (Steinberg & Pianta, 2006). The PDI has also been used in studies of teenage parents (Sadler et al., 2013; Slade et al., 2019), incarcerated parents (Sleed et al., 2018), parents with substance use disorders (Suchman et al., 2010, 2011), and parents living in a war zone (Isosävi et al., 2020).

Administering the PI and PDI

Administration Guidelines

Parents generally enjoy taking both the PI and PDI. Although there are some circumstances in which this is not the case (e.g., when custody is at issue, or when there are other sources of anxiety about being evaluated), most parents welcome the opportunity to talk about the child and about their experience of parenthood. Becoming a parent takes up enormous amounts of emotional and physical energy and changes one's life in such profound ways, and yet it is rare to be invited to talk freely and in depth about these experiences.

Although the interviews have a specified format, they are *clinical* interviews and should be administered in a way that is conversational and indicates that the interviewer is truly *listening* to the parent. This may seem self-evident, but in our experience, it bears repeating. The interviewer (who is in many instances the clinician working with the family) should do their best to create an atmosphere of safety and trust and to communicate warmth and interest. They should keep track of what the parent has already said. For example, an interviewer might say, "*I know you've talked about this a little already, but . . .*", when a question covers ground that the parent has already addressed. It is also important that the interviewer be careful not to impose their own way of thinking and understanding on the interviewee. The goal is to know how *the parents* see the child and themselves as parents. So often clinicians say things like, "*What I hear you saying is . . .*", reading between the lines, picking up on unstated thoughts and feelings, but it's best to stay with the parents' words and not make formulations during the course of the interview. It is also best to stay close to the language of the individual interview items, although there may be times when restating a question is, in fact, necessary—for example, when a parent's level of language comprehension requires it, or when the parent obviously doesn't understand what is being asked. It is also important to encourage a parent to expand on their answers when the meaning or circumstances are not clear; in our training sessions, we often make the point that "tell me more" are three of the most valuable words in an interviewer's lexicon. Extremely voluble parents need few such invitations, however, and may in fact need a gentle reminder to move to the next question. It is also important not to badger parents who are withdrawn and shut down, as they will often feel pressured and annoyed by repeated requests to elaborate on their answers. These basic clinical interviewing skills are essential if one wishes to get as "true" a sense of the parent as possible.

Recording the PI and PDI

It is often very useful to record interviews when possible, even when they are not being used for research. This allows clinicians to review the material on their own, as well as with supervisors and other consultants. Both can be enormously helpful. Although an ultimate goal is to train clinicians to *hear* the dimensions described below while simply listening to a parent, there are often so many things going on during an interview that having a record to review later can be enormously valuable and really deepen the work. Transcription is, of course, also very helpful in reviewing transcripts, but it is often costly and certainly not critical.

If interviews are being recorded, the parent's consent must be obtained. It is also very important to discuss the purpose of the recording with the parent. They may have many concerns about how recordings will be used, whether there is some "other" purpose to them (particularly if they have had any involvement with the law or child protection), and whether their privacy will be maintained. It is obviously important to allay these concerns as much as possible, and—when this is not possible—to graciously accept their decision to not be recorded. We would advise taking notes in such situations if parents will permit it.

Timing: When to Give the PI and PDI

We recommend giving the PI toward the end of the second or into the third trimester of pregnancy. Before 20–24 weeks, it is difficult to evaluate the parent's experience of impending parenthood; likewise, the parent's representation of the baby has yet to be developed and articulated. Once the birth is within sight and the press of reality is unavoidable, however, interviews are typically quite rich and clinically meaningful. The PDI, by contrast, can be given at any point after the child is born,[3] although, as Sleed and her colleagues (2018) point out, assessments made before the

---

[3] As we described in Chapter 4, the PDI has been used in research with parents of children up through adolescence. Here we focus primarily on its use with parents of children age 3 and under.

child is 2 months old tend to be less predictive of later outcomes.[4] Up until then, the parent is still just beginning to know the child, and it is hard to get any real sense of the relationship or how the parent might fare once things settle down a bit.

Aside from the question of the age of the child, the larger question is *when* in the course of treatment to administer the interview. This depends entirely on the context in which the interview is being used. It can be very helpful to administer the PDI as part of an intake process, that is, at the start of either a dyadic intervention (such as COS,[5] CPP, IPP) or a parent-focused intervention. It can also be given to a parent whose child is beginning individual psychotherapy; this provides the child's therapist with important insight into the parent's reflective capacities, as well as the quality of their representations of the child. Just taking the interview can be a kind of intervention; the parent may understand things in a new way, or struggle in ways they find illuminating. Administration at any point allows the clinician to evaluate strengths, as well as areas of pressing clinical need. One argument for giving it early in a treatment process is that taking the PDI can be a very powerful experience, one that bonds the parent to the clinician: *"I told you my story, and you heard me."* This positive valence can be of great value clinically.

If it is not administered at intake, the PDI can be given when the clinician wants to deepen their general understanding of a parent and the parent–child relationship. Although there may be good reason to test outcomes by giving the interview twice over the course of a treatment, we do not suggest giving it repeatedly. It is a substantial interview that evaluates—if you will—deep structures, and unless a parent has been in a fairly lengthy intervention (i.e., one that lasts at least 6 months and involves regular and ongoing meetings), one would not necessarily expect to see changes in its primary dimensions. And if given too often, it might well feel intrusive.

Finally, the PDI can be used *as part of* a stand-alone evaluation of a parent. For example, the PDI has been administered at the Anna Freud Centre as part of a broad and comprehensive evaluation regarding child placement and custody. Because neither the PDI nor the PI was designed for such purposes, however, they should never be used to make such decisions without supporting evidence from a range of other measures. They should always be one among many assessments in such complex and difficult

---

[4]Megan Chapman and Campbell Paul (Chapman, 2021; Chapman & Paul, 2016) have used the interviews with parents whose babies are in the neonatal ICU, with very interesting results.

[5]The Circle of Security Interview, which is administered to parents at the start of the COS intervention, is, in fact, an adaptation of the PDI (Powell et al., 2013).

situations. Nevertheless, they may well offer another and helpful view of the parent and their capacities.

Domains of Assessment

In the following sections, we describe various broad frames or domains for listening to or reading PIs and PDIs. The first domain is mentalizing: Is the parent capable of mentalizing, and if so, in what circumstances? When does mentalizing break down, and/or when is it absent altogether? The second domain is the quality of representations: What is their affective quality? How does the parent represent the child or themselves as a parent? And, finally, what is the clinician's (or interviewer's) response to the material presented in the PI or PDI? Each provides a particular framework that allows practitioners to identify areas of distress and clinical need and to listen for areas of conflict and "trouble." Both interviews can also be used to identify strengths that can be leveraged for change and growth. Once again, these are not distinct dimensions; rather, there is often considerable and important overlap between them. We wish to acknowledge here the work of Michelle Sleed and her colleagues (Sleed et al., 2021), whose system for the Assessment of Representational Risk (ARR) heavily influenced our thinking about the issues discussed in this chapter. The ARR system—which codifies many of the dimensions described herein—is used to score PDIs for clinical signs of representational risk. As such, it is a particularly useful adjunct to the PDI-RF coding described in Chapter 4.

Mentalizing Capacities

In this section, we focus specifically on how to listen for a parent's mentalizing capacities and/or their dissolution or absence during an interview. We begin by considering the degree to which they are able to give voice to thoughts and feelings. As we described in Chapter 4, this is not a mark of being able to mentalize; rather, it indicates that a parent has the requisite awareness of internal experience that underlies the three markers of PRF, namely, their understanding of the nature of mental states, the link between behavior and mental states, and the developmental or intergenerational nature of mental states.

A Language for Thoughts and Feelings

PRF on the PI and PDI is conceptualized as falling along a continuum from low to high (Slade, 2005; Slade et al., 2004b).

Parental Reflective Functioning Scale (PRFS)

Prementalizing

−1 Bizarre, hostile, or negative RF

1 Disavowed or absent mental states

The Foundations of Parental Reflective Functioning

3 Identifying thoughts and feelings

Parental Reflective Functioning

5 Average RF; reflecting on thoughts and feelings and their link to behavior

7 Complex or sophisticated RF

9 Exceptional RF

The first thing we look for in evaluating a parent's capacity to reflect is the use of words that connote an awareness of basic mental states, namely, thoughts, feelings, and intentions (Level 3). These are foundational to mentalizing. Do they use feeling words (e.g., *sad, happy, frightened*) or cognitions (e.g., *know, want, think*) to describe their own or the child's experience? The use of these words in a meaningful way indicates that a parent has begun to identify *subjective* experience; they are interested in what's *inside* and are beginning to recognize its importance. It is important to note that parents can, at times, *seem* to be describing feelings or thoughts, but a closer look reveals little true awareness of internal processes. For example, a father can say something like "*He just wants what he wants when he wants it.*" Although he is using the word *want*, he is likely not really thinking about the child's wishes; rather, the use of the term *want* seems more about behavior than a mental state. Likewise, a parent can use the words *I think* in a reflexive way—for example, they might say, "I don't think so," without any real evidence of *thinking*. These are, if you will, "throwaway" uses of mental state terms.

Words that describe feelings and thoughts are quite different in meaning, function, and valence from more behavioral terms. For example, a father might say, "*I'm a pretty laid-back parent, I don't get upset about very much.*" Here the father is using behavioral terms, which—although not troubling—tell us little about what is going on inside of him. Or, when asked to describe her child, a mother might reply, "*I think she's pretty cute . . . and she's nice.*" Even though the affective valence is positive, the mother is not describing anything internal to the child or to herself. Often clinicians mistake pleasing descriptions of the child (*"She's such a sweetheart"* or "*We have so much fun together"*) for reflective statements. Although, as we discuss later, affective tone is certainly important, it is not an indication of mentalizing. Neither of these examples—though benign—suggests that the parent is capable of reflecting. By contrast, a parent who says, *"I am just so excited about having this baby," "I love her so much," "She gets mad when I don't feed her on time,"* or *"I've been feeling so sad"* is able to recognize emotions and thoughts in the child or in themselves. These are the essential foundations of a mentalizing stance, though—as we noted earlier—not, per se, evidence of mentalizing or reflection. Clinicians often mistake the identification of internal states as evidence that a parent is mentalizing. Although these foundations (which Meins et al., 2001, would describe as mind-mindedness) are essential to its evolution, full PRF is more complex and dynamic and requires the capacity to reason about and make meaning of mental states.

The Three Markers of PRF

There are three clear markers for the emergence of PRF (Levels 5 and above), any of which signal that the parent is capable—at least in that moment—of making meaning of psychological experience. These are understanding (1) the nature of mental states, (2) the relationship between mental states and behavior, and (3) the developmental aspects of mental states. In order to describe a parent (or clinician, for that matter) as "reflective," one or more of these markers should be present in a fairly sustained way. But until they are sustained, and not—as we discuss in the following sections—"spoiled," we cannot really describe a parent as "reflective." Nevertheless, no matter how transient they are, we affirm these moments, support them, and invite the parent to expand on them.

Across all types of mentalizing, we look for the parent's curiosity about and interest in the child's experience or in their own motivations and actions: *"What's going on with you? With me?"* The parent is not certain; they wonder, they don't assume, they want to figure it out. We have described this mentalizing stance in previous chapters, and we can see it in PIs and PDIs, too. Often it is evident in a moment of "freshness," when a parent seems to figure something out for the first time, or in a moment of confusion giving way to clarity. It can also be evident in the parent's pleasure in making sense of the child, their delight in realizing that their efforts have led to increased closeness and intimacy.

UNDERSTANDING THE NATURE OF MENTAL STATES

Mental states, that is, thoughts, feelings, desires, and intentions, have various qualities. They are often opaque; rarely are our own or another's thoughts or feelings completely transparent. To get to know someone, we have to work to make sense of them, to guess at what they are feeling and try out various possibilities. We have to be curious. Some parents easily recognize that they cannot be certain about the child's internal experience: *"I'm not sure if that made him mad, but I think so."* *"Well, in a vague sort of way it probably makes her, you know, uncomfortable, I'm not sure exactly how."* Mental states can also be disguised. For example, when given a gift they don't actually like, the recipient proclaims, believably, *"Oh, I love this!"* And certain mental states are expectable or normative in certain circumstances. Thus a child's anxiety on the 1st day of school or before a visit to the doctor is to be expected. Finally, one mental state can be used to suppress or defend against another: *"Whenever we talk about that day, Miguel remembers the ice cream we had to celebrate his getting his tonsils out, and not the pain he felt when he woke up from the anesthesia. He seems to have pushed that all away!"*

UNDERSTANDING THE RELATIONSHIP BETWEEN MENTAL STATES AND BEHAVIOR

The second marker is the ability to see that thoughts and feelings can affect both behavior and other thoughts and feelings. At the most basic level, reflective parents understand that a child's behavior is meaningfully tied to underlying mental states. Thus, for example, a father understands that his daughter is crying and clinging because she hates it when she sees his suitcase and knows he is leaving for a work trip. Or a mother understands that her son is climbing out of bed and waking her up at night because he saw his dad hit her in a fight. Seeing behavior as *meaningful* is a radical shift from focusing on the behavior itself (getting the child to stop crying, stay out of the parental bed, etc.) rather than the feeling driving it. This awareness allows the parent to address the feelings and thus regulate the child. For example, *"I'm sorry, honey, but I'll be back in three sleeps! And I'll call you every night,"* or *"I know that was a scary fight you saw with Dad, but I'm OK and Dad's OK. He's still got to calm down a little. He went to Grandma's to sleep, but soon he'll come see us."*

PRF is also manifest in the parent's awareness of the separateness of minds and the dynamic relationship between one mind and another. The child and parent may have different perspectives on things. As Dr. Seuss put it in *Horton Hears a Who* (1954): "A person's a person, no matter how small." For example, the child might see the giant mud puddle as an opportunity for splashing and fun, whereas the mother might see it as a giant mess; their subjective experiences are potentially quite different. Reflective parents can also appreciate the fact that they (or the child) may have opposing thoughts and feelings (e.g., *"I love her independence, but I desperately miss her cuddliness and baby-ness"*) or that their thoughts and feelings will affect the child, and vice versa (e.g., *"I think maybe that because I was so unsure of myself and so afraid of really setting a limit with him, he picked up on it and kind of knew that if he just kept crying out for me to come take him out of his crib and let him sleep with us, I would."*). Here, the mother is acknowledging the impact of her insecurity on the child, as well as the impact of his unhappiness on her.

UNDERSTANDING THE DEVELOPMENTAL ASPECTS OF MENTAL STATES

There are many developmental aspects of mental states. They can change over time; sometimes they build and sometimes they lessen. Rarely does any emotion last at full intensity for a long time. Rather, it has an arc. Charlene, mother of a 10-month-old girl, clearly understands this: *"Sometimes she'll want to do something and I won't let her because it's dangerous, so she'll get angry. I may try to pick her up and she obviously didn't want to be picked up because she's in the middle of being angry and I interrupted her."* Charlene understands that her daughter not only is angry but is *in the process* of expressing her anger and getting through it; it can't just be shut down.

Mental states can also morph into other mental states over time. A loss can trigger sadness that then shifts into anger at being abandoned. Mental states are—by definition—dynamic rather than absolute. Along these same lines, mental states change over the course of development. A child's trepidation at the 1st day of school will shift as the child becomes more comfortable and familiar with their peers; what was a scary place full of strangers becomes a welcome joy. For a parent, understanding this can be so important. Nothing lasts forever, including the worst tantrums, and—sadly—the moments of sheer delight. But both will give rise to something new.

Ideally, these various capacities help the parent figure out who the child is and how their mind works; the parent has a model of the child's mind *in mind*. The child makes sense to the parent, and this understanding guides their response to the child (e.g., *"She has a really tough time with transitions because she doesn't know what to expect next, so we have to make sure she understands what's happening way in advance."*). In some instances, however, isolated bits of what appear to be mentalizing do not coalesce into a real sense of who the child is and how they are likely to respond across a range of situations. Thus *"my child hates transitions"* would signify a larger model of the child's mind only if the mother then described trying to figure out how to help the child manage transitions. Thus, unless we see evidence that a parent has a model of the child's mind that guides their behavior toward the child (as in the previous example), we should be cautious about thinking of the parent as reflective. PRF is only useful if it really guides the parent in their responses to and interaction with the child. Finally, mental states can have intergenerational effects. *"I think my grandmother always thought my mother was coming up short and was always disappointed in her. I had the same feeling when I was growing up: I could never do enough to make her approve of me. I was always doing everything but falling short. If my mother had felt better about herself, she might have been able to feel better about me."* This mother is tracking the transmission of mental states across generations.

The PI and PDI ask the parent to consider themselves, the child, and the emerging relationship from a number of vantage points. Some parents' mentalizing capacities are robust and stable across a range of contexts, although moments of instability are common and expectable (after all, parenting is a very high-stress endeavor, and some "trouble" is normal!). For others, the struggle to mentalize is far more tangible. Sometimes it shows up in more limited ways; in others, it pervades the entire interview. In the following section, we consider some of these variations and their particular manifestations.

Mentalizing Difficulties

Many of the parents we see clinically come to us, at least in part, because they have difficulty mentalizing. Thus we watch for areas in which a parent cannot mentalize or for signs that mentalizing processes break down or collapse under stress or distress. The clinician's work is to identify the nature and source of impaired mentalization and to work from there. To focus too much on PRF is to miss signs of its absence, which is where the clinical work really begins.

The forms of prementalizing we discussed in Chapter 5—overregulation (suppressing feelings), underregulation (being flooded with feelings), and dysregulation (freezing or becoming disoriented and dissociated)—are all signs that mentalization, at least in that moment, is failing, that the more primitive parts of the emotional brain are in charge. In reading a transcript line by line, we can often see the shift into flight, fight, or freezing from one line to the next. We can see a parent struggling to maintain their balance and perspective or falling into confusion and disorientation. Sometimes parents tend toward one or the other mode; some fluctuate between the two; and in some cases the parent's narratives break down altogether.

Difficulties in mentalizing are often manifest in various forms of what Mary Main and her colleagues described as "narrative incoherence." The assessment of coherence is central to a variety of coding systems, including the AAI classification system (Main et al., 1985), the system for coding RF on the PDI (Slade et al., 2004b), the ARR system (Sleed et al., 2021), and the Working Model of the Child Interview (WMCI) coding system (Zeanah et al., 1994). The reason for this is simple: When an individual's story "breaks down," when they lose the thread, contradict themselves, oscillate between points of view, or just stop making sense, *something* is going on. At times it is a struggle *not* to see, *not* to tell, *not* to feel or express thoughts and feelings that are experienced as dangerous, uncontained, or unregulated; in these instances, we see defenses hard at work (Bowlby, 1979; Main et al., 1985; Slade, 2000). At other times, the narrative is fragmented by raw affect. Here, defensive processes have failed. In either instance, the parent is unable to *monitor* (Main, 1991) their discourse or mentalize the breadth of emotional experience. A related way of thinking about this is that incoherence reflects a breakdown in higher level cortical functioning, with more raw, automatic "gut" responses of the emotional centers of the brain prevailing. This means that—from a clinical standpoint—disruptions in an individual's effort to tell their story are very meaningful and inevitably signal the need to look deeper: What is going on? Why has the speaker become incoherent at this particular point? Incoherence comes in many forms. As we describe later, incoherence sometimes signals avoidance of strong affect and at other times the relative failure to contain strong affect.

In the following section, we describe some of the mentalizing breakdowns we see when parents tend toward a concrete mentalizing mode or an intrusive one.

Concrete Mode

THE ABSENCE OF MENTAL STATE LANGUAGE

Some parents show little evidence of mentalization whatsoever and seem literally *unable* to attribute thoughts or feelings to themselves or the child. They have little language for mental states or mental experience; it is as if, when asked about their own or the child's experience, they keep coming up empty, choosing bland generalizations (e.g., "Fine") or simply answering "I don't know" when asked directly about affect. At the extreme, we see such difficulties in individuals with autistic spectrum disorders or cognitive impairments or who have been exposed to extreme deprivation or neglect. In these circumstances, interventions tailored to enhancing mentalization are unlikely to be successful. Rather, more concrete approaches will be required for some time.

DENIAL AND AVOIDANCE

In some parents, the relative absence of a language for thoughts and feelings reflects defensive efforts to push aside more difficult or painful emotional experiences. This can manifest in a kind of vague, nonspecific description of mental states, as in the following transcripts. The vague use of positive terms and the denial of negative affect in both transcripts actually reveal little about either mother's experience.

Here is an excerpt from the PI of a pregnant teenager. The mother, Gail, is 18 years old and 32 weeks pregnant.

INTERVIEWER: Pregnancy is usually a pretty complicated time in terms of feelings and ups and downs; let's start with the good feelings. What are some of the good feelings you've had during your pregnancy?

GAIL: (*long pause*) Um. . . . well I was happy to know that you're gonna have a baby . . . don't really know. . . .

INTERVIEWER: Have you had any more good feelings during your pregnancy, you're saying you were happy?

GAIL: Yeah . . . well, that is just a good feeling, isn't it . . . being happy (*laughs*).

INTERVIEWER: Can you think of a time when you felt happy, can you tell me about that time?

GAIL: I'm usually happy all the time anyway (*laughs*). Um . . . I dunno . . . I dunno (*laughs*).

INTERVIEWER: Take your time, just if there was a time . . . when you felt happy?

GAIL: When we went for the ultrasound, that was good, the first one because we went at 16 weeks because they didn't give us one at 12 weeks . . . yeah. . . .

INTERVIEWER: Why do you think you felt happy?

GAIL: Don't know, because it [was] realer then, like more real then. . . .

INTERVIEWER: OK. Have you had any hard or difficult feelings during your pregnancy?

GAIL: No. . . .

INTERVIEWER: No hard or difficult feelings during pregnancy?

GAIL: No . . . only that I'm getting stretch marks (*laughs*) and that's about it.

INTERVIEWER: OK, have you had any worries about the baby?

GAIL: No.

INTERVIEWER: Eh, have you had any worries about the baby or about how you would manage once the baby's here?

GAIL: No, I don't think so, I think I'll be fine.

INTERVIEWER: Or even in terms of like getting help with the baby, or financially or any kind of other circumstances you might be worried about?

GAIL: Don't think so . . . I'm not really a thinker (*laughs*).

Gail uses the word *happy* to describe herself again and again but nevertheless fails to convey any real sense of her internal experience and consistently denies negative affect. The passage ends with her remarking "I'm not really a thinker." This is quite striking and speaks to a real lack of access to her inner life.

Here is a passage from Ellie, the mother of a 9-month-old. Again, the "positive" tone ("*It's made me a better person*," "*Fine*," "*Good*") belies any genuine interest in her own or the child's experience, and again she denies any negative affect.

INTERVIEWER: And how has having Sofia changed you?

ELLIE: Um, it's made me become a better person. Some, made me grow up more. And, um, yeah.

INTERVIEWER: And do you ever feel really angry as a parent?

ELLIE: No.

INTERVIEWER: Do you ever feel really guilty as a parent?

ELLIE: Mm–mm [no].

INTERVIEWER: And, um, when Sofia's upset, what does she do?

ELLIE: Um, cries (*laughs*).

INTERVIEWER: How does it make you feel?

ELLIE: No way.

INTERVIEWER: And what do you do?

ELLIE: I just, um, turn to her.

INTERVIEWER: And does she ever feel rejected?

ELLIE: No.

INTERVIEWER: And when does Sofia need attention from you?

ELLIE: When she's hungry. She just fishes here (*gesturing to her breasts*). That means when she's hungry.

INTERVIEWER: And how do you feel?

ELLIE: Um, fine. I just give her, I feed her.

INTERVIEWER: And why do you think it's those times specifically that she needs help from you?

ELLIE: 'Cause she's hungry. (*Laughs.*)

Gail and Ellie deny even the most normal anxieties and instead opt for a kind of bland idealization that seems designed to avoid any deeper inquiry. As we show later in the chapter, idealization can function in other ways as well.

NEGATION

A parent's efforts to mute any discussion of complex or negative feelings can also manifest in negation, which reveals feelings or fears the parent does not wish to state directly.

INTERVIEWER: How did you feel when you found out you were pregnant?

BRIANNA: I was really happy and excited.

INTERVIEWER: Why do you think you reacted that way?

BRIANNA: Because we planned it, our baby wasn't not planned it was planned.

Here there is but a brief linguistic hiccup. "Wasn't not planned" is a double negative, leaving the reader to wonder whether Brianna might have, in fact, had mixed feelings about finding out she was pregnant. Indeed, she had taken four pregnancy tests before she "really believed" she was pregnant. The reader might also wonder whether Brianna felt shame in revealing an accidental pregnancy to the interviewer.

In the following passage, Nina seems to be trying very hard to suppress her feelings that her daughter is demanding, describing her child's positive qualities in the negative.

INTERVIEWER: Can you describe your child to me?

NINA: Um, I'd say pretty . . . a very good disposition, calm, not very excitable . . . I'd say she's very good for a baby.

INTERVIEWER: Uh-huh, what do you mean by very good?

NINA: Very good is she's not cranky a lot, it's not like she never wants to sleep, she's not always, you know, whining, she's pretty . . . you know, doesn't. . . . I mean she's demanding because any baby's demanding—

INTERVIEWER: Right.

NINA: —but she's not a hard baby.

INTERVIEWER: Right, how is she demanding?

NINA: Just because it takes, you, you have to spend every minute that she's awake, you really have to spend with her, being attentive to her.

SHIFT IN VOICE

Another common manifestation of an attempt to avoid talking about strong feelings is a shift in voice, typically from the first ("I") to the second ("you") person. This often occurs when a parent wants to put distance between themselves and feelings they are uncomfortable with; the shift in voice takes it out of the realm of "I" am feeling something, to "everybody" feels this.

> INTERVIEWER: Have you had feelings of just feeling needy or unsupported during your pregnancy?
>
> STELLA: Yeah, I think that's very common, though. There's, there's periods where you go through, where all of a sudden you feel incredibly dependent and you fear that your husband is going to die or to leave you or what are you going to do, uh, you know. And um, because of uh, there's a lot of that is not understood emotionally, there's not a lot of reading you can do or your husband can do to support you.

Here the mother is trying to minimize or normalize (and thus defend against) what sound like episodes of feeling utterly overwhelmed and terrified.

Intrusive–Hostile Mode

As we described in Chapter 5, whereas some parents attribute few thoughts or feelings to themselves or their children, others seem unable to see the child outside of their own thoughts and feelings. Often these are hostile projections, but we also see parents who are overly certain about the child's mental states or who see the child and/or themselves as utterly helpless, or who idealize the child at the expense of seeing the child in any holistic way. Thus, in contrast to the effort to defend *against* an awareness of mental states, this dimension reflects the press of thoughts and feelings that inherently make it difficult for the parent to see the child as a separate person.

HOSTILE–HELPLESS REPRESENTATIONS

Hostile mentalizing refers to moments in an interview when the parent attributes negative or malevolent intent to the child in the absence of any evidence that this is warranted (Lyons-Ruth et al., 2005; Terry et al., 2021). Luyten and Fonagy (2015) refer to this as negative automatic mentalizing; thus, when asked to imagine what the child is thinking or feeling, the parent's response is biased toward assuming the child's intent is hostile, and they seem unable or unwilling to see the child apart from their own projections. For someone prone to hostile or intrusive mentalizing, the world and the people in it are viewed as threatening and hostile.

The following is a transcript of Anjelica's responses to the opening questions of the PDI. Her child, Timmy, is 2 months old.

INTERVIEWER: Could you pick three words for me that describe your son?

ANJELICA: He's angry definitely.

INTERVIEWER: Hungry? Oh, angry.

ANJELICA: An-angry, an angry person.

INTERVIEWER: Okay. Why did you choose angry first of all, are there any examples or incid–?

ANJELICA: Angry because if he doesn't get what, uhh, he's feeding-time, he screams, he wants to, he wants to play. He has to be fed on time. So, that, that makes me angry, I feed him on time and even more it's just keep, keep him quiet for a while. That's how a lot of people describe him, he's an angry baby.

INTERVIEWER: Really?

ANJELICA: Yes, cuz he was born with a frown, when he was born.

INTERVIEWER: And what do you like least about him?

ANJELICA: Crying. (*Laughs.*) He just won't stop crying. When he cries I just want him to stop crying and I hate that point when he uses, when he uses my breast as a pacifier. He doesn't take a pacifier; I have to force him to take a pacifier. He just wants to fall asleep on my breast. He doesn't suckle, he just keeps it there. Like a pacifier. That's what I hate about him. To be honest, that's the least of it. Right now, he's hungry and he's fed, he's not hungry, I know he's not hungry; he just uses it as a pacifier now, just to fall asleep.

Admittedly, this is an extreme example, and exchanges like this would raise red flags for any practitioner, and particularly the possibility that the mother is psychotic. This is a dire situation that would require immediate attention. But let's deconstruct this passage a bit. To begin, Anjelica is not seeing her baby realistically. She has no sense of him or his needs. Her sense of him is dominated by her projected hostility, which overwhelms her experience of even the most mundane interactions. As such, she regards normative (and potentially quite pleasing) behaviors, such as the baby lying on her breast, as intrusive and invasive. Obviously, Anjelica's anger predates Timmy's birth and predates any actual experiences she might have had with him, but she seems to be using her conviction that he is angry and demanding as grounds for all of her own negative feelings toward him. It is so easy to imagine that—unless addressed—this essential antagonism will doom this child and this relationship.

Whereas Anjelica's conviction that her son is angry legitimizes her own anger, many parents have a more helpless reaction to the hostility they project into the child. For instance, a mother might say, *"He's just so angry.*

I don't know what to do. He's so fierce, and I feel he just wants to finish me off and destroy me. I can't cope. I just let him have his way." In this instance, the mother's perception of her child as aggressive terrifies her. By contrasts, Anjelica sees herself as a victim of her angry child, and yet she expresses her helplessness in rage. Hostility and helplessness are often two sides of the same coin (Lyons-Ruth et al., 1999a).

CERTAINTY

This is often another form of hostile–intrusive mentalizing. The preceding passage contains many examples of this, with Anjelica believing that she *knows* what her child is feeling. She is certain he is angry; there is no curiosity whatsoever. As a result, she feels assaulted by Timmy, which in turn justifies her feelings of hatred and rage toward him. It also sets up a power struggle, such that the mother sees herself as having to *submit* to the baby. This stance gives little room for learning about the other, for dialogue or discovery. And it can feel very intrusive and aversive to the child.

IDEALIZATION

This form of intrusive mentalizing can manifest itself in many ways. On the one hand, bland idealizations like those in the transcripts of Gail and Ellie above ("happy," "fine") are often efforts at denial. But some idealizations feel as if the parent's insistence that the child is "perfect" functions to negate any awareness of the child's actual experience.

In the following transcript, the mother's idealization stems from an earlier loss.

> INTERVIEWER: Yes, I see. What do you like most about Duane?
>
> DIDI: Everything. Yeah, I can't pick. I don't like to pick that I like this or like that, cause if I pick then I'm saying, "I don't like this about him or not." I mean if I like everything then there's no final picking which ones I like.
>
> INTERVIEWER: And what do you like least about him?
>
> DIDI: Nothing, I'm just enjoying my time with him, the time that I've got, 'cause you never know tomorrow, so. . . . I don't like to think I don't like anything about him. If he was five or something or six, seven, eight, then I can say what I don't like. . . . But even if he does something wrong, he's just learning. So, it's nothing bad, it's just (*inaudible*) in there. Doesn't know how to do it or not to do it.
>
> INTERVIEWER: OK, and could you choose three words for me again, this time words that reflect the relationship between you and Duane, the sort of relationship the two of you have?

DIDI: Special . . . and I don't know, love. Um, I don't know (*inaudible*). The love's covered everything. . . .

INTERVIEWER: That's OK, we'll just have those two. Um, special, why did you choose that, are there any examples or things that come to mind?

DIDI: Um, special, he is special. (*Laughs.*) He's the boy that I lost, so he is special to me, he's everything. I always look at him like that, you know, I don't know that's a special (inaudible) that God gave me another boy, so he's a special thing to me.

INTERVIEWER: So, he has replaced your last baby?

DIDI: Yeah, I think that. Even though, like, even though still that's on my mind, but at least I feel I'm given the chance to have a boy. That's a special thing to me.

INTERVIEWER: Yeah, OK. And love, why did you choose that to describe your relationship?

DIDI: I don't know, I just love him. I don't know. I don't know, I just love him. I don't know.

Sometimes idealization can feel brittle and fragile, as if they would shatter if pushed. Here we can sense the mother's desperate efforts *not* to talk about any difficulty; in so doing, the baby's individuality disappears. This makes him indistinguishable from her lost child, which is who she craves in her grief. At other times, idealizations can feel rigid and entrenched and as if no amount of pushing would dislodge them. Idealization is quite important clinically, for it signals the real absence of the capacity to tolerate negative feelings and can be just as significant an indicator of child abuse potential as indicators of hostility and anger toward the child (Young et al., 2018).

Other Indices of Mentalizing Difficulties

CONTRADICTION

In many instances, contradictions within an interview suggest a vacillation between avoiding and becoming overwhelmed by strong feelings. Sometimes the breaks in a parent's denial are manifest in a few sentences, and sometimes they are manifest in a sequence of responses.

INTERVIEWER: Can you pick three words to describe your relationship with your son?

DEIDRE: We're responsive, picking up on what the other wants and happy, laughing, laughter . . .

INTERVIEWER: Can you maybe now describe a time in the last week when you felt that you and Harry were clicking together? Uhm, like you were just together.

DEIDRE: Uhm. . . . Yes, yesterday, uhm. . . . He wanted to look out of the window, so we just stood for quite a while, quite a few minutes looking out of the window and I was just holding him on my lap, and he was very quiet, uhm, we were both just kind of occasionally pointing at things that we've seen and I'd say the words and he sort of showed me something that he was interested in. Just watching the people going by or the birds or whatever. There wasn't much kind of communication going on, but it was just very quiet and peaceful and it felt like he was really enjoying it and I was really enjoying . . . sharing what he was seeing and yeah. . . .

INTERVIEWER: How did that make you feel?

DEIDRE: Just very, very good.

INTERVIEWER: And what do you think he was thinking at that time?

DEIDRE: Uhh, how much he enjoys looking out that window, the view. . . . And, uhh . . . probably that he was really happy being held like that. He wasn't, uhm, in a hurry to get down and do something, or bored. He was quite happy to stay like that sharing his thoughts in a way.

INTERVIEWER: OK. That's lovely. Uhm, all right. So, on the opposite side: Can you now think of a time in the last week when you felt like you weren't, like you weren't clicking. Can you describe it to me?

DEIDRE: Uhm. . . . Yeah, over food. (*Laughs.*) Uhm. . . . Last week . . . I did get very frustrated with him. And I just shouted very loudly at him. Uhm. . . . He's going through the stage of, uhm, refusing everything, but then screaming 'cause he's hungry. Uhm . . . And screaming when I try to take the food away from him, but refusing to even touch it. And spitting and throwing the food and that kind of stuff. . . . And I did, uhm, slap him . . . that was definitely a bad mamma moment.

INTERVIEWER: Gosh. And how were you feeling at that time?

DEIDRE: Oh. . . . Really stressed and really angry with Harry. Because it feels like I'm putting so much . . . putting so much effort into trying to cook for him three times a day and find things that he will eat. And battling with him to even get him to touch them. And he's almost doing it deliberately to wind me up in a way. I think (*inaudible*) an anxiety thing that's going on, kind of his way of . . . getting more sort of attention is to . . . uhm, make me kind of dance attendance on him (*inaudible*).

Deidre's initially contained, measured, and generally positive descriptions of her relationship with her son contrast sharply with the descriptions of her powerful anger and loss of control. In a way that was surprising to the interviewer, Deidre's descriptions of their time together (which convey little actual sense of togetherness) give way to descriptions of dramatic trouble and conflict. Remembering the event, her defenses crumble. Incoherence is manifest in the contrast between the two opposed or incompatible representations of the relationship and reflects a struggle not to let her anger overwhelm the relationship. This struggle becomes all the more evident as the interview proceeds. This passage is also notable for its vivid negative affect; the language is extremely visceral and evocative, and one can feel the force of her anger in the very words she chooses. The last exchange, in which she describes her child as "deliberately" winding her up also provides a clear example of intrusive prementalizing, as she imagines his (presumably negative) intention to get her to "dance attendance on him."

NARRATIVE DISORGANIZATION

It is sometimes the case that, in reading or listening to a transcript, intense affect seems to overwhelm the parent to the point that the narrative becomes quite disorganized. In some instances, the parent is able to return to a mentalizing stance despite obvious moments of dissociation. In the following passage, we can see evidence of dissociation in the mother's description of a traumatic event, as well as in the telling itself. At the same time, we see her actively struggling to remain in the present, at the time of the trauma and as she retold it to the interviewer. Both dissociation and the struggle against it are tangible.

INTERVIEWER: Can you describe a time in the last week where you and Charisse weren't clicking, where you weren't on that same wavelength?

TANIA: Mm, OK. February 12th, um, my mother's brother, my mother's brother died on the same day that my son was killed in a car accident 3 years ago. OK, this past month my mother's brother just passed away, OK? He died February the 5th, my son was killed February the 5th, my uncle was buried February the 12th, my son was buried February the 12th, and they're in the same cemetery, you know, in effect they're two plots away from one another. So, um, that particular day I was having a very, very hard time getting myself together that morning, that Monday morning and I couldn't get myself together, cause it was like preparing for my son's funeral. I mean I knew this was my mom's brother, my uncle, but the only thing I could think about is my baby, Teddy, you know . . . because I'm, it was this beautiful day out, like it was, you know, and, you know, when I left out of there, I, I walked out the door and left Charisse in the house, you know, I didn't have, I had my suit on, I didn't have a pocketbook, I had slippers on, I didn't put my shoes on, because I couldn't think, you know, my mind was gone, you know, only thing I could think about, I got to go look at, you know, I'm thinking about Teddy, you know, that was it. I locked, good thing Charisse knows how to open up the door, you know, because, um, I walked out the door. My father came to get me, you know, I walked out the door, he said, "What's the matter?" I said, "Daddy, I'm having a hard time getting this together," you know. So he said, "Well come on." So now we walk off the porch, he said, "Where's the baby?" You know, I said, I said, "Look!" I says, "Look at my shoes!" You know, I have this real sharp suit on and slippers. You know, my baby's in the house, my pocketbook, my keys are in the house, you know, so he says, well, he said, "You know, maybe you shouldn't go," I said, "No, I got to go." You know. "I got to go," cause he was one of my favorite uncles, you know, I have to go, you know, but it was—

INTERVIEWER: So were you and Charisse not clicking that day?

TANIA: No, we were, you know, it seemed like she was kind of getting, she wasn't doing anything out of the ordinary, but every little thing was getting on my nerves, you know.

INTERVIEWER: So how did you feel during that? Like you say you were just kind of out of it?

TANIA: Out of it. You know, just out of it. It's like you just space out, you know, you know, you, they're talking to you, you hear them talking but you're not comprehending anything they're saying.

INTERVIEWER: How do you think she felt during that?

TANIA: Um, she knew something was wrong. And, um, it was like she was like cautious, like, you know, she like tried to stay out of the way and, um, this was one of the particular days where she was like real good, too. Quiet.

INTERVIEWER: She was real good, you said?

TANIA: Yeah, kind of quiet. You know, um, which when I yelled at her because she didn't pick up some toys, she says, "But I didn't put them there." You know, then I just realized I'm yelling at this kid for nothing. You know, so you know I had to step back and take a look at me. You know, so then finally my sister came and got her. You know.

Tania conveys both how dissociated she was on the way to her uncle's funeral *and* seems to dissociate somewhat in telling the story. At times, she seems to lose herself, as if reliving the moment. She offers a number of granular details, uses certain phrases ("February the 5th" and "February the 12th") over and over (both being forms of traumatized speech) and seems in the telling to reexperience both her disorientation and her distress at realizing she has frightened her baby. At the same time, she describes the way her own mentalizing had kicked in when she realized she has left the baby in the house unattended after scolding her for something that wasn't her fault. She was able to see her child's experience, calm down and take stock, and pull herself out of her dissociated state. The mother is also able to pull herself back from dissociating in retelling the story. At the beginning of the passage, she mentalizes the interviewer's need to understand the context for her response. She also uses the interviewer's questions as a kind of anchor. Such "aha" moments, when the parent finds their footing and sees themselves or the child in a different light, are crucial moments of therapeutic leverage. Expanding upon them becomes key to helping the parent become more regulated and more able to repair disrupted interactions.

In other instances, parents seem to lose track of the question or of the point they are trying to make. Here, Lucille's narrative becomes disorganized and confused, and the listener has to work hard to make any sense of it.

INTERVIEWER: And how do you think your relationship with him is affecting his development and his personality?

CHILD: Boy! (*Child is speaking in the background.*)

INTERVIEWER: He said "boy"!

LUCILLE: What did he say?

INTERVIEWER: It sounded like "boy."

LUCILLE: (*to child*) You said something? He says something else and then he can't say it. The only one he can say again is "bah." He used to say, "Ahoy!" Yes, it sounds like French babies do. And I don't know why he was saying that because I was not really speaking French with him and one day he started doing that. He was quite young, though. He was three or four months. Younger than babies usually start doing sounds. And he did that sound for many months until one day he found "bah" and the day he found "bah" he forgot the other. Because he couldn't repeat "ahoy" again. I would say, "ahoy" and he would say, "ahoy," and now he only does repeat "bah" but he doesn't repeat the others and he even forgot "ahoy." He looks at me like, "What's she talking about? What is that?" What was the question?

INTERVIEWER: Sorry, the question was, how do you think your relationship with him is affecting his development and his personality?

LUCILLE: Um, I don't know, but to be honest I feel a little bit guilty, like I spend too much time on the internet. I think I should be playing more with him and reading his books and doing things like this with him 'cause I think, how can he develop properly if he's sitting with his toys in his, in his rocking chair or with this, I think I should be talking more or singing him songs, ya know? I think I could be doing more, more development activities, like they say we are supposed to be doing more games and stuff. . . . Yeah, of course I feel a little bit guilty. I think, I'm not even working so I should be doing more for him, or start doing something more productive so, yeah. I don't know how this affects, but, on the other hand, he's not abandoned so that's, I mean, some babies they get very badly that their mothers put them in the child care, so they might get a lot of activities in the child care but then they are not with their mom and maybe he's benefiting a lot just being next to me. And if he cries or something, I just take care of him, so he's not like left alone crying or anything. But he doesn't like so much to be held. No. He gets up very easily.

This child is 9 months old; the mother keeps losing track of the question and veers off on a number of tangents as she responds to what is obviously a very loaded subject for her. She appears to be trying very hard not to describe neglect, although it is clear that she is leaving him to his own devices a lot of the time. It becomes evident as the interview proceeds that the child is quite delayed developmentally (which she hints at in her comments about his lack of language), making her neglect all the more concerning and the reasons behind her confusion and disorganization all the more apparent.

INSENSITIVE BEHAVIOR

A parent's report of insensitive behavior offers one of the most obvious clues that a parent's model of the child's mind is incoherent or fragmented by negative affect (Sleed et al., 2021). In the passages cited above, Lucille's neglect is obvious, and Deidre reports slapping her son in the face. Yolanda, in Chapter 15, reports leaving her child crying for over an hour without comforting him. Other instances can be more subtle: A father describes giving his young son the "silent treatment," leaving him to stew in his own unhappiness; a mother describes mocking her daughter's distress when she hurts her finger. These moments are very important indicators that—no matter how reflective a parent might seem in other ways—they are disregarding the child's experience when they respond insensitively or anomalously (Lyons-Ruth et al., 1999b) because they run counter to the parent's evolutionary role of protecting the child.

Affective Quality of Representations

The PI and PDI are often rich in affect, both positive and negative. The way these are both expressed and regulated within the narrative is, of course, inextricably linked to the capacity to mentalize. Nevertheless, it is useful to attend to the quality of expressed affect specifically.

Positive Affect

Just as we look for signs that parents can mentalize on the PDI, we also look for signs of genuine, unfettered expressions of happiness, delight, and joy. Recall that in Chapter 2 we described pleasure in connection as an essential aspect of a secure attachment relationship. One of the first mothers to ever take the PDI in the mid-1980s, Maritza's joy leaps off the page.

> INTERVIEWER: Can you choose five adjectives that reflect your relationship with Mari?
>
> MARITZA: Close, passionate, dependent, independent, terrific. Close, because I sense with her that I'm the closest person to her in the world. I probably never knew so much what was in another person's mind and understood so much another person as I do with Mari. I mean I probably never will again because a 3-year-old is more complex than a 2-year-old, and a 2-year-old usually has needs that you can reason out. I can figure out what it is that she wants, which is a wonderful feeling, so it's very close. Um, it's passionate because I just never loved anybody the way I feel about, the way I love Mari. I mean just sitting here thinking about her, I can feel tears welling up, and. . . . I lie in bed at night saying to my husband, 'Can you believe what she did today?' You know, I just can't believe it, and it's just, just a passionate kind of love, you know. I can't bear to be away from her, and I've been married for ten years, so I, you know, maybe I'll feel differently when she's ten, but I can be away from my husband for three days easier than I can be away from Mari.

Passages like these—quite coherent and full of authentic and heartfelt joy—are such important indicators of a parent's capacity to find pleasure in closeness and to experience moments free of conflict or ambivalence.

Pleasurable feelings can also temper more difficult times. In the following passage, Janie's excitement and joy about her child's upcoming arrival clearly mitigates the fear that she is also struggling with.

> INTERVIEWER: What do you think will be the hardest time in the first 6 months?
>
> JANIE: I'm not sure, probably when I first get her home, it'll be the most scariest, probably not hardest but be the most scariest—am I doing this right, am I doing that right? Even though I know my mom's there and she's had four kids and grandkids, she'll know everything, but it's just that bit of fear about her, is she all right, her breathing, when she's asleep, double-checking on her, and I think it'll be the hardest to try not to be as scared and not be as. . . . I can't think of the word, not be as frightened.
>
> INTERVIEWER: What was it like hearing the heartbeat?

JANIE: It was magical, like, yeah, it was magical, it was a miracle for me, really, it was really good. It was a good feeling.

INTERVIEWER: Would you say you have a relationship with her now?

JANIE: Yeah. I'll always talk to her and like my mom will always talk to her and say, "come out!" and like Mike will always then come and like sit down and talk to her and rub my belly. I know she can hear me, so we do talk to her quite a lot, especially when she's moving or when I get in the bath, in and out, I'll explain, "You're in the bath now," and so when I wash my belly, I'll tell her, "Oh, I'm cleaning my belly," umm, so I do have a good, like, have a relationship with her.

INTERVIEWER: What makes your relationship with her special?

JANIE: Because it's just me and her, she's like, it's special that I'm the one that's holding her 24/7, she's in my belly and she's growing off me and she listens to me and she knows everything I'm doing, she can tell when I'm upset and when I'm all right and when I'm being sick. And I can tell when she's very active, when she's not as active, and stuff, so it's like a special bond really that a mom has.

Although there is evidence of her anxiety later in the transcript, it seems clear that Janie has the capacity to experience the magic of the baby's presence, to feel powerfully connected to the fetus, and to access her own strength and the support of those around her. All of these will carry her through. For Janie, and indeed for many parents, pleasure in connection offsets or modulates the intensity and potency of the negative affects that are intrinsic to pregnancy and parenting. In this sense, the presence of genuine positive affect can serve as a protective factor against the inherent challenges of parenting.

Negative Affect

A primary sign of trouble, both in the ARR (Isosävi et al., 2020; Sleed et al., 2021) and HH (Lyons-Ruth et al., 2005; Terry et al., 2021) systems, is raw negative affect, notably fear, anger, and feelings of helplessness. As we saw in many of the passages cited earlier (e.g., Anjelica and Deidre), these can lead to affective dysregulation. Or as is the case in the following brief passage, it can break through in brief but intense surges, making it clear that intense affect lies just below the surface.

INTERVIEWER: Do you ever feel really guilty as a parent?

DIANA: A couple of times in the middle of the night when he's had a bad bout with teething and he wants to nurse a lot, he puts his little fingers in my mouth and he, I feel so guilty because all I want to do is just snap those little fingers up with my teeth, takes every ounce of control I have not to bite those little annoying fingers.

In this passage, the mother is making clear the great difficulty she is having controlling her rage. Her experience of nursing is filled with it. Although, of course, her guilt and effort to maintain control are good signs, the immediacy and power of her rage is quite evident. One could argue that there is at least a hint of mentalizing in her response (as she realizes that her feelings are making her want to bite the child's fingers), yet the intensity of her anger and her barely contained impulse to bite the child would mitigate against any of her response being indicative of reflection. It is hard to imagine that there aren't times when her rage leaks out—perhaps in rough handling, bodily tension, or "gentle" chews on the infant's fingers. All would be, of course, worrying. Sometimes breaks or disruptions in the narrative are very subtle and fleeting, and yet these are the signs that mark the way for us to explore further.

View of the Child

The nature of the parent's representation of the child is also vividly conveyed in PI and PDI transcripts. Maritza, above, describes her daughter Mari in a rich, textured way, taking pleasure in her daughter's many dimensions, her likes, her dislikes, her intensity, and her joys. When we finish reading the interview, we have a real sense of Mari and of their relationship. In the following passage, by contrast, we end up with a sense of Samantha's essentially negative representation of her unborn child. She pokes "it," shows little investment in her unborn child, and ends with the fear–certainty that the infant will be naughty and too difficult for her to raise herself. The baby will have to be disciplined by Samantha's own father.

INTERVIEWER: Would you say you have a relationship with the baby now?

SAMANTHA: (*pause*) Yeah . . . like I . . . don't really talk to it . . . I poke it a little sometimes. (*Laughs.*) I don't really talk to it.

INTERVIEWER: You don't really talk to it?

SAMANTHA: No, not really. Bobby talks to it more than me. (*Laughs.*)

INTERVIEWER: Can you think of two words to describe that relationship?

SAMANTHA: Um . . . I don't know . . . um . . . I don't know because it's not actually here . . . so . . . it feels weird just talking to my tummy . . . so, yeah, I just think it's weird talking to my tummy . . . weird. . . .

INTERVIEWER: Do you know the sex of the baby?

SAMANTHA: Yeah.

INTERVIEWER: How do you feel about it?

SAMANTHA: I don't really mind, I don't care what it is. (*Laughs.*)

INTERVIEWER: Do you have a preference either way?

SAMANTHA: No, I don't care.

INTERVIEWER: What do you try to give your baby now?

SAMANTHA: What do I give the baby now? Dunno . . . try not to annoy it too much . . . (*laughs*) or lie on it (*laughs*).

INTERVIEWER: What will your baby need from you after it's born?

SAMANTHA: I dunno. Love and food and stuff.

INTERVIEWER: How will you feel taking care of those needs?

SAMANTHA: Um . . . fine. . . . I think, yeah, I think it will [be] different when he's here 'cos I think it's weird just talking to my tummy, when he's here you realize that there is a baby. . . .

INTERVIEWER: Can you take a minute to imagine your child in the future, what kind of person do you imagine your baby's going to be?

SAMANTHA: Depends if he's naughty or not. (*Laughs.*) Eh. . . . Um . . . I'll make him get a job . . . that's it. (*Laughs.*)

INTERVIEWER: What's the ideal picture that comes to mind . . . when you imagine your child in the future?

SAMANTHA: Want him to be good, don't want him to be naughty . . . if he's naughty I won't be happy, I'll send him to live with my dad. (*Laughs.*)

In some instances, the representations are frightening and malevolent, with the parent seeing herself as a victim of the child. In Terry and her colleagues' (2021) study, "expectant mothers who received HH classifications represented themselves as malevolent and hostile, and/or frightened, helpless, or abdicating. Their fetuses were represented as hostile (e.g., as aggressors, as larger than life, as devouring of their mothers, and/or as destructive to their mothers), and/or represented as helpless or abdicating (e.g., as passive, fearful, or nonexistent)" (p. 66).

Sleed and her colleagues (2021) note that role reversal and enmeshment, as well as idealization, are signs of clinical risk, largely because the parent's view of the child is distorted. Main (Main et al., 1985; Main, 2000) described these same phenomena as signs of potential attachment insecurity. Enmeshment and role reversal both reflect some form of boundary dissolution, a failure to see that the child's thoughts and feelings and expectations may be different from the parent's. A mother might, for instance, insist that she and her toddler daughter are *"completely the same,"* often ignoring or minimizing signs of their difference. Role reversal reflects the failure to see the child *as a child*. A role-reversing parent might, for example, talk about the way his toddler daughter knows she should bring him his slippers and a beer after work or describe turning to the young child for comfort in times of distress.

View of the Self as Parent

As we emphasized repeatedly in the early chapters of this book, parents are evolutionarily primed to protect and comfort their children, to provide a secure base and safe haven for the child in times of distress and need. In addition, they are the first to provide the child with the experiences of deep pleasure and intimacy that will shape the rest of their lives. We can often deduce from the parents' descriptions of themselves as parents just how able (and willing) they are to serve as a secure base. Is this someone we can imagine the child turning to in a moment of pain? Or with whom they might feel great pleasure and closeness? The children of Charlene, Maritza, and Janie, whose transcripts we have cited previously, would in all likelihood be able to feel safe with and close to their mothers. Although there would, of course, be ruptures and times they were unhappy, these ruptures would be experienced against the background of pleasure and trustworthiness. By contrast, many of the other mothers whose transcripts we have cited would be confusing, frightening, overwhelming, and disorienting to the child. When we read a transcript and we hear the parent's struggles and intense affects and observe their defenses, what do we imagine it would be like to be that person's child, to be small and vulnerable and have this be the "stronger and wiser" person to whom they would turn in times of distress? Does that parent have the capacity to serve as a haven in the storm, or do they waver, disappear, or intrude and menace? Do they see themselves as "malevolent and hostile, and/or frightened, helpless, or abdicating" (Terry et al., 2021, p. 66), or as essentially capable and present?

The Clinician's Response

Just as is the case with clinical material, it is very important for the clinician to listen to their own reactions in when administering the PDI. A clinician can experience themselves as badgering the uncommunicative parent or as confused by a parent's incoherent response. They can also feel threatened for reasons that aren't immediately apparent, can feel overwhelmed and disoriented, frightened for the child, or physically depleted and unbearably tired and hungry after giving an interview. Sometimes it is just a gut reaction that something serious is amiss. For instance, it took the reader several reviews to locate her concern after administering this PDI:

MOTHER: Clicking? That day she got hurt probably five times, and she just kept falling, and kept tripping over her feet, and bless her heart, she was just trying, she's just trying to do these funny silly things to make me laugh, and I love it, and, and I felt bad that she was getting hurt, but it was just, it was fun, we were having fun together.

Here a response that seemed superficially OK raised an amorphous sense of concern and foreboding. The mother was talking about having a good time and connecting, yet she was describing the child's repeatedly getting hurt. A closer look revealed many other such instances in the transcript, all "disguised" by her pleasant affect and apparent sympathy for the child. It is very important to respect these feelings, to listen to the interview again, or to review it with a colleague or supervisor. In this instance, the odd juxtaposition of laughter and pain likely conveyed the contradictory realities faced by the child in everyday interactions with her mother. It can be helpful to ask the simple question, "*I wonder if this is the way the child feels?*" "*What does it feel like to be Mari? Timmy?*" Listening to the answers can be quite revealing and can guide the clinician in subsequent work with the parent. Of course, a clinician's reactions—feeling critical and judgmental, or "certain" of their interpretations—can also have to do with their own personal blind spots (e.g., not picking up on role reversal), their acute sensitivity to a given issue (e.g., becoming very dysregulated by any threat of abandonment), or their personal resonance with a parent's story (e.g., a parent or child's history being close to the clinician's own history). These, too, must be parsed out, usually within the context of supervision.

Summary

There are many ways to listen to a PI or PDI. And yet all of these frameworks point us to a relatively simple set of questions: How does the parent "see" the child and themselves as a parent? How does this affect their way of being with the child? And what might it feel like to be this child? Where are the ports of entry in working with this parent? Where are the signs of coherence and positive valence, and where are the hopes for connection and growth? Where are the struggles and disorganization? What bridges can be built between the parent and the child? Answering these questions requires attention to subtlety and nuance in the narrative and in the affects expressed. These are the questions that alert clinicians to the parent's pain and suffering and defenses against them, as well as to the parent's capacity for growth and transformation.

GUIDELINES FOR CLINICIANS

Mentalizing: Positive Indicators

- There is evidence of mind-mindedness (Meins et al., 2001): The parent uses mental state words.
- The parent understands the nature of mental states.
- There are efforts to mentalize or to reason about mental states and to understand the mental states that underlie behavior.
- The parent can think about mental states developmentally.
- The narrative seems for the most part organized and coherent.
- The parent recognizes and repairs incoherence.
- There are few, if any, breakthroughs of intense negative affect in the narrative.
- When the parent is defensive or negative affect intrudes, there are efforts at recovery.
- There is an awareness of the interviewer and a wish to collaborate and communicate.

Mentalizing: Negative Indicators

- There is little curiosity about or interest in the child's experience.
- The parent's narrative does not help the listener or the reader get a sense of the child's mind.
- The parent is focused on control and behavior.
- There are signs of denial/avoidance, bland idealization, negation, shift in voice.
- There are signs of hostility or helplessness in relation to the child.
- The parent shows evidence of certainty, idealization, or contradiction in describing the child or the parent–child relationship.
- The parent shows signs of dissociation and narrative disorganization.
- The parent describes insensitive, neglectful, or aggressive behavior toward the child.

Affect Quality: Positive Indicators

- Parent speaks about emotion in authentic, specific ways.
- There is generally a positive valence to the parent's narrative, such that even difficulties are seen within a positive framework.

Affect Quality: Negative Indicators

- There are instances of raw negative affect (fear, anger, sadness) in the narrative that seem fairly unbounded.

View of the Child: Positive Indicators

- Child is seen in a positive and coherent way.

View of the Child: Negative Indicators

- Child is seen as an aggressor or as helpless.
- There is evidence of role reversal, enmeshment, or idealization.

View of the Self as Parent: Positive Indicators

- The parent sees themselves as a caregiver, capable of providing a "stronger, wiser, bigger, and kind" (Powell et al., 2013) secure base for the child.

View of the Self as Parent: Positive Indicators

- The parent sees themselves as a hostile or helpless caregiver.
- The parent fails to protect the child from danger.

Clinician Reactions

- Having to try too hard to draw someone out, or shutting down, distancing.
- Having to try too hard to make sense, feeling overwhelmed and disoriented.
- The hair standing up on the back of your neck, feeling frightened or controlled.
- Concern for the child.
- Feeling punitive, judgmental, or "certain."
- Enabling, giving too much leeway.
- Feeling exhausted, hungry, dysregulated.

Part

IV

Clinical Applications
of *Minding the Baby* Parenting

In this section of the book, we illustrate the key principles of MTB-P using a series of case illustrations. Brenda, Yolanda, Genevieve, and their families[1] were seen in MTB-HV by an interdisciplinary clinical team and followed over a 27-month period from pregnancy to their children's second birthdays. In the first two cases, Brenda and Yolanda, we use session notes to illustrate many of the strategies we discussed in Chapters 10 and 11 and to give a flavor of the way the interdisciplinary team worked together. We also integrate mothers' responses to the Pregnancy and Parent Development Interviews in order to bring alive the phenomena we described in Chapter 13. In the case of Genevieve[2]—in line with what we discussed in Chapters 5 and 12—we focus more specifically on how both the nurse and the social worker addressed manifestations of complex trauma over the course of the 27-month intervention.

These cases illustrate common themes in many of the young families we saw. There was often a history of maltreatment, domestic violence, substance abuse, and previous child protective services involvement. And because so many mothers were quite young, maternal grandmothers tended to be quite involved, both in the lives of the babies and in the MTB-HV sessions themselves. For Brenda, Yolanda, and Genevieve, this

---

[1] All three are composite cases.

[2] See also Slade et al. (2017b).

involvement was painful and complex and to varying degrees impinged upon the parent–child relationship, as well as the clinicians' efforts to establish what they hoped would be transformative treatment relationships. Fortunately, the intervention helped Brenda and Genevieve disentangle themselves from their mothers enough to genuinely see and delight in their babies and lay down the foundations of secure attachment. For Yolanda, however, her mother's intrusions and undermining, coupled with her own extensive trauma history, made it very difficult for her to truly feel safe or to self-regulate. This was ultimately to have tragic consequences.

All three of the clinicians whose work we describe were fully endorsed infant mental health specialists or mentors and experienced reflective supervisors and were trained in child–parent psychotherapy.

Chapter

14

Brenda, Aidan, and Allie

Pregnancy: Getting to Know You

Brenda was a Latina whose family hailed from the Caribbean. She was 18 years old and in her 6th month of pregnancy when we met and began the process of getting to know each other and gathering her story. We began, as we always do, by creating an environment of safety and trust. This sets the stage for administering a range of assessments (e.g., health, psychosocial), as well as the Pregnancy Interview (PI) (Slade, 2003) and a genogram. All of this takes time and flexibility on the clinician's part. As we learned time and again in MTB-HV, the assessment process is not confined to the "intake" period but extends across the entirety of the intervention as the relationship deepens and the parent's story emerges over time and with increasing coherence and affective vitality.

When we met her, Brenda was living with her mother and her younger twin brothers; she planned to move in with her boyfriend, Aidan, before giving birth. He was 20, and they had known each other for nearly a year when she became pregnant. Brenda had graduated from high school and had a steady job in retail. She planned to take 8 weeks' maternity leave, at which point Clara, an older woman whom Brenda had known for many years, would take care of the baby during the day. Brenda expected Aidan to be an active, hands-on father and hoped that their complementary work shifts would enable the baby to always be cared for by either one or both parents and Clara. Brenda's mother and Aidan both worked long hours; as a result, the MTB-HV team rarely saw either of them.

Brenda was outgoing, lively, appealing, and very bright. She had taken good care of herself since the pregnancy was confirmed and now began nesting with great excitement. She was determined to do "everything right" (e.g., eating well, attending regular prenatal appointments, not drinking or smoking), and to have what she needed when the baby arrived. Brenda's general health was good. She projected a tough, no-nonsense demeanor, and it was clear that developing trust would take some time. The reasons for this became increasingly clear as we got to know her better.

Brenda had been born and raised in the United States; both of her parents had emigrated to the United States in their late teens. Brenda described her mother, Yvonne, as tough and critical, "*not* warm and fuzzy" and unlikely to be a "typical *abuelita*," namely, a warm, doting, or affectionate grandmother. She had used harsh discipline with all her children. Brenda's father struggled with substance use and disappeared from home frequently. Her parents often had violent physical fights and eventually had separated, leaving Yvonne burdened with the care of Brenda and her younger twin brothers. Brenda described her mother as bitter and angry and herself as an "angry" adolescent, fighting back against her mother's control and abuse.

Learning these elements of Brenda's history helped the team understand their experience of her as somewhat brittle and angry, ready to defend herself at any perceived criticism, fiercely independent, strong willed, and quite impulsive. But equally compelling, from the beginning, was her resilience: She'd had a job since the age of 14, had finished high school on time, and now had a secure full-time job. She was also very active in a local community center and identified several older female members of the center who might serve as "surrogate aunties and grandmas" to her daughter. And she was already protective of her baby, nurturing a vision of creating a family and a home. She "fell in love" with the baby at the first sign of fetal movement. These strengths and the capacity for emotional connection were to stand her in good stead in the hard times ahead. And they allowed her to trust the clinicians more and more as time went on.

Pregnancy Interview

In MTB-HV, the social worker administers the PI with the nurse present and listening. Brenda's PI was somewhat surprising in that her toughness was much less evident, as was the excitement she had first expressed to the team. Brenda could only go so far in describing her excitement or imagining the baby's arrival, and a general dampening and ambivalence characterized much of the interview. She alternated between describing herself as fearful or bored and apathetic. When asked how she felt when she found out she was pregnant, Brenda said simply, "*I cried . . . I was sad,*" and then—in explaining—became a little disorganized: "*I was kind of sad but I kind of knew it at the same time. So I didn't, it wasn't. . . .*" She was also afraid: "*I was scared most of it. I was scared most of it because of my*

mom. She always told us if we got pregnant, we had to leave the house."
As it happened, her mother did not kick her out, and her boyfriend stayed.
When asked what she imagined would be the most pleasurable times in the
first months of motherhood, all she could say was, "*When she gets here.*"
When asked why this would be such a happy time, she responded, "*Because
she'll be here.*" Most striking was her dread about the baby's health. She
was dogged by the fear that there was an anomaly the midwives might
have missed, something invisible on the sonogram but dangerous nevertheless. "*I can't see her anymore, so I don't know what's going on inside of
me, and they don't check the placenta specifically. Like they don't look
at it.*" (The social worker clarifies that Brenda hasn't had an ultrasound
recently and asks Brenda why she's upset despite the midwives' reassur-
ances.) "*They don't know she's OK, because they're not actually looking at
the baby. They're just hearing her heartbeat and measuring how it's going
to grow. Everything could go perfectly fine and she . . . still something
could be wrong with her. Like what if the, the umbilical cord is around her
neck or something? They don't. . . .*" Only when she felt the fetus move
did she begin to feel better.

Throughout the PI, she tended toward vague and general characteriza-
tions, seeming somewhat unhappy, frustrated, and generally "*bored.*" The
same ambivalence that had characterized her description of her pregnancy
was evident in relation to her mother. On the one hand she described herself
as frightened of her mother, yet on the other hand she also described her
mother as her "*best friend,*" "*because I go to my mom and tell her anything.*" It was clear that this was a fraught relationship. At the end of the
PI, parents are asked what three wishes they would have for their child in 5
years' time. The clinical team uses the answer to this question throughout
the intervention to remind mothers of their own goals and wishes for the
child. Often this can be very orienting and empowering, particularly at
times of crisis. When asked this question, Brenda responded: "*Um, I don't
even want her to grow up. I don't want to think about 5 years old.*" When
gently prompted, she replied, "*I want her to trust me and be able to count
on me and feel safe . . . to have two parents living together. And I want
her to go to school and have good grades.*" Then, to the social worker's
surprise, she added, "*And I don't want her to always be getting into trouble. . . . I don't want her to give me as much headache as I give my mom.*"
That she had such hopes for her daughter was a very positive sign. However,
her overall PRF score was only a 2, indicating a general lack of even the
most rudimentary reflective capacities. She could not really describe any of
her own feelings or imagine her daughter or her experience. Nor could she
reflect on any of the traumas that had consumed so much of her childhood.
She approached criterion for the designation as Hostile–Helpless, largely
because of the amount of fear that emerged on the interview.

The Genogram

Several weeks later, the social worker and Brenda created a genogram, which offered more clues to understanding the complexities of Brenda's emotional life and of the tragedies that were her family's legacy. Both parents had immigrated to the United States to escape the harsh poverty and violence of their home countries. Both had lost their fathers at a young age and had raised their own children with few resources and opportunities. As she completed the genogram, Brenda turned pensive. She began to wonder out loud about her parents' childhood experiences and hypothesized that maybe some of the things that happened to them explained why they were *"such screwed-up parents."*

The social worker used this moment, when Brenda had let down her guard, and seemed open to reflection, to draw her out some more.

> SOCIAL WORKER: Tell me more about your parents being "screwed up," Brenda.
>
> BRENDA: Well, you know, my mom was so angry and strict, and my parents were always having these fights, and my dad, well, he was just gone. He could be sweet but most of the time he was high. This (*gesturing to the genogram*) makes me think about . . . they both had it pretty rough.
>
> SOCIAL WORKER: Yeah, they really did . . . it kind of makes sense that they struggled raising you and your brothers.
>
> BRENDA: Yeah, it kind of scares me . . . what if I screw up, too? I don't want to, but . . . and then Aidan's family is a mess, too—his mom was a drug addict, and his dad was never around. His grandma raised him—she's amazing, though. I love her.
>
> SOCIAL WORKER: It's kind of like traveling without a road map, or not such a great road map . . . I'm glad you and Aidan have his grandma in your corner. . . . What do you think you're afraid of?
>
> BRENDA: Well, I don't want to be like my mother—she's so angry, and she can get violent. And I want to be around. My dad was just never there when I needed him. I already love this baby so much, and Aidan is really excited, and he wants to be a good dad. I don't know . . . I just don't want the baby to feel like I did growing up.
>
> SOCIAL WORKER: And what was that?
>
> BRENDA: Well, I guess scared . . . and . . . when I got older . . . pretty angry. . . .
>
> SOCIAL WORKER: Can you imagine the kind of parents you'd like your daughter to have? What kind of parents would you have wanted for you and your brothers growing up? Can you think of any words to describe them?
>
> BRENDA: (*concentrating*) Well, sober for sure. Not fighting in front of us kids. More patient, like my mother never listened to us, we could never have

feelings. If we didn't do what she said, she would hit us. I got hit a lot 'cause I'd stand up for myself. I don't want to hit my daughter . . . ever. I want us to be able to talk.

SOCIAL WORKER: So you want your daughter to be able to tell you what she thinks and feels.

BRENDA: Most definitely. I want her to trust me enough to come to me when she needs me or if she's in trouble. I told Clara I was pregnant before telling my mother. I don't trust my mom at all because I never know how she's gonna act.

SOCIAL WORKER: That must be hard for you now even as a young adult, but as a little girl that must have felt scary. . . . What about your father? Where is he in all of this?

BRENDA: It's just a struggle for him to stay alive and stay sober. He's back living with my grandma now, and I look at him and he looks so sad and beaten down. I can tell he regrets things, like he failed his kids, even though he'll never say it. He was actually happy about the baby. Unlike my mom, who basically said, "Oh, well, it's your life and you deal with it."

SOCIAL WORKER: Wow. That's hard—that must make you feel pretty alone. But maybe this is a sign of hope for your dad. You know, for many grandparents, a grandbaby is like a second chance to maybe be better parents than they were with their children.

BRENDA: Yeah, that makes sense.

SOCIAL WORKER: So, I think what you're telling me is that you think good parents should be sober, available, able to talk with and listen to their children without being physically violent, reliable, and trustworthy.

BRENDA: Right, exactly, oh and loving, you know like cuddles, hugs, and kisses. I so wanted that when I was little, and I can't wait to cuddle with my daughter!

SOCIAL WORKER: These are all beautiful qualities. . . . Your baby is so lucky to have a mom who is thinking about the best ways to love and raise her even before she's born.

BRENDA: (*blushing and appearing more open and vulnerable*) You really think so??

SOCIAL WORKER: I know so. . . . You could easily say, "Look how my parents were, and I turned out fine." But instead, you're recognizing that your daughter will be a child with her own needs and wants. The fact that you are already so invested in developing as healthy a relationship as possible with her says more than you know. Intentions are huge.

BRENDA: (*smiling shyly*) It feels good knowing that.

In this passage, the social worker was doing a number of things. First, she judged that Brenda felt safe, regulated, and trusting enough to have a deeper conversation about her experience as a child and her hopes for herself as a mother. The social worker also helped Brenda put into words some of the ways she wanted to create a different sort of childhood for her daughter, one in which she felt safe and loved. But it remained difficult for Brenda to imagine some of the darker feelings she might have as a mother and to fully describe her own childhood abuse. As we were to learn more and more fully as we came to know her, the vagueness and contradictions of the PI, as well as her general sense of foreboding and danger, were signs of the larger story that Brenda could not yet tell.

Prenatal Visits with the Nurse

It was in a conversation with the nurse only weeks before giving birth— long after the social worker had completed the psychosocial assessment, the PI, and the genogram—that some of the starker details of Brenda's story emerged. Clearly, this was made possible by her coming to trust both clinicians and to feel safe enough to tell her story without becoming dysregu- lated. In this instance, Brenda and the nurse had already met many times, and the nurse had been impressed by Brenda's diligence about taking care of herself and the baby throughout her pregnancy. She went to all her pre- natal appointments and couldn't wait to show the nurse the ultrasound of her little girl. They were sitting together on a couch at her mother's home, which was cluttered but clean. The nurse began talking about nutrition. What were her favorite meals, and who did the cooking and shopping at home? "My mom. But she usually brings home food already made. She's not always home because of her work." Brenda then explained that she had often been expected to cook for her parents growing up. "And I had to clean, too. I would get hit if the house wasn't clean. I never knew when she'd start throwing punches. I was used to it, but when I was 14, I'd had enough. I was pretty big. I showed her my fist and said she better stop or I'll stop her."

As is not uncommon in MTB-HV, Brenda had disclosed these experi- ences to the nurse rather than to the social worker. It might have felt too hard to tell the social worker because of all the feelings it would evoke in that context. This is one of the many values of an interdisciplinary team. The nurse wondered how best to respond to what Brenda had told her, newly concerned about Yvonne's involvement with the baby, worried for Brenda's safety, and knowing all too well how these experiences would make parenting a challenge for Brenda. She used this moment to help

Brenda imagine the sort of mother she would like to be, and so returned to the hopes and wishes she'd described in the PI, siding with the part of her that wanted to create a different experience for her own child.

> NURSE: Wow—that sounds hard, not knowing what your mom was going to do next.
>
> (*Brenda nods.*) I remember one of your wishes for your own daughter was to trust you and know that she could count on you. (*Brenda nods again.*) I wonder what that would look like. How will you show her that you'll be there for her?
>
> BRENDA: I don't know. . . . That's a good question. I guess I wouldn't lie to her and I'd show up when she was upset. And I wouldn't hit her.
>
> NURSE: So she'll feel like you are a safe mother to go to!
>
> BRENDA: Yeah—not like my mom!
>
> NURSE: Sounds like you are really thinking about how you would like your daughter to have a different experience than you did growing up.

In this passage, the nurse supported Brenda's desire to be a present, loving, and trusted mom. At the same time, hearing the extent of the violence in Brenda's childhood home made clear just how important it was to listen for signs of reawakened trauma as delivery approached. The nurse was keenly aware that Brenda's experience of her mother's violence might well lead to her own struggles with anger and aggression.

The couple found an apartment just weeks before the baby was due. In one of the last visits before the baby's birth, the parents excitedly showed the nurse the bassinet they had purchased. The nurse used this as a moment to bring up sleep safety and shaken-baby syndrome. This was a standard part of the nurse's prebirth meetings, but she felt it was particularly important to review in light of Brenda's history of maltreatment. Brenda remembered a television show in which a parent had injured their baby, but she couldn't imagine ever doing so. "*I mean, I get mad at my boyfriend and push him sometimes when he bugs me, but I wouldn't hurt a baby!*" The nurse noted that Brenda was hitting her boyfriend, confirming some of the team's concerns about Brenda's potential for violence. To Brenda, she said, "*I know it's hard to imagine harming a helpless infant. But during the first 6–12 weeks of life babies often cry up to 5 hours a day. I don't think any parent means to harm their tiny baby, but not knowing how to console a baby and being very tired can make staying calm very difficult.*" Brenda listened quietly, clearly open to hearing more. The nurse asked Brenda to think about what her body felt like when she got angry and then introduced a simple stress reduction exercise aimed at helping Brenda become aware of building tension before she lashed out. They role-played her being exhausted by the new baby and needing help and came up with a plan to call Clara, who Brenda felt would be available to help without judging her.

As the birth approached, the home visitors wondered when and how the ghosts in Brenda's (and Aidan's and her parents') nursery would make themselves known. Up to that point, she still struggled to put words to her feelings, although there were many signs that intense feelings were brewing. Brenda was actively struggling with her anger, but at the same time she was exploring her childhood relationships in a new way. And she was working hard to imagine herself as a more reliable, safe, and loving mother. Although there were relatively few signs of RF on her PI, these began to emerge more clearly as the intervention took hold and the team met with her consistently throughout the third trimester of her pregnancy. Though both clinicians had their concerns, they were also heartened by Brenda's openness to them and by the many signs of her resilience.

Allie Arrives

Allie arrived on time, and the birth was long but uncomplicated. Brenda and Aidan were both over the moon about the baby. For the first 6 months postpartum, things seemed to go smoothly.

Postbirth Visit with the Nurse

Brenda invited the nurse to visit soon after giving birth. Entering the house the nurse observed that the new mother's face was relaxed as she calmly breastfed her infant. She smiled as she greeted the nurse, who asked about Brenda's labor and delivery. Brenda said it was long, but all worth it because the baby was *"perfect!"*

NURSE: Look at how she's gazing into your eyes!

BRENDA: I love the way she looks at me when she's breastfeeding. I wonder what she's thinking?

NURSE: It's hard to know! What do you think?

BRENDA: Maybe. . . . "Who is this person who gives me yummy food?"

NURSE: Yes! "It makes me feel warm and safe when you hold me, Mommy." (*Speaking for the baby*)

Although Brenda had few words to describe her feelings toward the baby, she was tender and responsive to the infant's cues and open to thinking about baby's experience. These were important signs of her sensitive care-giving. The nurse made note of these to Brenda throughout the visit, highlighting the connection between the mother and baby as Brenda read her baby's cues. At one point, the baby became fussy. Brenda gently held her close, rocking her until she was consoled. The nurse pointed out the baby's responsiveness and obvious sense of comfort and safety. "*Look at how she molds into you! She feels so safe with you.*"

Two months later, however, the nurse witnessed a painful scene between Brenda and her mother, who came by with some laundry she'd done for Brenda. Yvonne dumped the unfolded clothes onto Brenda's bed and—as she left—described the apartment as an "*f-ing mess.*" The nurse waited a moment and then turned to Brenda. "*How're you doing?*" Brenda looked down at her lap and said, sadly, "*My mom told me the baby wasn't dressed warmly enough and that she was too skinny.*"

NURSE: Hmm . . . that's hard to hear. What do you think?

BRENDA: (*glancing at Allie*) She seems okay to me. I think my mom is mad that I'm breastfeeding 'cos it means she can't take Allie if she can't feed her.

NURSE: That makes a lot of sense to me . . . what a good observation. And you really wanted to breastfeed.

BRENDA: Yeah. I mean it's supposed to be best and make her smart. And I think she is smart and growing.

NURSE: Yeah, remember that she'd gained just the right amount of weight at your last clinic appointment, and that she's starting to grow out of her clothes!

BRENDA: (*Turns away to get a diaper. When she turns back, she makes eye contact with Allie. The baby responds with coos as she wiggles and smiles.*) I guess she's happy! She's so funny. Are you learning to talk?

NURSE: It looks like she's saying, "Hi Mom! I really love the way you take care of me!"

The nurse affirmed her effort at mentalizing ("*I think my mom is mad that I'm breast-feeding*"), highlighted the ways mother and baby were genuinely and happily connecting, and supported the mother in her own decisions and wishes for the child. Brenda was, in fact, doing beautifully, and the baby was clearly thriving.

Visit with the Social Worker at 9 Months

By the time of this visit, things had begun to tilt toward the negative. The social worker arrived for her regular visit to find Allie happily squealing and laughing as she crawled around the room. When asked how things were going, Brenda replied that she was exhausted from keeping up with her. She was tired and irritable. *"I'm happy to see her growing, but I miss when she was a baby, when I could just cuddle her all the time."* The social worker agreed: *"It is hard when they move around so much—a lot of parents feel sad to lose that sweet time."* She then asked whether there was a way Brenda could catch up on her rest. Maybe she could nap when Allie napped, or perhaps her mother could stay with the baby while she slept? Brenda sagged: *"I'm not getting much help."* The story spilled out. Aidan was so in love with Allie at first, but now he was more interested in going to clubs and hanging out with his friends. Brenda was very angry with him and very lonely. None of her friends had children yet, and they were off doing their own things. Her mother rarely visited, and when she did, she spent most of her time criticizing Brenda's mothering and housekeeping skills. Brenda was so disappointed that her mother showed so little interest in Allie. She was the opposite of a doting grandmother.

Now nearly a year into the intervention, the team had learned more and more about the abuse Brenda had suffered at her mother's hands and how violent the fights between her parents had been. Keeping this history in mind, the social worker suggested that as much as she *knew* who her mom was, a part of Brenda might have hoped she'd be more loving and involved with Allie. Maybe she'd be a better grandma than she'd been a mom. Brenda acknowledged that it was in fact very hurtful, because she was at a point in her life where she *"needed a mom"* to help her be a mom. The social worker simply affirmed this: *"It can be so sad to realize you don't have the mother you need."* Then, in an effort to side with Brenda's resilience, she reminded Brenda that even in pregnancy she had known she wanted to be a different kind of mom to Allie. She could be loving and giving in ways her mother couldn't. And perhaps she could get some of the support she needed from Clara, who both supported her mothering and doted on Allie. The social worker then returned to the question of Allie's motility, which was wonderful but overwhelming for Brenda, who worried that the baby would hurt herself or put something in her mouth while crawling around. The fear that she expressed on the PI (of her being harmed) had returned. This led to a discussion of what Brenda could do to make sure the space was safe for Allie to explore freely. Here and in many other ways, the social worker was trying to help Brenda create a new narrative about the kind of mother she wanted to and could be. The social worker then returned to Brenda's relationship with Aidan.

SOCIAL WORKER: You said he's not helping . . . what's going on?

BRENDA: *(tightening with anger)* He has so much freedom, and I have none! He's so immature and clueless—I get so angry at him. He helps with money, but he comes and goes as he pleases. It's so unfair!

She then reluctantly told the social worker that she had slapped and pushed Aidan a number of times when he came home after staying out late. The social worker immediately linked this to her feelings:

SOCIAL WORKER: Sometimes you just get so mad you lash out . . . how does Aidan respond?

BRENDA: He just leaves the house until he calms down.

SOCIAL WORKER: How does that make you feel?

BRENDA: (*her face clouding over*) Abandoned. And it's just like what used to happen with my parents, my dad walking out. (*tears sliding down her cheeks*) I can't believe I'm acting like my mom.

SOCIAL WORKER: (*mirroring her distress*) You must've felt so confused and frightened when your parents would fight and your dad would leave the house. Sometimes those scripts are the ones that stick even if we wish they wouldn't.

The social worker then turned her attention to Allie.

SOCIAL WORKER: Where's Allie when you and Aidan are fighting?"

BRENDA: Oh, it mostly happens at night. She's asleep.

SOCIAL WORKER: (*pushing a little*) Do you think she realizes things are different sometimes?

BRENDA: I don't think so . . . she's not around most of the time.

The social worker quietly accepted Brenda's reply but gently added that babies can be more aware of things than we realize and that, even though they can't tell us about their feelings, sometimes changes in their appetite, level of activity, or sleep pattern is their way of telling us that they are scared or worried.

BRENDA: Do you think Allie can tell if something is wrong?

The social worker knew this question signaled a critical shift, from denial to reflection.

SOCIAL WORKER: It's certainly possible . . . and you know she could have some of the feelings you had as a small child when the people you relied on most were angry and one of them left. I know how much you love Allie and want her to feel safe. Let's keep an eye on how she's responding, and maybe we can think about finding some better ways to communicate with Aidan. Maybe he'd even like to join in that discussion."

Brenda agreed. What was striking in this session was that, despite how much difficulty she was having and how unsupported and alone she was feeling, Brenda trusted the social worker, and together they reflected on what were some very painful feelings about her mother, her partner, and her relationship.

Visit with the Nurse at 9 Months

When the nurse visited a week later, things were getting worse. Brenda found herself crying "for no reason," not sleeping well at night, and wanting to sleep all day.

> BRENDA: (*watching as Allie put everything she touched into her mouth*) Why can't she just leave things alone?! (*She was too irritable to see things from Allie's point of view.*)
>
> NURSE: It's really hard to keep all the small things out of her reach now, isn't it? But she is too young to remember not to put them in her mouth.
>
> BRENDA: I know, but she's driving me crazy! (*turning to Allie*) Why are you so bad? Can't you make it easy on me? It's hard enough on me dealing with your father and your grandmother! (*Then, to the nurse*) Look! Now she's crawling away from me! It's like she won't listen, and she doesn't want to be with me now that she's big.
>
> NURSE: Is that what it looks like to you—that she's crawling away from you? Let's watch. I wonder what she will do next.
>
> (*Allie crawls over to the couch and tries to climb onto it. She loses her balance and falls, startling herself. She quickly looks to her mother with tears starting and crawls back into Brenda's lap for a hug.*)
>
> BRENDA: I guess you still need me sometimes, don't you?
>
> NURSE: She does need you! Even though she's growing older and trying new things—like babies do— that is one reason she is crawling further away— to learn about new things. But she's also keeping track of where you are, where she can come back to, if something worries or upsets her. She comes to you because she knows you will accept her and comfort her. You're safe and make her feel secure.
>
> BRENDA: (*Smiles shyly and nods.*) That's how I want her to feel.
>
> NURSE: I bet she also brings things to you to look at when she's excited about a toy or something she's found.

BRENDA: Yeah, you're right. She does that, too.

NURSE: So, she knows she can come to you to share things she's enjoying, and she knows she can come to you when she needs a hug.

BRENDA: That's a good thing, isn't it? That's good to know.

The nurse noted that—likely as a function of an emerging depression—Brenda was lapsing into prementalizing, attributing malevolent intentions to Allie. She reviewed the symptoms and causes of depression with Brenda, underlining the fact that these feelings are not uncommon after a baby is born. They discussed possible medication and therapy, and Brenda agreed to an appointment to talk to the midwives. They prescribed an antidepressant, and the social worker increased her visits to weekly in order to address Brenda's depression and anger therapeutically.

Allie Turns 1

As a toddler, Allie was animated and very social, and Brenda clearly adored her. When the nurse visited, Allie would take the baby doll from the toy bag and feed it with a bottle, then put a book on her lap and "read" to the doll. This despite the fact that her mom was still depressed and that things with Aidan were very rocky. The nurse actively supported Brenda's delight in her daughter, her curiosity about Allie's development, her capacity to plan and to follow routines, and her wishes for the future. Again and again the team saw that—even when things were really tough for Brenda—her connection to Allie was solid, loving, and full of pleasure for both of them. Allie was classified as securely attached when she was seen in the Strange Situation at 14 months.

Visit with the Nurse at 15 Months

A few months after Allie's first birthday, the nurse received a call from Brenda asking to have their visit at her own mother's home. She had separated from Aidan and moved back into her childhood bedroom with Allie. No explanation was offered for the separation. Brenda told the nurse that Allie saw her father frequently and that she would set up FaceTime when Allie asked for Papa. The nurse asked Brenda what Allie's response had been. Brenda was not able to put words to her daughter's or her own experience. Although her symptoms of depression had lessened, she shied away from exploring her disappointment in her failed relationship and move back to her parent's home.

Up to that point, Allie was walking and saying a few words. She would seek out her mother if hurt or worried and was playful and open to the nurse on her visits. Despite the conflict between her parents, multiple moves, and her mother's depression, Allie was on track developmentally and was doing well. The nurse hypothesized that the young parents were able to keep the baby's emotional, as well as physical, needs in mind, allowing Allie to feel a sense of stability throughout the changes. But this latest move and the loss of her father were clearly taking a toll on her.

NURSE: Allie seems quiet today.

BRENDA: Yeah, I'm not sure why. She's been like that lately. She's not sleeping too well, either.

NURSE: There have been so many changes in her life in the last few weeks.

BRENDA: Yeah, lots of things have changed, you know, with me moving back to my mom's and going to work and having her dad move somewhere else. Come here, Little Allie. I wish you could talk and tell me what's going on! (*Brenda hugs the little girl, who smiles up at her.*)

NURSE: That is a lot—for both of you! Look at that smile when you gave her a hug. You could tell what she needed even if she couldn't tell you in words.

BRENDA: You need a hug, honey? You trying to tell me you need me? It's been hard, I know . . .

NURSE: It sure has. And you're watching her behavior and noticing changes so you can figure out how she's feeling. You've really thought a lot about Allie's feelings this whole year in spite of everything that's happened. You've also taken care of yourself. You are taking the medication and moved out of an unhappy situation. That helps both of you.

Visit with the Social Worker at 18 Months

Brenda canceled several visits with the social worker after breaking up with Aidan, so Allie was nearly 18 months old when they met again. Brenda told the social worker the story of their breakup. Things had fallen apart after an intense argument that escalated in front of a very frightened Allie. Both parents knew at that point they would be better off apart.

SOCIAL WORKER: Oh, Brenda, I'm so sorry. That sounds really hard. And scary.

BRENDA: Yeah, it was really bad.

SOCIAL WORKER: It sounds like it was. . . . How does it feel to tell me?

BRENDA: I couldn't tell you. I'm so ashamed that we argued like that in front of Allie. We've talked about my anger so many times. And my childhood, but

I just lost it completely. I was so angry. I just saw red. There I was, acting just like my mom did. (*Tears up.*)

SOCIAL WORKER: It's so hard. . . .

BRENDA: And now everything just feels so chaotic. We had a good routine, and now it's so hard to keep to any schedule. And Aidan and I have to figure out how to do this together. We're still both so mad.

SOCIAL WORKER: How do you think Allie felt seeing you fight?

BRENDA: She was scared. But she's so young, she won't remember, she'll be fine.

SOCIAL WORKER: Well, she's a pretty sturdy, happy little girl, but you know, the nurse told me that she hasn't been sleeping, and that she's been having a hard time saying good-bye at day care.

BRENDA: Yeah, that's right. . . . Allie's not sleeping, and she seems exhausted. She's usually such a happy girl, but it just feels like she's different now. She's been so clingy. I'm exhausted, too.

SOCIAL WORKER: Can you tell me more about how she's changed?

BRENDA: You know, she was starting to learn words, and she's walking better, so she was more confident, kind of fearless, it was so funny to watch her play. She thought she could take on the world (*laughing*).

SOCIAL WORKER: (*smiling*) I know what you mean. She's just a joy to be with! She loves to explore.

BRENDA: Right! And now it's like she doesn't want to do anything but be in my lap or up under me. She's also not using her words as much. Instead, she just whines for everything. It's hard to be patient, but I don't want to be harsh with her 'cause she seems so sad!

SOCIAL WORKER: You're both having a lot of strong feelings, and—as bad as you feel—you're paying attention to her feelings, too. That can be so hard. You know, it might be she's missing her dad?

BRENDA: It's possible. But I mean she does see Aidan a few days a week and on the weekends. I guess I figured she wouldn't notice the difference since she's a baby, you know?

SOCIAL WORKER: Even though Allie can't say to you, "Mom, I don't understand why Daddy isn't here anymore and it makes me sad and scared," she may be feeling this way. It might feel different to Allie that her dad isn't home anymore when she goes to sleep at night or wakes up in the morning. Babies and toddlers express their distress with behavior, sometimes even with changes in eating and sleeping, since they don't yet have the language. Does that make sense?

BRENDA: So, maybe she's not sleeping at night because maybe she's scared or missing her father being home?

SOCIAL WORKER: Well, we can't know for sure, but it's possible. It does seem like there's a very good chance that she's having a hard time adjusting to the changes in your family, just like you and Aidan are, but that she's expressing this in different ways. I am wondering if her clinginess is a desire to stay close to you.

BRENDA: The nurse said that, too. . . .

SOCIAL WORKER: It would make a lot of sense. From her perspective, she already has one parent she doesn't see as regularly anymore. She may think keeping you close will keep you from leaving her.

BRENDA: Well, that would explain why she's been giving me such grief at day care. She used to be so happy to be there, and now she cries every morning when I drop her off.

SOCIAL WORKER: What's that like for you?

BRENDA: Really hard! It took me so long to trust anybody with her, and when things finally start going well, she falls apart. I feel guilty, like I should just stay with her, but I have to work.

SOCIAL WORKER: These are always such hard choices for moms, and you're also going through a separation from Aidan so it's really hard!

In this long and difficult conversation, Brenda and the social worker explored many complex and difficult elements of her current situation. Brenda was ashamed, afraid, overwhelmed, and didn't see a clear path forward. She could acknowledge her own pain but needed the social worker's support to see Allie's. It was so painful to be repeating her own past in such a stark way and so deeply disappointing not to be able to create the family life she'd hoped to. Her trust in the social worker allowed her to explore each of these areas without defensiveness and to feel and tolerate the complexity of it all. The social worker moved from observing to mirroring to reflecting and hypothesizing throughout the conversation. The social worker also continually pointed out her strengths, her resilience, and her commitment to her little girl, who, though she was regressed, had so much going for her.

By the time graduation approached, Brenda had established a stable routine for Allie and herself. Both were clearly feeling much better. She had grown in her ability to read the child's cues with fewer misattributions (of rejection or aggression). Allie was very verbal and playful, sweet, and charming. And she was a cuddler. Brenda and Aidan had a stable coparenting plan in place and were cooperating in raising Allie. This sometimes meant Aidan coming over to see Allie at Brenda's family home, which—although she didn't like it—worked out OK. She knew how happy it made Allie to see him. It was clear that in so many ways Brenda had succeeded in giving Allie the sense that she was loved and that her mom was truly emotionally present, all important protective factors during the turbulence of the child's young life.

Allie and Brenda Graduate

Parent Development Interview

A research assistant administered the PDI just as Brenda and Allie were about to graduate from the program. The vagueness and contradictions so apparent on her PI, as well as her significant difficulties putting her feelings into words, were much less apparent. Whereas she scored in the low range of PRF on the PI, the PDI made it clear that she had become much more able to think about her own and her child's feelings. Her responses were also considerably more organized; she was forthright, coherent, and open about her feelings. Often this is communicated on the PDI by the structure of the responses themselves. In Brenda's case, nearly every sentence was clear, to the point, and relevant to the question at hand. When asked for three words to describe Allie, she answered, "*She's smart. She's funny, and she's friendly.*" All were absolutely true.

Brenda's pleasure in her daughter was palpable throughout the interview. She adored her, and it came across vividly in the PDI, as it had in home visits. When she was asked to describe a time when she and her daughter were "clicking," she replied:

BRENDA: Well, like yesterday morning . . . we woke up. She woke up, she woke me up because she climbed into my bed. She kept telling me, "Good morning, Mommy," and rubbing my hair. So we were just laying there, and she was giving me a kiss and I was giving her a kiss, and we were just playing.

INTERVIEWER: How did you feel?

BRENDA: I felt good. . . .

INTERVIEWER: What made you feel good?

BRENDA: Like, I don't know, just to hear her, just to hear her laugh, and she keeps telling me "Mommy, I love you," so it just feels so good. My baby.

INTERVIEWER: And how do you think she felt?

BRENDA: Loved. I don't know. I know she feels that I love her because she knows that I love her. She does.

This was one of many passages in which Brenda described them happily snuggling and cuddling. This was what she had hoped for in pregnancy and what she had so missed in her own childhood.

Needless to say, her own struggles with anger had hardly disappeared. Yet she saw her daughter as helping her be more patient and less quick to anger: *"After I had her, and I started to realize that she was picking up on our bad habits and the fighting and all of that, I grew up a lot. Like, right now, her dad'll come here. Um, he'll try to argue with me. I'll rarely exchange words with him because I don't . . . I can't say that I don't, I do sometimes. But I don't do it as much, and I try not to—I try to watch what I'm going to say, even though I'm angry, but . . . sometimes it doesn't work. Well, I do try (laughs)."* The fact that she could laugh at herself and recognize that she was still struggling was so important.

She also realized that her anger frightened her daughter. When asked how she thought Allie felt when she got angry as a parent, she replied, *"I don't know. I feel like, because of me and her father's past, she's already seen me really angry. So when I yell at her, I know it kind of scares her a little bit because of what she's seen me and her dad put each other through. So, I know she gets scared."* She returns to this later in the interview when asked whether Allie had had any setbacks in her early life: *"Yeah . . . I feel like when she saw me and her dad yell, and all of that. For her, I kind of feel like, I don't know . . . like because now if anybody in the house argues, she starts to yell and cry, and she gets scared. Even if we're like play fighting, or somebody is like yelling out of excitement, like—like we're, we're loud when we talk sometimes. She gets . . . she gets scared so she starts to cry."* Clearly, Allie was deeply affected by her parents' fights, but Brenda was no longer denying it. And Brenda responded to her daughter's fear by reassuring Allie that she was safe and loved.

It was clear from the PDI that Allie had her own struggles with aggression—she could (like all toddlers) pinch and hit—but these seemed within the typical range. And her tantrums were big ones. Brenda described these as the times that she felt most overwhelmed and angry herself. But she managed to control her temper by walking away or taking some very deep breaths. Again, their shared pleasure in each other seemed to balance and soften their inevitable conflicts and was clearly the dominant force in their relationship.

Brenda still struggled with her fear that Allie would come to harm. *"I'm, like, any little thing. I want to run to the hospital with her because that's my baby. So, I'm like, I don't know. . . . I'm just all up in, and I feel like sometimes I'm overinvolved in her, but sometimes I feel like it's the best thing to do because anything that happens to her, it'll, like, kill me. I don't know, I haven't found a way to live without her, well, I shouldn't have to find a way to live without her, it's just, she's just—I don't know . . . it's weird, like I just want to be with her 24/7. I don't know."* Nevertheless, her pleasure in so many aspects of their relationship and in seeing

Allie's many strengths—sociability, intelligence, warmth, and humor— overshadowed and softened her most difficult feelings.

Clinicians' Responses

Brenda was a fighter whose emotional and psychological robustness gave the clinical team hope that she and her daughter would thrive even in difficult times. The clinicians believed in Brenda's capacity to be a good-enough parent and were invested in her success. Despite multiple obstacles, including a broken relationship with her daughter's father, bouts of depression, family dysfunction, employment instability, and legal troubles, Brenda always managed to maintain a positive relationship with her daughter. She was attuned to her little girl and thought about her experiences and feelings. Brenda was also open with the clinicians about her shortcomings and expressed remorse when she made mistakes. She seemed to feel emotionally safe enough to fully be herself with the clinical team. This gave the team confidence in Brenda's competence as a mother, as well as her ability to ask for support when needed. Brenda's emotional safety in the therapeutic relationship seems to have been transferred to her daughter. By age 2, Allie was a confident, verbal, curious toddler who felt free to explore her world knowing that her mother was never too far away.

Summary

Both the social worker and the nurse, throughout their many sessions over the 27 months of the intervention, continuously balanced support and affirmation on the one hand with gentle pushes toward reflection and affect tolerance on the other. They helped Brenda discover her story; this narrative provided coherence for what had been so much chaos and distress. As evidenced by the security of Allie's attachment, as well as Brenda's improved ability to mentalize on the PDI, both mother and daughter benefited greatly from this approach. The affirmation and emotional presence of the clinicians were critical to Brenda's feeling safe and regulated and to her feeling trusting enough to reflect upon her painful history and painful feelings in the present. Brenda was then able to build on the many strengths she had and to provide enough of a secure base for Allie that she could really thrive. Although Brenda could still be quite angry and impulsive, anger had not invaded her relationship with Allie, and she had succeeded in being there for her, in understanding her, and supporting her. Brenda took great care not to frighten Allie. They had the kind of relationship she had hoped for.

Despite the many stresses in her life and her frightening and abusive child-hood, Brenda was able to find her strengths and the pleasure in deeply loving her daughter. She was blessed with a keen intelligence, and Allie was—from the start—an enormously appealing, easy baby. She was easy to love. This made the transition to mothering the real and present Allie much easier than it would have been had she been a more difficult baby. In this, Brenda was blessed as well.

Allie and her mom always attended the MTB-HV reunions, which were held yearly in an outdoor park. What the clinicians saw year after year was a happy, confident, and delightful young girl and a happy, confi-dent mother. Their delight in each other was palpable. Life was not neces-sarily easy, but their relationship was a source of comfort and stability for them both.

Chapter

15

Yolanda, Manny, and Mildred

Pregnancy: Getting to Know You

There are obstacles to progress that even the most practiced clinicians cannot overcome. In this chapter, we describe the painful and difficult outcome of our work with Yolanda and her son, Manny. Like many of the young women we saw over the years, Yolanda came to us with a very significant trauma history. Whereas some parents were able to disclose, process, and at least partially work through traumatic experiences once they came to trust us (as had been the case with Brenda), Yolanda's age, the nature of her trauma, as well as her complex family situation made this virtually impossible.

Yolanda was a shy, pretty young Afro-Latina who became pregnant in her mid-teens. Her partner was only intermittently present and was largely uninvolved with her or the baby. She had been raised in several foster families after being sexually abused in her biological family and had only recently returned to live with her biological mother, Mildred. The team learned of her sexual abuse history from her child protection worker; Yolanda herself was quite unable to talk about any of these experiences. Fragile in every sense of the word, she could not tolerate any discussion of her past and would readily dissociate and "disappear," requiring great skill on the part of the clinicians to bring her back. What was evident from the first was how very much Yolanda just needed the clinicians' attention and care. She was painfully shy, and she was frightened. She seemed so alone, and indeed it seemed clear that her mother—who had failed so many times to protect her—did not see or hear her. In stark contrast to what was to follow after the baby was born, Mildred attended only a few of the 15 prenatal

325

appointments we had with Yolanda. She adopted an attitude of "you made this mess, now you deal with it" and left Yolanda to cope on her own.

Initial Visit with the Social Worker

When the social worker first met Yolanda, establishing safety and building the relationship was at the top of her mind. Yolanda already had a lifetime of experience with social workers and with being evaluated. Talking with a social worker often led to another placement. This made it likely that Yolanda would feel threatened meeting the social worker for the first time. Indeed, she looked down, spoke in short sentences, and seemed generally uncomfortable. Picking up on this, the social worker began to create a new frame: She was there to help with the pregnancy and get ready for the baby's arrival. She was not there to evaluate Yolanda's fitness as a parent. Yolanda seemed surprised. This was a different kind of social work from what she had experienced in child protection or residential hospital settings. *"I didn't know social workers worked with pregnant ladies or knew anything about babies,"* she said. Yolanda began to relax as she realized that *she* could ask questions and that the social worker was there to provide information that she very much needed. The social worker explained that it could take a while for them to get to know each other and for Yolanda to feel comfortable, and—in a radical shift from what Yolanda was used to— she asked permission to inquire about her family, how she grew up, school, and the things that had happened to her. The social worker reassured her that she wouldn't be asking all of the questions at once, but that they'd have these conversations as they got to know each other. She invited Yolanda's agency and partnership in the process.

The two of them began by talking about the things Yolanda enjoyed doing in her spare time. She liked school, was doing well, and wanted to continue. She liked reading and coloring books; coloring made her feel calm because all she had to do was color neatly to make a nice picture. The social worker offered to bring a few coloring books and colored pencils to their next visit so they could color together while they became more acquainted. Yolanda agreed. They then agreed on a convenient time for their next visit, and the social worker showed her how to program the time into her phone. She also agreed to take Yolanda to a local consignment shop to buy maternity clothes.

From the beginning, the social worker established the frame of safety: *"I'm here to help, and I'm here to understand."* Yolanda sensed that this social worker was different from those she had seen in the past: She was curious, interested, and helpful. And she was responsive to Yolanda's pace and to the issues that mattered to her. This was a critical hedge against Yolanda's potential defensiveness or withdrawal, promoting regulation.

The social worker also responded to the fact that—as a young, traumatized parent-to-be who had been betrayed by adults so often—Yolanda needed a lot of concrete support. Taking a more active role was essential to building safety, helping her feel regulated, and establishing trust. After this first session, Yolanda likely felt heard and supported in a new way and had new tools to help her feel less overwhelmed and more agentive. As she gained confidence, the social worker would help her do more on her own. We could only imagine, from the little we knew of her life story, how chaotic, alone, and neglected she must have felt inside.

Pregnancy Interview

The social worker administered the PI 2 months before the baby was due. Though 7 months pregnant with her son, Yolanda was a teenage girl, excited about the things teenage girls are excited about: going back to high school, seeing her friends, and so on. And also like a teenager, she had little sense of what parenthood would actually be like and expected to go to school "*like a normal kid*" with only a little more to juggle. It took her a long time to accept that she was pregnant. When asked about the moment she found out she was pregnant, she said simply, "*Oh, it was not a good day.*" She was shocked, and simply didn't believe it. It took months for the reality to sink in.

SOCIAL WORKER: When did you first really believe you were having a baby?

YOLANDA: When I heard the heartbeat. I mean, I seen my stomach getting big. I just thought I was getting fat, so I was just like, maybe it's not a baby in there. But then when I went for my first, um, when I went to hear the baby's heartbeat and I heard it for the first time, that's when I—it took, like, almost two, like three months for me to actually believe it. And I got to hear his heartbeat and I cried. I was always sad. . . . I, I don't know . . . I mean, I didn't know. The midwives told me it was normal for me to feel sad.

SOCIAL WORKER: Why do you think you felt sad?

YOLANDA: I don't know . . . I don't know . . . everything about everything. Looking in the mirror made me sad because I was getting big.

Consistent with her age and the degree of her prior trauma exposure, Yolanda couldn't articulate what made her sad. Her style was to push things down and try to keep moving. However, there were times during the interview that her feelings broke through. This tended to take the form of her contradicting herself within the course of a couple of sentences or falling into a kind of helpless state.

SOCIAL WORKER: Do you have any worries about the baby?

YOLANDA: So I really didn't have any worries. But when he didn't move for, like, 2 days, that's when I was worried.

SOCIAL WORKER: What do you think will be the hardest times in your baby's first 6 months?

YOLANDA: The crying . . .

SOCIAL WORKER: Why?

YOLANDA: Because I want to . . . I think I'd, like, I'd want to think everything bad, like, is he, like, I don't know. Probably calling the doctor every 5 minutes, worrying, like, if I did something wrong, or if he's hungry, but I know if he's hungry or if he needs to get changed, or something like that. I don't know, I just. . . ."

Her feeling of being overwhelmed and helpless came through when she was asked whether she had a relationship with the baby yet; she said yes, but then struggled to put words to it. "*I don't know. I don't know everything. I know, like, I don't know . . . because he's not here, so I really wouldn't. . . . I just know what things he likes and what things he doesn't. And I know when he hears my voice or my mom's voice it makes him happy. He starts moving around a lot. That's pretty much all the stuff I really know.*" The helpless refrain of "*I don't know*" repeats throughout the transcript.

Contradiction and conflict laced her descriptions of her relationship with Mildred. Allusions to Mildred's anger and inclination to violent outbursts were quickly contradicted. "*My mom was fine. She don't yell. She doesn't yell like that. Only if, well, technically, at me, because I'm older. But she would never yell at an infant.*" She unconvincingly described their relationship as "*closer,*" but then puts this in a larger context: "*Because I depend on her for a lot of stuff. Before, I didn't want to depend on her. I wanted to be, like, on my own, but now, I have no idea how to raise a, like, baby, so I depend on her a lot.*" As the team was to learn over the upcoming months, Mildred was in fact very difficult: controlling, restrictive, angry, critical of Yolanda to the point of cruelty. Yolanda had been rebelling against her mother's control and struggling to be more independent when she became pregnant. But in the early months of getting to know the clinicians, Yolanda resorted to more benign descriptions of her mother's anger, such as "*jumpy,*" "*going overboard,*" and "*a little upset,*" "*it wasn't like my mom was going to hit me.*" She acknowledged there would be conflict, imagining, for example, that her mother would want her to let the baby cry at night, while she would want to comfort the baby. "*I just won't be able to.*"

On the more positive side, she brightened when she talked about taking care of herself and thus her son.

SOCIAL WORKER: What do you think you give your baby now?

YOLANDA: Well, before I didn't never drink milk like that, so I drink a lot of milk. I drink, I eat a lot. I could actually go for hours without eating, and now I have to eat, almost like every five minutes, because if I don't, it hurts.

SOCIAL WORKER: How do you feel about taking care of the baby's needs?

YOLANDA: Oh, that's, actually, it came easy to me.

SOCIAL WORKER: What will he need from you?

YOLANDA: I'm planning on breastfeeding. So, I have to eat healthy. I know that. . . .

SOCIAL WORKER: How do you think you'll feel taking care of those needs?

YOLANDA: I don't mind. I want to do it.

This was what we would try to capitalize on.

The Genogram

Yolanda had a very difficult time completing a genogram. Although some of this had to do with her age, it had much more to do with the extent to which she had blocked out all memories of the past. She responded to nearly all questions with a shrug of her shoulders and "*I don't know.*" She knew little about Mildred's family history or relatives and wasn't sure where Mildred had grown up. Yolanda had no memory of her father and hadn't had any contact with him since she was removed from home at age 2. Mildred never mentioned him.

Visits with the Nurse: Developing a Labor Plan

In her visits with the nurse, Yolanda began to discuss how frightened she was of giving birth. She hated going to her prenatal appointments and found the pelvic exams painful. The nurse gently encouraged her to tell her more, thinking of the ways that Yolanda's history of sexual abuse might affect her reactions to bodily sensations during pregnancy and delivery (see Chapter 11). Yolanda described being unable to catch her breath on the exam table; lying flat and exposed made her feel panicky. "*I don't know. It feels like I'm going to jump right out of my body, but I can't move.*" Her midwife had been very calm and tried to help her relax, but Yolanda found it impossible to do anything but stiffen up, which caused more discomfort. The nurse and Yolanda came up with a plan: Yolanda would raise her hand and signal the midwife to stop when she became fearful and stiffened. This would give her time to take several deep breaths. They role-played how Yolanda might ask for information about the procedure and practiced breathing techniques to help her regulate when she stiffened in fear.

At their next appointment, Yolanda filled the nurse in on her most recent prenatal visit and acknowledged that the midwife had been very responsive to her request to stop when Yolanda was overwhelmed. She also wondered why the midwife had to look *"down 'there' . . . I mean the baby is in my belly, not there."* The nurse offered to show Yolanda some pictures about how her body was changing as the baby was growing over the 40 weeks of pregnancy. Yolanda agreed. They then turned to a discussion of labor. The nurse asked Yolanda what she had heard about the experience.

YOLANDA: (*eyes wide*) I hear it's gonna be really hard and hurt a lot. I'm scared and I think I might freak out.

NURSE: You sound worried you might have a hard time and you might freak out. Tell me more about that.

YOLANDA: (*speaking quickly and obviously upset*) I've heard that you have to have a needle in you that makes your legs numb so you can't walk. It sounds scary. And what if I scream or want to get off the table? Will the nurses get mad? Will they think I shouldn't keep my baby?

NURSE: Those are a lot of worries. It sounds like you think of one thing that's scary and then you think of another and another. Does that sound right?

YOLANDA: It sure does! Sometimes I can't even sleep. My mind is going, going, going.

NURSE: (*leaning forward and using a quiet, calming voice*) That sounds really hard. And tiring!

YOLANDA: (*Whispers.*) Yeah.

NURSE: (*after pausing to let Yolanda sit with her feelings*) I'd like to tell you about the things that might happen when you get to the hospital so you know why a woman in labor might have an epidural or another procedure. But I also want you to know that many moms get scared and some scream. The nurses understand and no one will take away your baby if you cry and yell.

YOLANDA: (*Answers tentatively and takes a deep breath.*) Really? OK. . . .

NURSE: Let's start with ways you can help yourself with all those frightening thoughts that keep you from sleeping well, OK?

YOLANDA: (*Takes another deep breath and nods, her body relaxes a little.*) Yes. That would be good.

Over the next few weeks, Yolanda and the nurse developed a labor plan, but every step was difficult. The nurse described in detail the various stages of labor, from the onset of contractions to her water breaking, describing the positions she'd be in during the labor, and when forceps or other measures might be necessary. She walked Yolanda through the decisions she might need to make regarding pain management, anesthesia, and the like. And they practiced a variety of techniques to manage her fear and her pain: deep breathing, relaxation, and mindfulness. By helping Yolanda think through and anticipate the stages of labor as well as the feelings she was likely to have throughout the process, the nurse aimed to empower Yolanda at a time that she was likely to feel helpless and retraumatized.

The nurse, like the social worker, was focused throughout on building their relationship, listening, being curious, and wanting to understand. She praised Yolanda's efforts to take care of herself, empathized with her fears, and highlighted even the smallest successes. Although the "ghost" of Yolanda's sexual exploitation was always in the room, she could not discuss it directly. The nurse tried to address how her bodily memories were affecting her ability to tolerate obstetric exams and would—if not addressed—intrude unbearably during labor. She continuously assessed what Yolanda knew and understood and tried to provide the information she desperately needed to feel more competent and able: how her body was changing, how the baby was growing and developing, how important it was for Yolanda to take care of herself, what the labor would be like, what the baby might need after he was born, and so on. The nurse slowly helped the young mother bring the baby into focus, making him more and more real. Though lost in so many ways, Yolanda was bright and eager to learn. The nurse tried to normalize her fears and vulnerabilities and to keep in mind the ways her history of sexual abuse and abandonment were coloring so much of her experience of the pregnancy and impending motherhood.

Manny Arrives

The team visited Yolanda shortly after she came home from the hospital. She had made it through labor beautifully, and though she acknowledged that it had been terrifying, she was so proud to have come out the other side and to have a beautiful baby in her arms. The midwife had applauded her grit and bravery throughout and honored all of their prearranged signals and plans without missing a beat. Despite this very good news, the team could not help but notice that Mildred was suddenly very much present, and not in a good way. Thus began a tragic but perhaps predictable set of events that was to culminate in a very different outcome from the one Yolanda and the team had hoped for.

Postbirth Session with the Nurse

At the first visit after Manny's arrival, the nurse found Mildred sitting close to her daughter as the baby nursed. Yolanda was looking into the distance and holding the baby awkwardly and slightly away from her body. The grandmother, who had listened to the midwives talk about the benefits of breast feeding, insisted that her daughter breastfeed for at least several months. However, the new mother was very uncomfortable with the baby on her breast and was clearly not taking any pleasure in the activity.

> YOLANDA: Look—he keeps moving his head. He's saying he doesn't like it.
>
> NURSE: I see the baby really trying to find your nipple. It does look a little like he's shaking his head. Many babies have to figure breastfeeding out, and he is learning how to find your milk.
>
> YOLANDA: (*Frowns, sighs.*)

The nurse sensed that Yolanda was unable to hear the information and reassurance she was offering her and hypothesized that her arousal level was high. She thought about how to approach her. She knew that adolescents, especially those with a history of sexual abuse, often find the needs of the baby and the intimate touching during breastfeeding triggering. So, in an effort to offer Yolanda permission to try another mode of feeding, the nurse stressed that building a positive relationship was more important than the *mode* of feeding.

> NURSE: When you're relaxed, you communicate safety and security. If you don't like breastfeeding, he can feel just as safe and secure if you bottle-feed him.
>
> MILDRED: No, I want my grandson to have the best. Yolanda decided to have this baby. She needs to do the right thing now that she is a mother.

Yolanda looked defeated. The nurse was uncomfortable with the tension but aware that the mother needed the grandmother's support. She searched for ways to repair the situation and help Yolanda enjoy her newborn. After the baby after was fed and alert, she helped Yolanda sit holding the baby face-to-face.

> NURSE: Look how he is gazing right at you!
>
> YOLANDA: Can he even see me?
>
> NURSE: Yes! He can see you and he can even try to imitate you. He is learning from you. Let's try something.

The nurse asked Yolanda to make an "O" with her mouth and then wait to see what her son would do. The baby imitated Yolanda's facial expressions.

YOLANDA: Oh wow! How did he know to do that?

NURSE: Your baby was born wanting to know you! When you connect like this—holding him and playing quietly—you are both getting to know each other.

Moments of gentle play between mother and child, supported by the nurse, brought them both pleasure and became a foundation for their relationship. But Mildred continued to undermine Yolanda in a number of ways.

Visit with the Social Worker at 3 Months

Manny was about 3 months old and thriving. Things were not easy for Yolanda, however. Although she was working very hard at becoming a new mother and trying to keep up with her studies, her mother had quickly taken over caring for Manny and continually criticized Yolanda's attempts at soothing and attending to him. The social worker arrived for her visit to find that Mildred was out running errands, so the visit would take place just with Yolanda and the baby. Yolanda was feeling very confused by the advice her mother had been giving her. She wanted to pick Manny up and hold him when he was crying, but Mildred insisted that she would "spoil" Manny if she held him too often and that he only needed to be held for feeding, bathing, and diapering. The social worker could see that Yolanda's sense of competence as a mother was very fragile, and she was already concerned about Yolanda's mental and emotional well-being after labor and delivery. Yolanda constantly feared she would do something wrong and trigger her mother's censure.

Yolanda mentioned that Manny needed a bath, so the social worker offered to help.

SOCIAL WORKER: It's so nice how you have everything organized for Manny ahead of time. That will make the bath time go easier for both of you.

YOLANDA: Yeah, I remember reading that I should do that, and then you told me having the bath stuff out makes it easier, too.

SOCIAL WORKER: Ah, so you remembered! (*smiling*)

Yolanda: Yep. (*Shyly giggles.*)

SOCIAL WORKER: Manny looks so relaxed! It's almost as if he's thinking, "Mommy, you are being so gentle with me, and I know you'll take good care of me." (*Speaking for the baby*)

YOLANDA: He likes baths, but I don't get to bathe him as much as I want because I always have homework to do, and my mom doesn't think I do it right.

SOCIAL WORKER: Well, you certainly have a lot to juggle! What does your mom think you are doing wrong?

YOLANDA: She thinks I am too slow.

SOCIAL WORKER: Hunh, what do you think?

YOLANDA: I mean I just don't want him to cry, and if I take my time, I feel better, and he won't fuss as much.

SOCIAL WORKER: You know that's a really good observation! You're paying attention to how you and your baby feel. It sounds like you recognize that if you don't feel rushed, the bath time is better for the baby.

YOLANDA: Yeah, that's right, and my mom just wants me to hurry up and get it done. It stresses me. Manny is still so tiny and I haven't held little babies before like my mom has. I need to take my time so I don't drop or hurt him.

SOCIAL WORKER: That makes a lot of sense. You want to protect your baby and keep him safe. Very natural feelings for a new mom.

YOLANDA: I just want to take care of my baby the way I think is best. I listen to the pediatrician and you and the nurse. And I read a lot. My mom thinks I don't know anything but I do.

SOCIAL WORKER: (*wondering how to validate Yolanda without undermining Mildred, even though she does not agree with Mildred!*) That must be frustrating for you to learn so much and not be able to use it. You know quite a lot! I remember when we first met and one of the things you said was that you didn't know anything about babies, but look how much you know now!

YOLANDA: Yeah, I guess I do know more stuff now.

SOCIAL WORKER: Believe it or not, this happens all the time with new mothers and their mothers. Sometimes grandmas forget that their daughters are capable of taking care of their babies. I wonder if there are some times during the day where maybe you have time alone with Manny and you have a chance to follow your own instincts about taking care of him?

YOLANDA: I never thought about that. I do have time alone when I feed him when my mom goes out. Maybe I could just do what feels natural without hearing my mom's voice in my head telling me I'm wrong.

SOCIAL WORKER: That's a great idea. Manny will let you know in his own way what he needs. Remember we talked about his different cries and how he tells you when he's hungry, tired, or ready to play? It's almost like dancing. You and he will communicate with each other and get into your own special rhythm.

YOLANDA: Yeah, I remember. That kinda makes sense.

SOCIAL WORKER: It can be so hard in these early months, but you are doing a good job with Manny. He's healthy, growing and he's learning to trust that you will be there for him when he needs you just like you want him to.

YOLANDA: (*looks up at social worker with pleading eyes*) Really??

SOCIAL WORKER: (*Makes direct eye contact with warmth.*) Really.

YOLANDA: (*smiling and shyly bowing her head*) Thank you!

Nursing Visit at 6 Months

Midway through his first year, Manny was very active and into everything. Mildred insisted that the house be neat and everything put in its place and regularly harangued Yolanda about cleaning up after the baby. She was not to leave anything of the baby's around. Mildred made no attempt to child-proof anything, and there were breakable objects, knickknacks, house-plants, and stacks of DVDs within easy reach. Yolanda was tense all the time and followed Manny everywhere, cleaning up after him. Now in her junior year, she was also trying to keep up with her schoolwork. She often put him in his high chair while she worked. But it frustrated them both: He wanted to get down and explore, and she wanted peace.

The nurse wondered how to help Yolanda grow in confidence and competence. When they met, she would bring a bag of toys, sit on the floor, and encourage Yolanda to observe and wonder what her baby was thinking. Manny, who had little experience with playing, would crawl over to the TV remote or take clean diapers out of a basket. Yolanda found this very annoying.

NURSE: I know it's frustrating. Does he see you with the remote or diapers?

YOLANDA: Oh, yeah! I'm always looking for a show on TV that's OK for the baby to watch. And it's obvious I'm always reaching for a diaper. (*Laughs.*)

NURSE: Why do you think he chose those things?

YOLANDA: I don't know why he chooses those things instead of the toys you brought. Maybe he wants to get into the things I'm doing?

NURSE: (*reframing*) Yep! He really wants to be like you so much! You're so important to him. You are really the model of who he wants to be as he grows. He can't really tell you because he doesn't have words for it, but he can show you that he wants to be like you.

YOLANDA: So he's not just being bad and messing with things?

NURSE: What Manny is doing today is exactly what children do at his age. They learn by imitating. He's a smart cookie!

YOLANDA: Huh! I should tell Mom!

Hoping to defuse the tension between Yolanda and Mildred, the nurse began to include Mildred more intentionally in home visits. She drew attention to the ways Manny was learning new skills by exploring his surroundings and imitating the adults around him. On one occasion, she asked Mildred what it had been like for her when she was once a new mother. Mildred talked about how she wasn't sure what to do and how hard it was to have to learn everything all at once. She laughed at some of her own mistakes; Yolanda had never heard Mildred talk like this and laughed along. Soon afterward, the nurse noticed that Mildred had allowed Yolanda to set up a small toy kitchen near the dining room table where the toddler could imitate his grandmother cooking.

Manny Turns 1

As he entered his 2nd year and became proficient at walking and running, Manny was always on the move. Mildred had not yielded in her insistence on order, and it seemed as if her rules inhibited Manny's exploration and interrupted his play on a regular basis. Indeed, Manny seemed uninterested in playing with the toys but ran from one end of the house to the other, pulling things down onto the floor. There seemed to be little routine in his young life, and interactions with his mother still revolved around Yolanda following and cleaning up after him. Manny's frustrations had become all-out tantrums: falling to the floor, kicking, and crying. He was classified as disorganized in relation to attachment in the Strange Situation. Yolanda was very unhappy. She felt tyrannized by her mother's rules. She had to be home directly after school, was not allowed to bring her son over to her friends' homes, and her being able to do anything was contingent on her getting high grades. She seemed (re)traumatized, and we saw increasing signs of depression, apathy, and withdrawal. It was very hard for her to be emotionally available to her son, who clearly found her emotional distance, as well as the lack of structure and predictability, very disorganizing.

Mildred continued to send Yolanda mixed messages about her role in Manny's life. One minute she would criticize Yolanda's parenting skills, saying that she had no control over Manny and was too young to raise a toddler. The next she would berate Yolanda for wanting to do normal teenage things like attend her senior prom, insisting, "*You had this baby, he's your responsibility. There's no prom for fast girls who get pregnant.*" This left Yolanda in a constant state of confusion. When she tried to assert parental authority, her mother would immediately step in and take over. When she tried to be a normal teenager, Mildred would accuse her of being an irresponsible, unfit parent.

They continually struggled over Mildred's inability to tolerate any form of disorder. She expected the living room in their relatively small apartment to remain spotless, with all of her delicate figurines and houseplants untouched. This was hardly an ideal living situation for a curious, mobile toddler who needed to explore his environment. Despite multiple attempts by the home visiting team to educate the family about toddler development, safe exploration, and childproofing and to negotiate ways of making the home safer for Manny, Mildred insisted that he must learn to *"know better"* than to touch her valuables. She even went so far as to refuse to move a houseplant known to be poisonous out of his reach. As we discuss subsequently, that marked a most unfortunate turning point in Yolanda and Manny's relationship.

Session with the Nurse at 13 Months

In a session shortly after Manny's first birthday, the nurse arrived to find Yolanda somewhat withdrawn and Manny wandering around aimlessly. She decided to see whether she could find a way to engage Yolanda in play.

> NURSE: Tell me about your day with Manny. What do you enjoy doing together?
>
> YOLANDA: I don't know. Just the usual, get him dressed, feed him, give him a bath.
>
> NURSE: Uh-huh—all the things that need to get done! What do you two do together during the rest of the day?
>
> YOLANDA: (*clearly not very engaged in the conversation*) You know, hang out. Sometimes he'll look at his toys and throw them around. Sometimes I turn on the children's channel and he likes to dance to the music. That's good 'cos then I can clean up his stuff before my mom comes home.
>
> NURSE: (*picking up on Manny's pleasure in dancing*) He likes to dance? What sort of music does he like?
>
> YOLANDA: (*still not showing enthusiasm for the visit*) Yeah—he'll dance to anything, really.
>
> NURSE: (*Realizing that Yolanda is still very disengaged, wonders whether talking to Yolanda about her own feelings would be an entry point.*) What's it like for you to have a toddler now?

YOLANDA: (*looking up at the nurse for the first time*) It's tough! It was so much better when he was a baby. He's always whining or getting mad for no reason. Why does he have to do that? He's got everything he could want—nice clothes and toys—everything!

NURSE: You're wondering why he gets so upset?

YOLANDA: Yeah! It just makes my life so much harder.

NURSE: It is hard when he gets so frustrated and upset! What do you think that's all about?

YOLANDA: I have no idea! What does he have to get upset about? If I had all those things—clothes and nice stuff—I would be happy.

NURSE: Sometimes when babies, and even older people, can't find a way to say what is going on for them, it feels really frustrating! You feel like that at times?

YOLANDA: Like not having the words for what I feel? Yeah—like when my mom says I can't go to the school dance unless I get better grades. I get so mad I can't think.

NURSE: It is hard to think when you are really angry. What helps you when you feel that way?

YOLANDA: Sometimes I just go in my room. Just, you know, to be alone. I take some deep breaths, maybe listen to some music. It helps me calm down a little even if I'm still mad.

NURSE: (*Noticing that Manny has found his sneakers and is trying to put them on with no success, says to him*) You really wish you could do that all by yourself! I can see it's tricky and a little frustrating.

Manny looks at the nurse and tries again. The nurse refrains from offering help right away, wanting to see how Yolanda supports her son.

YOLANDA: (*frowning*) Oh boy—here it comes. He's gonna get angry!

NURSE: (*moving closer to Manny in case she can help diffuse the child's frustration if his mother cannot*) I bet you are right. (*To the child*) That looks hard. (*To Yolanda*) He really wants to do something that isn't working out. What would help him right now?

YOLANDA: (*watching her son*) Hmm . . . I have no idea.

Yolanda seems to feel helpless and resigned in the face of another of her son's tantrums. She sighs loudly. Manny looks up at his mother and imitates her sigh. Surprised, Yolanda smiles, and they both laugh.

NURSE: I guess taking a big breath helps with big feelings for both of you!

This vignette highlights how difficult it had become to engage Yolanda and how she seemed to be slipping back into the helplessness and withdrawal we had seen in pregnancy. In a visit with the social worker several weeks later, everything came to a head, marking a turning point in our efforts to support Yolanda and her son.

A Visit with the Social Worker at 14 Months

When Yolanda opened the door, Manny was wearing nothing but his diaper and crying loudly.

> YOLANDA: (*looking frustrated and exhausted*) Hi.
>
> SOCIAL WORKER: (pleasant, calm tone) Hi there, Yolanda! How are you?
>
> YOLANDA: I'm all right. (*Sighs.*)
>
> SOCIAL WORKER: It looks like I walked into a rough moment. My friend Manny's not happy. Did I interrupt something?
>
> YOLANDA: No, you didn't. He's been impossible all day. We didn't sleep much last night, and he won't take a nap, but he's been fussing all morning.
>
> SOCIAL WORKER: Wow, that does sound rough! (*Then, taking care of Mom first*) How have you been holding up?
>
> YOLANDA: I'm just really tired. All day I run after him to try and keep him from making a mess because I don't want to hear my mom's mouth. But he gets so mad when he can't touch what he wants, or I make him stop playing.
>
> SOCIAL WORKER: So, you feel pressured to keep up with him every minute to make sure he doesn't ruin anything of your mom's, because then she will be angry with you.
>
> YOLANDA: Right, exactly. . . . Can you help me get him dressed?
>
> SOCIAL WORKER: Sure, I'd be happy to! (*She distracts and entertains Manny while Yolanda dresses him and his mood slowly picks up. He is no longer distressed and beginning to show a faint smile.*) Aww, how's that, Manny? Do you feel better now? "Thank you, Mommy, for taking care of me even when I fuss."
>
> YOLANDA: (*smiling at him*) Are you gonna give Mommy a break now? He's so cute but he's so demanding. (*She lets Manny get up to walk around the living room now that he is dressed.*)
>
> SOCIAL WORKER: Hmm. Can you say more about that . . . demanding?
>
> YOLANDA: Well, when he was little, I felt like I had more control, you know? He couldn't move around as easily, and now he's so quick! Plus, my mom used to like him more when he was a little baby. Now she treats him like he's

in the way, and I really don't like that. He's not bad, he just likes to touch everything, you know, explore.

SOCIAL WORKER: Makes sense! You are so right, Manny isn't being "bad." He is actually doing exactly what toddlers should do, and that is play, explore his environment, and learn about his world. What would it feel like to be able to have Manny roam around and explore safely?

YOLANDA: Relief, I wouldn't have to worry all the time. Here it's like my mom, well, she doesn't say it outright, but she's always talking about how nice her things would stay if she didn't have a kid around all the time.

SOCIAL WORKER: (observing that Yolanda hanging her head) What does it feel like to hear her say that?

YOLANDA: Like she doesn't want us here.

SOCIAL WORKER: Oh, Yolanda, I am sorry, that must be hurtful.

YOLANDA: It used to hurt my feelings, but my mother used to always say how I kept her from living her life when I was a kid, so I'm used to her saying stuff like this.

SOCIAL WORKER: (noticing that Manny is chewing something) Did you give Manny something to eat?

YOLANDA: No.

SOCIAL WORKER: I think he's chewing on something.

YOLANDA: Wait, let me see. (She goes over to Manny, who is standing by a tall houseplant. She puts her fingers in his mouth and pulls out what appear to be bright green leaves.) He ate some of my mom's tree! (fear in her voice)

SOCIAL WORKER: That plant might be poisonous. I wonder if we should call poison control just to be safe. Don't panic, it might be no big deal, but it can't hurt to call, right?

YOLANDA: Will I get in trouble?

SOCIAL WORKER: Oh, no! Toddlers and small children are always getting into things. I mean we were right here with him and turned our heads for just a moment. These things can happen. Why don't we call together and see what they say?

YOLANDA: OK, can we do it together?

SOCIAL WORKER: Of course.

Manny did ingest a small amount of the poisonous tree the team had previously recommended be removed from the house. Poison control recommended that he be seen immediately, and Yolanda took him straight to his primary care provider. He had no symptoms at all. Yolanda's caseworker at the Department of Children and Families was informed, and Yolanda was not penalized in any way as the incident was an accident, immediate medical attention was sought, and the issue was resolved. However, Mildred blamed Yolanda and called her a "terrible mother" for "almost killing" her grandson.

This was the last straw for Yolanda, who left home a few weeks later to move in with her new boyfriend. Mildred filed a report with child protective services accusing Yolanda of abandoning her son. Yolanda was too defeated to contest Mildred's charge, and Mildred was eventually awarded custody of Manny (despite MTB-HV's recommendation to the contrary). Yolanda was offered supervised visitation. Although these were regularly scheduled, the conflict between Yolanda and Mildred often interrupted these visits. The MTB team continued their work with Yolanda and Manny and worked directly with Mildred.

Graduation from MTB

Parent Development Interview

A research assistant administered the PDI when Manny was 22 months old. Yolanda was living about a 15-minute drive from Manny and Mildred. Unsurprisingly, the PDI was concerning on a number of levels. On the one hand, Yolanda painted a very positive picture of her relationship with Manny, some of which seemed quite heartfelt and authentic.

> YOLANDA: I love spending time with him. I love being with him. I love everything about him. Um . . . I don't know . . . he gets away with a lot. (*Laughs.*) That's all . . . but he just, you can't be mad at him.
>
> INTERVIEWER: And are there other things about him that you really like?
>
> YOLANDA: Just his smile. He has the cutest smile and he likes to learn new things. I like teaching him so when he learns one thing, he likes to say it over and over. He likes to show people that he learned something, so—I love that he learns—he loves learning. So it's good.

She was clearly so proud of him and of herself for being able to read his signals and pick up on his cues. She emphasized again and again how very close they were.

Yet these positive representations were filled with longing and anger that she and her son were separated, despite the fact that they were "*the same.*" When asked about a time she and Manny "clicked," she gives a fairly chaotic answer:

> YOLANDA: I took him to the library and he likes books, so I showed him the little kids' books and he read his little books and I read my little books and he would follow me. He wanted to do everything I wanted to do, run the computer. I showed him how to use the computer. Showed that he was really close to me. So we spend a lot of time together. I gave him a bath. We were standing in the bath. He, he was eating. My son loves fruits. I love fruit. I like grapes, strawberries, all of that. He loves the same things I like, so I cut his up and I eat one and he eats one, so we're like, we look like twins eating the same at the same time. It was cute.

She jumps from one activity to the next and focuses on how similar they are, this being the evidence of their "clicking." When asked if there is ever a time they don't click, she draws a blank. She cannot think of a time of "trouble" between them; she is never, ever mad at him. She never feels angry, guilty, or needy as a parent. Negative affect toward anyone but Mildred is intolerable. She is trying so hard to hang on to what's good. Sadly, Manny seems to be having a very rough time. He has terrible tantrums: *"He'll scream really loud. He has a set of lungs on him, so he'll scream and scream really loud, or he'll hit."* The following passage gives a good feel for how much Manny is struggling, how confused he is about the situation he's in, and how much difficulty Yolanda is having making sense of him.

> INTERVIEWER: When he's upset, what does he do?
>
> YOLANDA: He screams. (*Laughs.*) Or he'll cry. But he'll go to me if he cries, or he'll go to my mom if he cries, or if not, he'll just run. He'll run, or he'll try to hide, or he screams a lot. A lot.
>
> INTERVIEWER: How does that make you feel?
>
> YOLANDA: Confused, like I don't understand why he's screaming like that so much because you have to hear him scream. I mean, it, it's loud. And I ask him, Why are you screaming? What's wrong? And he just, he just gets frustrated. He don't want nobody to touch him. He's like me. He doesn't want nobody to touch him. He doesn't want to come near nobody when he's mad, so he, I- I- he screams a lot.

Manny clings to her when she arrives and falls apart when she leaves. As is evident in the bald contradiction in the following passage, she cannot bear to see how much pain he is in.

> YOLANDA: He was happy that I was with him. He was happy at the time because he didn't want me to leave, and I had to go because I had to come back home. He had a hard time watching me leave, so he had fun.

The conflicts with Mildred are ever-present, and there are so many moments in the interview that make clear the ongoing war with her mother: Who knows him best? For instance:

YOLANDA: Because I know, I know exactly what my son likes. I know what he doesn't like. I know, my mom does, too. But I'm his mother. I have this in, I know when there's something wrong, and my mom doesn't really have that instinct like me, because he didn't come from her. But I know when there's something wrong with him, and I know when he's faking and I know when he's not, but my mom doesn't really have that. That instinct. She just thinks I'm going to fail at everything but she never gives me a chance to try.

The following passage, late in the interview, expresses these deep conflicts so clearly.

INTERVIEWER: When you were not together, when you were separated, can you think of a specific time?

YOLANDA: Oh, that's my worst feeling is not being with him. Um, I remember going more than like three days without seeing him, and it was hard. And I was always calling my mom and always listening to his voice, and it's just hard not being there, so when he sees me again after like three days go by, he will not let me go. He will cry, and he will scream, and he don't want to go to sleep because he doesn't want to close his eyes and see me leave, and so it's hard not being with him. So seeing him every other day, he gets used to it, to seeing me.

INTERVIEWER: OK. What kind of effect does it have on your child when you're separated?

YOLANDA: He is sad. I can tell it makes him sad, and it makes him anxious. He wants to be with me. He doesn't want to be with my mom. He wants to stay with me when I'm there. So I could tell it bothers him, so we try to keep it constantly, constantly, constantly.

INTERVIEWER: Um—what kind of effect did it have on you when you were separated?

YOLANDA: It makes me sad. Makes me really sad, and I feel like he needs me, and I can't be there, so it's hard. It makes me feel sad.

It becomes painfully clear how displaced and hurt Yolanda feels, and how hard it has become for her to see Manny with any regularity at all (despite her attempts to paint a more hopeful picture).

Summary

This heartbreaking story is one that infant mental health practitioners are sadly familiar with. Clinicians (and their supervisors) hope that some of what they have tried to build and support will "stick" as parents move forward with their lives. At the same time, they come to accept that toxic stressors—in Yolanda's case, prior sexual and ongoing emotional abuse (namely, complex trauma), the lack of any familial support, and her young age—can and do fundamentally undermine the development of a robust "enough" attachment relationship. Brenda, whom we described in the previous chapter, suffered a great deal of physical abuse as a child, but she had lived with her mother all her life, and somehow both parents had communicated their love for her. She was bright and feisty, and she was resilient. She had an angel in Clara, and she was already 18 when she became pregnant. Her child was secure in relation to attachment, and she became more reflective over the course of the intervention. She was able to process some of her early experiences of abuse with both clinicians. Yolanda suffered much deeper wounds and had no angels. And though the home visitors filled this role transiently, Mildred's continuing assaults on Yolanda's fundamental sense of herself made it impossible for her to fully take in what the team had to offer. Her child was disorganized in relation to attachment, and he seemed quite chaotic and disrupted at age 2. Yolanda had only become slightly more reflective. In the end, Mildred turned against the MTB team, making it all the harder for Yolanda to have anything at all to cling to. As we mentioned in Chapter 1, one of our analyses of the RCT data showed that mothers with the highest levels of trauma and the fewest familial, educational, or economic resources were most likely to have disorganized children. And although they might look somewhat more reflective, they were still struggling mightily at the end of the intervention.

Yolanda needed more than we could give her. Had we been able to ensure that Manny and Yolanda stayed together and/or been able to diminish Mildred's toxicity and possibly help Yolanda find a safer place to live, things might have gone better. But given her age, how profoundly insecure and disorganized she was when she came to parenthood, the extent of her mother's emotional difficulties, and the utter lack of any family resources, we were thwarted. In some communities, there might have been others willing to step in, or there might have been a residential setting that would provide Yolanda and Manny the support they needed to thrive on their own. But sadly, it was not to be. These are the families that we—and so many others—find so difficult to help. This is a challenge for the next generation of infant mental health providers and other practitioners working with young families.

Chapter

16

Genevieve, Jared, and Jimmy

In this chapter, we describe our work with Genevieve; her husband, Jared; and her son, Jimmy. Like many of the parents we have described throughout this book, Genevieve was struggling with multiple sequelae of early and prolonged trauma, and in many respects she met the criteria for complex trauma disorder. As we outlined in Chapter 5, trauma has a profound impact on the body, both the corpus itself *and* the brain. It also has a profound impact on parenting. Recall that the symptoms of complex trauma—"depression, anxiety, self-hatred, dissociation, substance abuse, self-destructive and risk-taking behaviors, revictimization, problems with interpersonal and intimate relationships (*including parenting*), medical and somatic concerns, and despair" (Courtois, 2004, p. 413, emphasis added)— are best viewed as *proxies* for underlying posttraumatic adaptations.

van der Kolk (2014), Courtois (2004), and others note that working with complex trauma necessarily balances stress and distress regulation on the one hand and alliance building on the other. As van der Kolk (2014) puts it, interventions must combine "top-down approaches (to activate social engagement) with bottom-up methods (to calm physical tensions in the body)" (p. 86). Establishing safety, quieting the body (and thus regulating the stress response system in a variety of ways), and establishing a trusting therapeutic relationship are crucial to the emergence of thinking, remembering, and mentalizing (i.e., cortical processing). To use the terms we have used throughout this book, building the relational foundations of reflection—safety, regulation, and the relationship—is essential to progress.

Genevieve

From our first meeting, Genevieve showed signs of a range of posttraumatic adaptations to a childhood filled with violence and fear. We worked in a variety of ways to address these adaptations and their sequelae for her and Jimmy. As we hope to make clear, she made a good deal of progress over the course of the intervention. She stabilized and her baby stabilized, and she was able to protect them both from violence and upheaval. And yet—as is manifest in the PDI collected at the point of her graduation from MTB-HV—she had work to do to more deeply process what had happened to her. Fortunately, her work in MTB-HV prepared her for this next stage of her and the family's healing.

Background

Genevieve joined MTB-HV when she was in her third trimester of pregnancy. She and her husband, Jared, were both in their early 20s. Genevieve, who was African American, had been a college student prior to becoming pregnant and planned to return to school after having the baby. Jared was intermittently employed. Genevieve's parents were in her life on a daily basis.

Genevieve's complex family history was a mosaic of poverty, trauma, physical and emotional abuse and neglect, alcoholism, and violence. She was the firstborn of two children. Her father was a severe alcoholic, and her mother beat her frequently as a child. Genevieve often had to intervene in physical fights between her parents. Neither parent was in any sense able to meet Genevieve's needs, either as a child, an adolescent, or a young parent. Her father was, in all but the physical sense, absent, and her mother, Estelle, was manipulative and controlling at best, and cruel at worst. Throughout Genevieve's childhood, Estelle's willingness to help her daughter in any way was contingent on Genevieve's ceding to her control. When Genevieve decided to marry Jared despite her mother's protests, her mother told her, "*Well, you are stupid, and you are gonna get exactly what you deserve, 'cause he's a bum.*"

Although Genevieve was capable of verbalizing traumatic incidents from her childhood, she idealized her parents and could not acknowledge their role in or contribution to her childhood of deprivation and hardship. This idealization rarely wavered, despite chilling disappointments, and she connected her self-worth to how much she could please them. She would blandly insist: "*My parents provided a home, and I had what I needed,*" as she struggled to please everyone. Her mother often demanded that she shop and prepare meals for her, despite the fact that she had a new baby and was quite overwhelmed. Estelle treated Genevieve like a servant, and

Genevieve found it nearly impossible to say no to any demands, no matter how unreasonable. She was the "good daughter" to her parents and the "good wife" to her husband. Unsurprisingly, her inability to put her own needs first often left her feeling overwhelmed and depleted.

Genevieve had wanted to have a baby since the day she and Jared were married, when she was 19. Jared did not feel ready for fatherhood, however, and expressed a great deal of ambivalence about becoming a parent. Like so many of the fathers we worked with in MTB-HV, he, too, had suffered repeated traumas as a child and chafed at the constraints of a committed relationship. When we met Genevieve, she made it clear that she and Jared had struggled throughout the pregnancy. He often drank too much, and—reading between the lines—we suspected both domestic violence and infidelity. Genevieve suffered from severe anemia during pregnancy, but she refused iron pills and eventually needed intravenous iron several times during the last months of the pregnancy. This added a layer of medical complexity to what was already a very stressful time in this young woman's life.

Pregnancy Interview

Genevieve described her reaction to discovering she was pregnant as happy shock. Like so many of our mothers, she couldn't believe she was pregnant, even though she and Jared had been trying to get pregnant for several months. Jared was shocked and happy, too, and actually brought home a second pregnancy test to be sure. Her mother bought a third pregnancy test. Genevieve was happy and excited, and once she heard the baby's heartbeat and saw the ultrasound, she began to believe "*it's really happening.*" When she was asked about hard feelings, she responded, "*feeling alone, and not having the support that I wanted from my husband.*" She became somewhat incoherent as she described finding herself pregnant and without the option to "*not be pregnant or walk out.*" She had no choice but to face the responsibility, which—given Jared's own difficulties and inability to fully commit to the pregnancy—left her feeling alone. She talked about how hard it was for her to "*feel out of control,*" worrying about the baby's health or about how she would balance caring for her baby and going to school. But, throughout, she made an obvious effort to minimize her worries.

Despite the fact that she had already begun to describe her fraught family relationships to the social worker, these were completely denied on the PI. When asked how she dealt with her loneliness, sadness, and feeling out of control, she replied, "*Talk to my family, my parents. Always. I know that they love me unconditionally, and they support me no matter what. That they only want the best for me.*" When asked how she imagined she'd be like her mother as a parent, she did not waver in her idealization: "*You know, I hope I'll be like her, like, in the way that she's . . . caring and she just supports us and she does whatever we need. She'll get it for us. She really wants us to be happy and independent.*" When asked if there was anything she feared repeating of her experience with her parents, she simply said, "*No.*"

The only chink in her armor came when she described her mother as sometimes "*too much of a friend. . . . Like she wants to have a friend. Sometimes, instead of, I don't know, being a mother and giving advice like a mother, she just thinks more like that she was my friend. Like when I was younger, she would let me get away with a lot of stuff because I think she was acting more like as if she was my friend.*" This seems to be a tolerable way to talk about her wish that her mother could've been more of a secure base. As we will see, this theme recurs in the PDI.

One very positive sign was that—despite the marital turmoil throughout her pregnancy—her delight about the pregnancy was palpable. She described her relationship with the fetus as "*incredible and amazing. . . . I love him, you know, and he's so a part of me. I think sometimes I forget how a part of me he is. Like if I'm sad or if I'm crying or if I'm upset, he'll kick me (laughs) and I just feel so good.*" These feelings were to anchor her in the difficult months ahead and to provide critical leverage at points throughout our work with her. When asked to describe her hopes for her son, she replied, "*I hope he'll be nice and calm. (Laughs.) And respectful and playful. We'll have a respectful family.*" Later, when asked to describe three wishes for her son at age 5, she replied, "*I'd want him to be healthy, respectful, and caring.*" Notably, she repeated the word "respectful." This was the only clue that disrespect had been a feature of all of her significant relationships up to that point. It was also a clue to how deeply she wanted to have a "respectable" life.

Jimmy Arrives

Following a smooth, healthy labor and delivery and a positive birth experience, both parents found themselves smitten with their beautiful baby boy. Although a successful breast-feeding relationship was established between mother and baby, pediatric well-baby checks 6–8 weeks postpartum revealed diminished growth and less than expected weight gain. Despite efforts to increase milk production and to protect the breast-feeding relationship, Genevieve became discouraged and gave in to her mother's pressure to switch to formula feeding.

Genevieve's hopes for a happy family and the euphoric feelings between the couple did not last. During the early months of Jimmy's life, marital tensions mounted, and both Genevieve and Jared felt their needs were unmet. Couples' counseling sessions with the MTB social worker focused on creating space for increasing healthy communication and exploring how the demands of parenthood affected the relationship and each spouse's expectations of the other. The team also offered to link Jared with services for anger management and alcohol treatment. Nevertheless, physical confrontations between the couple escalated. Jared's drinking increased, and he cheated on Genevieve. Her feelings of rage, betrayal, shame, and powerlessness undermined her sense of competence as a wife and mother, and she described feeling intensely sad and fatigued, unable to take pleasure in the daily activities that she previously enjoyed. At this point, Genevieve met criteria for postpartum depression and was prescribed a selective serotonin reuptake inhibitor (SSRI). In addition, she presented with various somatic complaints. Nevertheless, she had difficulty making and keeping health appointments for herself.

Fortunately, Genevieve did maintain Jimmy's pediatric visit schedule reasonably well. The feelings of love she had first described in pregnancy sustained her. And Jimmy's temperament was social, low key, and content for much of the first 6 months of his life. His "easygoing" disposition proved to be adaptive given the volatile family system he was born into. By 8 months of age, however, Jimmy appeared to have poor eye contact and low energy. He was still having difficulty sitting on his own and had not tried to roll over. Assessment with the Ages and Stages Questionnaire (ASQ; Squires et al., 2002) revealed delays in gross motor development that warranted a referral to early-intervention services. The team shared their concerns with Genevieve about Jimmy's development, yet she was unable to prioritize her son, given her own depression and rumination over her failing marriage. We then lost touch with her for several months. Phone calls and texts and letters went unanswered, as our concerns grew.

Genevieve Returns

Genevieve found her way back to MTB after a terrifying incident with Jared. The couple had agreed to separate after she learned of another of Jared's affairs, and she decided once and for all that her marriage was over. However, Jared's reaction to her beginning divorce proceedings was brutally violent. He came to the apartment drunk and enraged and physically attacked her. She was able to free herself and call the police, and he was arrested. Genevieve pressed charges, obtained a restraining order, and filed a motion in court that Jared only be allowed access to their son through supervised visitation.

Genevieve explained that she'd been out of contact for months because she had felt too embarrassed to tell the clinicians what had been going on, worried that they would be disappointed in her and judge her for her current circumstances. The team reassured her of their nonjudgmental support (starkly contrasting her own mother's response), and Genevieve reengaged with MTB and agreed to increase the frequency of home visits with the nurse and social worker. She had double the usual number of visits during her second year in the program. Her treatment involved a layering of interventions designed to address her needs for safety and support, more peaceful sleep, better nutrition and an exercise plan for weight loss and management, education regarding safer sex and access to long-term contraception. We also worked to increase opportunities for pleasurable interactions with her baby, and to create a safe space to explore her feelings about her role as a mother and how her life and relationships had changed. The clinicians also encouraged her to spend more time outside with the baby. Genevieve finally consented to a developmental assessment for Jimmy, who began physical therapy with an early intervention program soon afterward and made steady progress.

The second year of the MTB intervention revealed that the explosive confrontations between Jared and Genevieve had deeply affected Jimmy. Based on some of Jimmy's play, the clinical team began to suspect that the child had seen his father pushing and hitting his mother on more than one occasion. The social worker explored the impact on Jimmy of witnessing the violence between his parents and helped draw some parallels between Genevieve's own early childhood narrative and Jimmy's plight. This work fueled Genevieve's motivation to obtain a long-term protective order against her husband, to follow through with the divorce, and to continue fighting for supervised visitation as the only means of contact between Jared and Jimmy. It also helped her to think more deeply about how she could regulate her own feelings and learn to communicate in more assertive, modulated ways. She was also able to finally acknowledge that some of her early experiences with her parents had, in fact, been traumatic, letting go of some of her idealizations of her childhood. We learned more about her history of severe physical abuse at the hands of her mother and of her terror of her father when he was drunk and violent. Supporting Genevieve in putting her experiences into words in a safe, nonjudgmental context eventually led to recommendations and referrals for both Genevieve and Jimmy for more intensive therapeutic intervention. Genevieve's trauma as a domestic violence survivor and her need to control her own anger required more specialized care, as did Jimmy's need to have developmentally appropriate, relationship-based play therapy to recover from his own traumatic experiences.

Over time, Genevieve evolved into a mother engaged in caring for her child's needs. Jimmy's developmental progress and his increasing ability to communicate verbally and interact with his mother helped Genevieve feel more competent and confident. This newfound give-and-take exchange in the attachment relationship enabled Genevieve to become more emotionally available for her child. Jimmy's attachment to his mother was secure in the Strange Situation Procedure (SSP; Ainsworth et al., 1978) at 14 months.

As graduation drew near, Genevieve was acutely aware that it would soon be time to say good-bye to the MTB team. Although this was difficult, for the first time she had the experience that relationships can end in a positive, caring way. She was also able to see the end of her work with MTB as the mark of a new beginning for her as the mother of a healthy, playful, inquisitive toddler. Genevieve also noted that she emerged from the past 2 years "stronger" and with a clearer focus as she worked to build a better future for herself and her son.

Genevieve and Jimmy Graduate

Parent Development Interview

The PDI, administered after graduation by a neutral research assistant, revealed a young woman who clearly adored her son and who was proud of finding her way through a very tough time. It was clear that she took great pride in her mothering and in the many ways she was good at taking care of him, setting reasonable limits, and comforting him when he was distressed. At the same time, it revealed her clinging to an airbrushed picture of Jimmy's childhood, their *"beautiful, happy life,"* and the idea that little of what had happened affected him. It also revealed to a striking degree her continued idealization of her parents. This despite the fact that she had made progress in acknowledging how painful her childhood had been in her work with the clinicians; all nuance was gone from her PDI, however. There was no mention of Jimmy's difficulties, of her own depression, of the severe domestic violence that could have easily cost her custody of Jimmy. Their home was *"full of love . . . a happy environment."*

Genevieve's descriptions of her relationship with Jimmy were overwhelmingly positive; unlike her descriptions of her family, these felt more coherent and authentic. In myriad ways, she described herself as a trusted secure base: *"I just couldn't have asked for a better bond between us. I think that he really does trust me. And every time he's hurt, he looks for me . . . just like, every time he's hurt or he's not feelin' . . . he's just uncomfortable, whatever, he'll look for me. I'm the only one that can calm him. And I love that, I really do."* When asked what brings her joy as a parent, she remarked, *"So many things. I don't know. Seeing his face every day, kissing him goodnight, just . . . it's such a joy being able to see this little boy everyday grown up and really be his own person and know that I influenced him in every way. You know? Like . . . it's beautiful."* The MTB team worked hard to affirm and support the powerful positive feelings she had for her child.

Likely as a result of our sustained support of her efforts to be present for Jimmy, we saw the emergence of mentalizing on the PDI; she scored 1½ points higher on the RF scale at graduation than she had during pregnancy. When asked to describe a moment that she and her son weren't "clicking," she remembered a time when she had been too sick with the flu to care for Jimmy and had had to stay at her mother's house.

> GENEVIEVE: I had to stay at my mother's house, because I felt terrible, I was sleeping all day. And I would wake up, and say, "Jimmy, come here!" And it's like "No! . . . I want my grandma!" He didn't really want me. But I guess it was because I couldn't, I wasn't devoting as much time as he's used to. So he was upset at me, but he got over it.
>
> INTERVIEWER: How did you feel?
>
> GENEVIEVE: Well, terrible because I'm so used to comforting him, and I'm so used to him giving me all this love. But I understood where he was coming from. I knew it was because he was upset.

She understood his behavior in light of his feelings of being ignored and hurt and could respond accordingly.

Genevieve found it very difficult to identify any negative feelings she might have as a parent, and she consistently minimized her own distress, except in relation to her ex-husband. she viewed him as the sole cause of her anger and distress. When asked to describe a time in the preceding week when she felt angry as a parent, she replied, "*I can't think of one,*" and quickly turned to her anger at Jared and the pain she felt over Jimmy's time with his dad. She denied that her angry feelings had any effect on Jimmy: "*I don't think they affect him too much, only because I don't let it. Like, I don't, it's not his fault. It's just the situation, and I don't let it affect my son at all. Like, ummmm. I don't get angry in front of him. I don't. Uh-uh. I'll go walk away, or, you know, go to the bathroom or something.*" As she had found it difficult to see how powerfully Jimmy had been affected during the height of her struggles with Jared, she saw him as unaffected by the few negative feelings she was willing to acknowledge. When asked whether Jimmy might ever feel rejected, she responded: "*I would say no. I hope not. I really do.*" Her wish to have it be so is palpable. And yet there are moments of contradiction when she is able to briefly describe her anxiety and his hurt. When asked whether she ever worries about him, she replies, "*If I worry about him, I worry about how much pain he is in. Every time . . . like, he's with anybody else, I'm always like, 'Oh my gosh, is he OK?'*" In an unguarded moment, she describes her son as quite a "*handful,*" throwing himself on the floor, throwing things, really screaming and melting down: "*He really shows when he's upset. Phew. You know he's upset.*" But for the most part she has a good deal of difficulty seeing his struggles.

Interestingly, the theme of potential role reversal that emerged in the PI emerges even more clearly in the PDI. She describes their relationship as loving and provides the following as an example of their loving relationship: "*Like, he's only 2. He's really young, but if I'm like stressed or crying or, you know, he's just, he'll come over and he'll give me a hug or he'll give me one of his laughs. And like, he knows, like everything's going to be OK. This is what Mommy needs. She needs love and I love her.*" Speaking for the baby, she sees him as knowing it is his job to take care of his mom. She likes most his being the little man of the house: "*I like . . . he's such a helper. Like, if I'm sweeping the floor, he'll come with the broom, too, and he'll help me sweep. And he's all . . . everything is, 'Can I help? Can I help?' And I love that about him. I really do.*" And in an almost spooky repetition of her own struggles with her mother, she noted that: "*I really think that when I get older he's gonna cook and he's gonna clean for me. I'm like, I got this? You know what I mean?*"

But what is most striking in the interview is her continued idealization of her parents. When asked to provide three adjectives to describe her childhood relationship with her mother, Genevieve replied, "*Honest, trust, and friend.*" At first she has difficulty coming up with any examples of these adjectives and can't think of anything. Then, she talks about her early childhood: "*It was so loving, so nice, so honest.*" When asked to provide an example of her mother being a friend, she says, "*She's always been my friend. Me and my mother always had a great relationship, always. I knew I could go to her for anything, for anything, anything. You know, and she's not—it's not a friend, like, you know, she doesn't care what you do or whatever, you know. Still, but I, I, I love her and. . . . .*" [*Interviewer:* "*Is there a particular memory you have of her being a friend?*"] "*Um, just going shopping together and just . . . everything.*" Thus her example of closeness is a neutral and not intimate time spent together. When she is asked later how she wants to be like and unlike her mother as a parent, she replies, "*I wanna be like her in the sense that I want the love. I feel loved by her always or whate— . . . um, and she's just a great person. I really— she helps me with everything. I couldn't ask for a better per- . . . a parent.*" The one hint that this closeness is freighted comes when she says, "*I tell my mom everything. I feel guilty about it.*" Here she implies, quite indirectly, that her mother *needed* her in a way that made Genevieve feel obligated.

The PDI reveals in a rather stark way how much work Genevieve has ahead of her. The idealization of her parents, as well as her relative difficulty tolerating negative affect (both born of trauma), will, until they loosen and become more flexible, make her more vulnerable, both as a parent and as a person.

Genevieve and Complex Trauma Disorder

Diagnostically, this young mother really didn't "fit" most DSM criteria for PTSD, nor did she consistently meet criteria for an anxiety or mood disorder. Instead, she presented with multiple symptoms of depression, anxiety, and interpersonal problems throughout the first 12–18 months of the intervention, with symptoms shifting and manifesting in different ways over time. She did, however, meet many of the criteria for complex or developmental trauma disorder, specifically poor self-regulation, minimal tolerance for negative affect, poor impulse control, dissociative tendencies, and a tendency to abuse substances, particularly alcohol. Further support for this diagnosis came from the chaotic nature of her daily life, which included family *and* community violence; the role she adopted in her family as "pleaser," combined with her intimate interpersonal relationship struggles; and her overall internal dysregulation. It is useful, in this regard, to consider Genevieve's clinical presentation in light of the seven essential posttraumatic adaptations of complex trauma and to describe the clinical strategies used to address them.

Alterations in the Regulation of Affective Impulse— Anger and Self-Destructiveness

Genevieve's depressive, immobilized affect masked a simmering rage. At the end of her first year with MTB, it became evident that she was drinking more heavily when she wasn't with her baby and inviting random partners into her life. Genevieve also shamefully admitted to an incident in which she confronted her husband outside of his parents' home and assaulted him. She was arrested. Genevieve described this incident as the "lowest of her lows" and struggled with reconciling this image of herself with the image she aspired to project to the outside world and, most importantly, to her son. She worked diligently with the MTB team in mindfulness exercises, learning the difference between aggressive and assertive behavior, and pausing before taking action to think through other ways of responding.

Alterations in Attention and Consciousness— Amnesia and Dissociative Episodes

We saw many instances of dissociation in our work with Genevieve. For example, she reported that when she attacked Jared, she felt as though she were outside of her own body watching herself hit and punch him. In the months that her marriage was deteriorating, she reported frequent experiences of losing track of time, losing track of where she was in space, feeling disoriented and lost. She would sometimes seem to dissociate in sessions when discussing her interactions with Jared.

Alterations in Self-Perception—Chronic Guilt and Ongoing Feelings of Shame and Low Self-Worth

After Genevieve's return to MTB, we learned that her months-long "disappearance" was driven by her own shame and humiliation. Her persona as "the good one" became tarnished following her repeated makeups with Jared and her final assault and arrest. "*I was just too ashamed to see you guys,*" she said. "*You both think I am so smart and good, and look at what I have done, I got arrested for doing something so stupid. I wasn't even thinking about Jimmy. I was just so angry, and Jared isn't even worth it. I was supposed to finish college, be more educated, and have a good life. What happened to me? How could I sink so low?*" Reframing Genevieve's actions and helping her understand the feelings that drove them was key in helping her separate what she had done from who she was and who she had the potential to become. Making mistakes did not make her "*bad*" or "*unworthy.*" This was an important parallel for Genevieve, who, as a mother, would need to contain the growing pains and mistakes of her own son.

Alterations in Perception of Perpetrator

Genevieve's perceptions of Jared changed almost daily. He was a "*monster,*" a "*drunk,*" "*irresponsible,*" and "*useless,*" yet he was also the father of her child, the man she loved, and the husband with whom she so desperately wanted to craft a marriage and family life. Genevieve vacillated between wanting to make it work and knowing she couldn't stay in the marriage. Our work was grounded in allowing Genevieve safe space to explore these highly conflicted feelings without judgment, to bring her thoughts back to her baby whenever possible (e.g., wondering with her how Jimmy felt when he saw his parents fighting, being curious about how Jimmy made sense of his dad's absence and the new visiting arrangement), and to gently challenge the disconnection between the sense of self-worth she aspired to and how self-destructive she was in relation to Jared. It is important to note that Jared was not the only perpetrator in Genevieve's life, although it was much harder for her to see the depth and breadth of her parents' neglect and emotional abuse.

Alterations in Relationships to Others, Including Parenting—Trust and Intimacy Issues

Genevieve endured a great deal of what appeared to be manipulation, coercion, and violation in her marriage before filing for divorce, a pattern of revictimization that mirrored her childhood experience with her parents. She resumed sexual activity during the earliest postpartum weeks to appease Jared and continued to engage in an intimate relationship with him after they had separated, knowing he was unfaithful. Genevieve was desperate to believe that if she could keep the family together, Jimmy's childhood could only be happy and carefree. When gently challenged with alternative views on how a home riddled with verbal and physical conflict could affect a child's well-being and development, Genevieve would react defensively, change the subject, or simply shut down and disengage. When the MTB team gently observed her resistance to exploring this territory, Genevieve finally admitted that she could not tolerate the idea of her child being frightened or unhappy, despite knowing deep down that at times this was a reality. She desperately needed to believe that Jimmy was OK, because admitting otherwise would be a reflection and confirmation of her shortcomings as a mother. Her high hopes for herself mirrored the hopes the team held for her, and the sense of promise unfulfilled permeated the therapeutic relationship. The team created a "holding space" (Lieberman & Van Horn, 2008) for Genevieve to forgive herself and strive to be a more responsive, nurturing mother.

Somatization and/or Medical Problems

Although a very attractive young woman, Genevieve became obese following her pregnancy and struggled with sleep deprivation, depressed mood, and anxiety. She was aware that she was not herself and rarely felt healthy or energetic, yet she simply could not manage her own medical needs. She was able to articulate concerns about being depressed and feeling a lack of energy or pleasure in her life, but when the MTB team coordinated appointments for her to see her medical provider, she would deny any symptoms or problems. The MTB team then literally took Genevieve by the hand and accompanied her to her appointment with a list of concerns and "spoke for Genevieve," giving her the words and language she needed to describe what was ailing her. Following a physical exam and prescription of medication for her depressive mood and sleep deprivation, Genevieve began an exercise routine and changed her eating habits. By the time Jimmy reached his second birthday, Genevieve was reporting better quality of sleep and improved mood. The change in her confidence and overall well-being radiated in her smile and the delight she could now express in being with her son.

Alterations in Systems of Meaning— Hopelessness and Despair of the Future

When Genevieve began her relationship with MTB, she was an ambitious young woman determined to complete her college education and develop a meaningful career. When she lost sight of her goals and her sense of competence, feelings of hopelessness and despair became intense. Genevieve felt low, like a failure, and a poor example for her son. She was desperate not to end up like the women in her community who had multiple children with different men and relied on the government for support; she saw herself and the life she and Jimmy would have differently. As we prepared for graduation and a healthier, more emotionally stable Genevieve emerged, she decided that if she could survive the past 2 years, she could certainly complete school. She registered herself for the spring semester following her graduation from MTB.

Establishing Trust as a Central Goal of Treatment

Courtois (2004) describes the establishment of a safe clinician–patient relationship and a focus on rupture and repair as proceeding in stages, with a lengthy first stage of relationship building as crucial in *preparing* patients for the more common treatment for trauma symptoms, namely, psychotherapy and medication. The failure to focus on safety and the relationship and moving in too quickly on trauma processing hardens defensiveness and precludes the development of the capacity to reflect on one's own experience without fear and dysregulation. Thus a stage "devoted to the development of the treatment alliance, affect regulation, education, safety, and skill-building" (Courtois, 2004, p. 418), as well as self-care and self-compassion, is essential. This is analogous to what we have described as building the relational foundations of reflection before working more dynamically. Addressing trauma without crucial supports in place exposes the patient to unnecessary harm and the potential for retraumatization. This then paves the way for what Courtois calls the "middle stage," which is generally undertaken when the client has enough life stability and has learned adequate affect modulation and coping skills; in other words, when the relational foundations of reflection have been established. At this point, the individual is able to begin processing "traumatic material in enough detail and to a degree of completion and resolution to allow the individual to function with less posttraumatic impairment" (Courtois, 2004, p. 418). It is at this point that meaningful dynamic work (i.e., remembering, feeling, and understanding the roots of one's suffering or making sense of family relationships), becomes possible.

We would add to this that, when working with traumatized individuals *who are also parents,* this stage is essential to their being able to provide a secure base for the child and to developing the capacity to reflect on the child's experience. That is, "keeping the child in mind" (Slade, 2002) is impossible until the parent feels safe in the therapeutic relationship and in their body. Our work with Genevieve very much followed this pattern. For nearly the whole of the intervention, we worked on establishing and maintaining the alliance and providing a secure base for Genevieve to make sense of her emotional life, to regulate her intense negative affects, and to think about life beyond the chaos of the moment. At the same time, mindfulness, breathing exercises, and body scans were used to build self-regulation skills and assist her in stabilizing herself emotionally when she became distressed. A range of supports for self-care included nutritional counseling, birth control, linkages to her medical home, and so on. As her body became less alien to her, she began to settle. Only when she felt safe and regulated could she attend to Jimmy's very real developmental and emotional needs, and the child began to thrive.

Courtois (2004) notes that many patients will not disclose their traumatic experiences for a very long time; in some instances—despite a good relationship with the clinician—specific working through of trauma may not occur at all. However, the capacities for connection and regulation may be adequate for functioning to stabilize. This was entirely consistent with our experience implementing MTB-HV with Genevieve, as well as many other parents; some mothers would only disclose traumatic experiences as they approached graduation, or would only unburden themselves to the neutral research assistant collecting data after they had said good-bye to the clinicians. Nevertheless, the consistent focus of the program on safety, regulation, and relationship allowed them to stabilize, to function more effectively in a range of situations, and to keep themselves and their children in mind.

Some complex trauma survivors will not be able to move beyond establishing safety, regulation, and trust during the lifespan of a typical therapeutic relationship. Nevertheless, this work greatly improves the trauma survivor's quality of life and functioning. In Genevieve's case, the treatment phase only began as she was ending her relationship with MTB, and it was only her recent traumatic experiences with Jared that she could process. She was never really able to work through her own traumatic family history, name her feelings about these experiences, or identify how they might have been connected to her current circumstances as a young adult. At best, she was able to draw some basic parallels between witnessing violence between her parents as a child and Jimmy's witnessing his parents' violent marriage. The team recommended individual psychotherapy for Genevieve at graduation in hopes that the work she had done in MTB-HV would make it possible to move on to deeper work.

The Clinicians' Experience

The constant need to shift focus and contain many of Genevieve's intense feelings left an indelible imprint on the clinicians, who at times found themselves in the same grip of rage, helplessness, and hopelessness that plagued

Genevieve. The personal strengths that the team saw early on, namely, intelligence, insight, thoughtfulness, curiosity, and a willingness to learn new things, gave them high hopes for her development both as a young woman and as a mother. And the feelings of disappointment that ensued left the clinical team feeling unpleasantly surprised and depleted. This "hazard of caring" for a young mother and baby who had such great potential for better outcomes, yet remained in such peril both physically and psychologically, put each clinician at great risk for burnout and vicarious trauma (see Chapter 8). Indeed, the team showed signs of vicarious trauma at times and found the work with Genevieve intersecting with their personal and professional lives in complex ways. Both the nurse and social worker experienced physical symptoms such as chest tightening or headache prior to home visits; they also felt extreme fatigue upon leaving the home. Both found themselves worried about Genevieve's and Jimmy's safety. They listened anxiously to local news broadcasts, a feeling of panic rising whenever a story about a domestic dispute or murder in Genevieve's violent community aired. There were also moments of conflating Genevieve's experiences with what the clinicians were experiencing personally, which likewise altered the way the team perceived their expectations and hopes for Genevieve, as well as their own sense of competence as helpers and healers in her life.

During these times, the clinicians used clinical and reflective supervision to understand Genevieve diagnostically and dynamically, to make meaning of the feelings triggered by their relationship with Genevieve, and to plan next steps and strategies for intervention. When the team felt that they were failing or were unable to make repairs in the therapeutic relationship, the supervisory relationship provided containment for the clinicians in a way that paralleled the accepting, affirming, nonjudgmental holding space the clinicians themselves provided for Genevieve. The supervisors validated the clinicians' fears for Genevieve's safety and their feelings of helplessness when she temporarily disengaged from the program. And just as the team reminded Genevieve again and again how important she was to her son, the supervisors reminded the clinicians of their transforming role in Genevieve's life.

Chapter

17

Embracing Complexity

In this final chapter, we briefly review what we see as the main "take-aways" from this volume and consider some of the broader implications of the MTB-P model.

MTB began as a home visiting program, and, indeed, many of the examples in this book are drawn from our 20 years' experience working with parents and children in their homes. But the development of MTB-P grew out of our realization that the same principles that guided us in our home visiting model could be applied to a range of clinical settings, such as clinic-based infant–parent or child–parent psychotherapy (Lieberman et al., 2015), group interventions, health care practice (Ordway et al., 2015), or mental health consultation in classrooms and schools. The MTB-P approach is not tied to a particular discipline or form of intervention; rather, it can inform a range of interventions across a range of disciplines.

The Relational Foundations of Reflection

From the very beginning, we saw MTB as a reflective parenting program, meaning that it was based in the principles of attachment and mentalization theories and that one of our primary goals was to increase the reflective capacities of the parents we were working with. But as the program evolved, our understanding of our mission evolved and deepened. We realized that enhancing *parents'* reflective capacities was dependent upon the establishment of the relational foundations of reflection (RFR; see Figure 17.1). These are (1) safety from threat and danger, (2) the capacity to regulate states of arousal, and (3) an openness to relationship. We

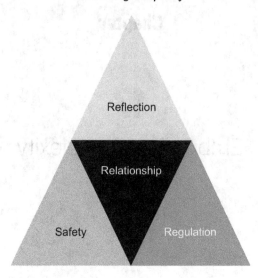

FIGURE 17.1 The relational foundations of reflection.

conceptualized these as building upon each other from the ground up, with safety and regulation essential to and reciprocal with the development of a relationship. We represented the interrelationship of threat, arousal, and the capacity for closeness and attachment using the interlocking triangles of the RFR pyramid.

We used the RFR pyramid for several reasons. The first is that it provides clinicians with a guide for assessment. Where is the parent on the pyramid, where is the child, and where is the clinician? Where must the work begin? The pyramid, as such, represents a process that experienced clinicians engage in all the time, gauging the parent's or child's level of threat, level of dysregulation or defense, and capacity for connection. It provides a framework for intervention. What techniques and strategies do I have at my disposal that will help build capacity from where the parent or child *is*? The RFR pyramid also graphically represents phenomena well described in the many literatures we reviewed in Part I. Threat, fear, and dysregulation are at the heart of attachment disruptions and failures of mentalizing, and as such they must be addressed before more secure relationships and genuine reflection can emerge. This is true for parent–child relationships, clinician–parent–child relationships, and indeed all relationships.

These relational foundations are particularly important for highly stressed and traumatized families who are vulnerable—by virtue of their everyday structural stresses, as well as the long arm of childhood trauma—to *prementalizing,* namely, defending against (too little) or flooded with affect (too much), in self-protective states of fight, flight, or freezing. These stances, which we understand as failures of affect regulation that arise from an abundance of threat, preclude true closeness or intimacy, and instead lead to a range of relational disruptions. They are often the focus of our work, where we begin and where we try to loosen well-entrenched defenses and the manifestations of an individual's fight to survive. What we are striving for (and what can often be so difficult to achieve) is for parents to stay, as much as possible, in a reflective space, where they can experience their feelings but at the same time think about and regulate them in a playful, authentic way. These are the relational foundations of reflection or mentalization; the more stressed and challenged parents are, and the more they struggle with the effects of current or past trauma, the more critical these relational foundations become.

To a large extent, we have focused throughout this book on working with parents. Although we are very concerned with children and their wellness, we see the parent as the conduit to the child. We reach the child *through* the parent. In Chapter 8, we used the concept of nested mentalization to describe the layers of "holding" (Winnicott, 1965) and reflection necessary for the child to flourish, with the supervisor holding the clinician, the clinician holding the parent, and the parent holding the baby. Our "arms" extend around the parent and child, and the supervisor's arms extend around the practitioner and the entire family. Although many practitioners recognize this intuitively, there remains today insufficient focus on the complexities of working with parents, who we must reach if we are to change the fundamentals of the child's experience.

Pleasure

A careful reader will note that—throughout this volume—we have pointed again and again to the important role of pleasure. There is great pleasure— both for the parent and infant—in becoming attached, in feeling deeply connected to another human being. There is pleasure in meeting the child's needs and in watching the child flourish. There is pleasure in loving and being loved. And there is pleasure in mentalizing, in "seeing" another in a way that deepens connection and makes intimacy possible. This is as true for the clinician as for any other actor in the clinical situation. For a whole host of reasons, pleasure has been all too absent from our thinking about relationships and what helps them grow. One of the most important elements of Alicia Lieberman's concept of "angels in the nursery" (Lieberman et al., 2005a) is the notion that the recovery of pleasurable memories can mitigate the impact of even the greatest pain. Likewise, the concept of "buffering" that is central to so much of the ACE and toxic stress literature implies that pleasure, delight, and warmth go a long way to dulling the impact of trauma and other environmental stressors. Good clinicians *know* this in their bones and look for every opportunity to help a parent engage with that pleasure—to laugh, to play, to snuggle, to name their hopes for their unborn child, to in so many ways awaken the systems in the brain that mitigate and soften negative affect.

The Mentalizing Clinician

Over the course of developing MTB-HV and training a diverse array of clinicians, we learned that the most critical aspect of any mentalization-based approach is the mentalizing capacity of the clinician, the capacity to be curious, to wonder, and to ask, in a variety of ways, "What's going on?" *This* is the agent of therapeutic change (Suchman et al., 2012). Parents' progress "up" the RFR pyramid depends upon the clinician's capacity to work from the top of the pyramid as much as possible. The clinician models reflection even in the most charged moments, providing a "zone of proximal development" (Vygotsky, 1980) for the parent or caregiver. This can, as any clinician knows, be very difficult, for parents' own pain and the defenses they have erected against it can be very activating for even the most seasoned clinicians. We fear for a parent's safety, for a baby's safety, for a parent's health or a baby's health. We may feel threatened when parents defy us or fail to change in the ways we wish they would or feel they *should*. And we, too, can become defensive, controlling, and too focused on teaching or "doing." When both the clinician and the parent are threatened, ruptures are inevitable. What is most important is to realize and acknowledge when we have been activated and to step back and try to reestablish our own reflectiveness. The only way parents are going to develop the capacity to reflect in a difficult moment, rather than react, is if they first feel they can trust us to provide a safe context for difficult feelings, that we can hear these feelings, name them, and tolerate them. They must also trust that we will not react by becoming threatening ourselves—judging them, fearing them, wanting to control them—at which point we become triggers, too.

We see a reflective stance as, by definition, an antiracist stance. As clinicians, we begin with the humility of not-knowing, of appreciating the limits of our own understanding. From this perspective, we build bridges while at the same time appreciating and celebrating difference. This makes true human connection possible; our shared humanity challenges the inequalities that are baked into care systems and societies at large. Reflective approaches mitigate the fear that one will not be heard or known. They challenge the assumption—usually based on long experience with care systems—that one will be criticized, implicitly or explicitly, and that one's perspective will not be taken seriously. They challenge the expectation of being dehumanized and rushed through a process without attention to one's particular needs and concerns. And they violate the assumption that one is not worth the care that comes with privilege.

Setting Expectations and the MTB-P Approach

We began MTB-HV with the goal of supporting health, mental health, and attachment by enhancing parental reflective functioning. But we learned that parents will not necessarily become adept at mentalizing over the course of an intervention. Hopefully, however, they will develop the skills to name and recognize their thoughts and feelings and to recognize those of the people around them. In any event, our gold standard for any intervention's success is *not* the development of full PRF. Our and others' research (e.g., Huber et al., 2015; Paris et al., 2015; Sadler et al., 2013; Fonagy et al., 2016) suggests that it is particularly those parents who have the "furthest to travel," who begin an intervention without any language for their inner lives, and who are prone to prementalizing and other primitive forms of self-protection who are most likely to benefit from this approach. Reflecting or mentalizing helps parents quiet storms of affect, make it through a rough patch because they can see the bigger picture, and calm themselves enough to find a way out of a deeply distressing situation. We see this when parents begin to summon a little perspective, to access what they know in a moment of panic, to *see* the child, to settle down and listen. And, as they become more regulated, they can experience a wider array of feelings, including hope and joy. Understanding this takes away the pressure on clinicians to achieve the "outcome" of PRF and allows clinicians to meet the parents where they are, which is the only place they can be!

Guidance and Concrete Support

The MTB-P approach does not preclude providing concrete support, information, or guidance. Doing so can be essential to establishing safety and regulation and to building a relationship that is based on the parent's being heard and understood. What distinguishes this approach from more psychoeducational or behavioral approaches, however, is *how* such support is given. *Directives*—particularly coming from a privileged professional who is likely of a different race and class than the parent—can be experienced as demeaning and disrespectful, potential invitations to shame and defensiveness. As such, balancing reflecting and directing is critical. As we hope is evident in our clinical examples, taking the time to hear the parent out, to repair ruptures, to hold their feelings and understand their thinking and cultural practices creates a very different context for the exchange of information and the offer of genuine help.

Many early-intervention models offer guidance, education, and support without engaging the parent's reflective capacities. But knowledge that is offered without an opportunity to learn it *from the inside out* (Suchman et al., 2017) cannot be internalized in a meaningful way and used to support parents' agency and autonomy. To return to the central message of Part II, by attending to threat and dysregulation, by building on the relationship we have developed with parents, by being willing to repair when we've gotten it wrong or have threatened the parent, we create the foundation for increasingly complex reflection and the development of a sense of competency and confidence as a parent.

Interdisciplinary Practice

MTB-HV was an interdisciplinary intervention, with nurses and social workers or family therapists working together to provide integrated and coordinated care. Thus what parents often experienced in other settings as distinct, uncoordinated, and fragmented systems were unified in their work with us. As we learned again and again, there was tremendous value in having health care and mental health providers working side by side. The pairing of nurses and social workers worked particularly well. Nurses provided critical health care and developmental guidance, and social workers provided both therapeutic and concrete support, facilitating access to resources and helping to navigate complex and seemingly impenetrable social systems. Working *collaboratively* allowed clinicians to provide what Osofsky and Lieberman (2011) refer to as a "seamless web of care." On the one hand, the ability to practice in this way is—in today's economies—a luxury. On the other hand, many view interdisciplinary work as an "innovative" practice and, as such, one to be strongly encouraged across a range of systems (Roney et al., 2021; Tomasik & Fleming, 2015). In this sense, it may one day well be considered a best practice for delivering care to young children and their families. From our perspective, collaboration among health, mental health, and other providers is essential, regardless of one's particular discipline. Once we appreciate how challenging it is for highly stressed, underresourced, and often traumatized parents to coordinate what are often fragmented, dysfunctional, and often dehumanizing health and social service systems, the value of interdisciplinary collaboration becomes crystal clear.

We have, throughout this volume, focused *both* on infant mental health and health practitioners, specifically nurses. We do this because we see the assessment of threat, the establishment of regulation, and relational engagement as essential to most, if not all, clinical encounters, regardless of the discipline of the practitioner. As we described in Chapter 11, the discussion of a range of health matters benefits greatly from creating a reflective space in which knowledge can be shared and truly integrated, where threat and dysregulation can be mitigated (Theede, 2018). We see the RFR model as transdisciplinary and applicable to a range of intervention approaches. Above all, it is an antidote to clinical approaches that fail to use the relationship to leverage change.

Expertise

In our view, developing *expertise* in one's area is an essential aspect of diversity-informed reflective practice. In recent years, the notion of expertise has come under scrutiny because of its association with the abuse of power, colonialism, and paternalism (Nucha Isarowong, personal communication, January 5, 2022). And yet, as we emphasize throughout this volume, we believe that the development of expertise—in its various forms—is essential to good clinical practice. The expertise that clinicians gain in their discipline, beginning with their education and building over the course of their careers, makes them better able to perform their given roles. Whether it is an appreciation of relational dynamics and defenses, knowledge regarding the impact of trauma, or the signs of developmental delay or potential illness, knowledge expands our reach. Across a range of domains, the more we know, the more helpful and trustworthy we can be (Allen, 2022). There is also our "skill in being human" (Allen, 2013), expertise in reaching people, connecting with them, knowing when and how to speak, to remain silent, to make eye contact, to allow for distance. Some clinicians bring elements of this expertise to their work from day 1, but even this skill builds with experience and training. These points should be self-evident, but they bear emphasizing.

In Chapter 8, we described the supervisory relationship as one path to the clinician's growing expertise. The supervisor, with many years of clinical practice under their belt, ideally has much to teach the supervisee; as such, supervisors are the midwives to the development of the supervisees' craft and discipline. From the supervisees' perspective, there is great value in learning from the supervisors' accumulated clinical experience and knowledge, in appreciating the wisdom that "elders" have *in their bones*. This is why we place such emphasis on *clinical* supervision as a necessary and critical accompaniment to reflective supervision. This is where, for example, nurses learn how to make an assessment and determine treatment options and where social workers and psychologists learn about interpersonal dynamics, about defenses, and about how to work therapeutically. These are the kinds of expertise that make transformative work possible.

Clinical Hypotheses

In Chapter 10, we described the value of the clinicians' offering their own knowledge and expertise to parents in the form of hypotheses. Clinical hypotheses, of all kinds, depend upon clinicians' ever-expanding knowledge base and deepening education about people, about the body, about development, about dynamics, about pathology and psychopathology, and about the clinical process. Without these, they are without critical tools to genuinely help. Clinicians scaffold or encourage the parent's understanding by offering their own thinking. The clinician has the tools to go beyond *"I wonder what this feels like for you"* to *deeper* reflections: *"I wonder whether that reminds you of when you were a little girl."*

We focus on hypotheses for a set of interlocking reasons. Mentalization-based treatment (Bateman & Fonagy, 2004) was developed—at least in part—as a challenge to classical psychoanalytic notions of the clinician as "expert" in the patient's experience: *"I am the expert, and I know what you feel, think, need, or know."* Rather, the mentalizing stance is one of curiosity, humility, and seeking to understand: *"I am an alien. Teach me what I need to know to understand you."* Although (as should be obvious to anyone reading this book) we wholeheartedly agree with this perspective, we also believe that clinicians have the potential to expand the parent's (or child's) understanding with what they can offer by way of knowledge or expertise. Recall the case of Sandy, the woman in Chapter 8 who was so angry at another woman's spreading lies about her. Rather than trying to engage the mother in why she shouldn't go out and fight the perpetrator, the clinician might have wondered (based on her knowledge of dynamics, of human behavior, and of this woman's history) *why* this was so incendiary for Sandy and begun forming a series of clinical hypotheses. She would begin with mirroring: *"This must be so humiliating,"* *"You try so hard to be a good mom, and do the right things, and she's making you out to be something else."* Had Sandy agreed, the clinician could begin to expand these slowly: *"You have this feeling a lot, I know, that people don't see you for who you are, that they don't recognize you."* These kinds of hypotheses, which go beyond mirroring and wondering and are based on the clinician's clinical experience and knowledge, can be very organizing for the parent (or child) and pave the way toward deeper understanding.

In our role as supervisors, we have at times found clinicians reluctant to move from mirroring and wondering to developing clinical hypotheses. Some of this has to do with mistaking hypothesizing for "directing" or imposing one's perspective on a parent or child. And some of it has to with a lack of confidence and, perhaps, of experience and skill in clinical formulation. This is where a focus within supervision on developing a range of clinical hypotheses becomes so important. The more we know, the more we can bring different perspectives and knowledge to bear, the more our hypotheses are likely to lead to genuine growth and change. It should go without saying that, in any context, knowledge that is delivered without an invitation to reflect is often an imposition and not a tool for personal and professional growth. Neither knowledge nor expertise should be experienced—by parent, child, *or supervisee*—as a bludgeon, or, to put it another way, a tool of oppression. But knowledge offered within the safety of a relationship, with an invitation to make meaning and integrate, can be enormously helpful.

Mental Health Challenges

We have made the point throughout this book that mental health challenges are known sequelae of structural stresses, systemic racism, and childhood trauma. As such, the more that families struggle with these realities, the more important it is for those who work with them to be reasonably knowledgeable about symptoms, diagnosis, and potential treatment options and to be able to create a therapeutic environment in which understanding and compassion can flourish. It is equally important that practitioners have a basic understanding of dynamics and defenses, for these are the processes most disrupted by early childhood trauma. Although this is a tall order, and many will argue that it is not within their scope of practice, we believe that such tools are critical to keeping families engaged in interventions and to *really* helping them. The well-documented success of CPP (Lieberman et al., 2015), which is a *psychotherapy* intervention grounded in both dynamic and trauma theories, is a case in point. The families who most need help drop out of more behavioral and psychoeducational programs at high rates. "Light touch" often means "no touch." This is a pressing problem for infant mental health practitioners and educators in a time of shrinking resources and limited funding. But it is a problem we cannot ignore.

The COVID-19 Pandemic

The COVID-19 pandemic has raged throughout the years we have been writing this book. It is unlikely to truly wane until the latter end of the decade (if we are lucky). This natural (and human-exacerbated) disaster has changed the lives of billions of people worldwide; it has also had a disproportionate and dramatic impact on the families with whom many of us work. Vital economic, social, educational, health, and mental health systems broke down as the pandemic spread; even today, in 2023, many of these systems are still struggling to recover. The pandemic hit racially and structurally minoritized families living in poverty, in close quarters, and with little access to quality health care very hard; they were far more likely than their more privileged neighbors to be infected and more likely to die (Magesh et al., 2021). Already-stressed families lost access to intervention services at a time when rates of child maltreatment and domestic violence were driven up by the effects of social isolation and economic collapse (Brown et al., 2020; Bullinger et al., 2022; Tso et al., 2022). The loss of services for children who were developmentally delayed was especially catastrophic (Slade, 2020).

The pandemic has had a dramatic impact not only on the families with whom most of us work but also on the way interventions are delivered. In the face of the collapse of multiple systems, a range of programs—home visiting programs, infant mental health programs, health clinics, early intervention, and other consultation services—quickly pivoted to telehealth. It was a rapid and stressful transition, but with creativity and persistence on the part of both practitioners and families, dyadic and triadic work was possible (Alvarez, 2021; Mayers, 2021), across a range of modalities (Davis et al., 2021). In MTB-HV, home visitors worked very hard to find creative ways of establishing additional in-person contact (conducting visits from the street, with the parents in a window or on their front porches; leaving supplies on the doorstep; and working double time to assess families' needs and link them to desperately needed resources). Across a range of programs, despite multiple bumps in the road and with their only (or primary) contact being through phones, iPads, or other fallible and often frustrating devices, fragile bonds were maintained. For many families, these lifelines were absolutely vital. The work was altered, but viable.

Today, in 2023, although many practitioners have returned to in-person care, for some families—namely, those who are geographically dispersed, living in neighborhoods with high rates of infection, or who prefer virtual to in-person sessions for a variety of reasons (availability of transportation, etc.)—telehealth has become the modality of choice. Some practitioners also prefer telehealth, again for reasons of convenience, safety, and so on. Overnight, what had been largely unthinkable in 2019[1] became a normal and acceptable way of working. We are just beginning to learn how these rapid changes in service delivery have affected home visiting and other interventions with parents and young children. The "key ingredient"

---

[1] Though it is important to note that telemedicine (Ekeland et al., 2010) has been practiced in various forms since the mid-1990s.

in psychotherapies of all kinds, and likely in many forms of health care delivery, is the therapeutic relationship (Holmes & Slade, 2018; Wampold & Imel, 2015). But in this time of expanding virtual service delivery, how do we think about the development of online relationships (Bashshur et al., 2016; Fernández-Álvarez & Fernández-Álvarez, 2021)? The process of forming a meaningful relationship with someone you have never met in person will inevitably be different from forming a connection in person. In many instances, it may be challenging. This is likely especially true in the kinds of work we have described throughout this book, when clinician and parent and/or child must cross the multiple divides of race, class, and other forms of privilege and difference, or when problems are particularly severe and acute.

A recent issue of the *Infant Mental Health Journal,* edited by an international team of infant mental health practitioners (Brophy-Herb et al., 2022), presents evidence from around the world that telehealth provided a critical lifeline to families and children during the pandemic. In a special section on home visiting, edited by Mary Dozier, researchers document the viability of tele-home visiting, with many interventions continuing without substantial attrition or loss of fidelity (Dozier, 2022; Roben et al., 2022; Rybińska et al., 2022). What is unclear at this point is how the shift to telehealth will have affected *intervention outcomes.* We know that telehealth will work, but we don't know how effective it will be. How will outcomes be affected by the loss of live, real-time observation? It takes great effort to replicate the home visiting or clinical context virtually, to observe both parent and child, to pick up subtle fluctuations in the interaction, and to move beyond the practical to the more personal and internal. So much can be and is hidden from screens in child–parent work. And how will outcomes be affected by the loss of personal, human contact between practitioners and families? There is much scientific evidence of the body-to-body and brain-to-brain resonance that takes place when people are in close contact (Di Pellegrino et al., 1992; Feldman, 2015); all these factors have been linked to therapeutic change (Blanck et al., 2019; Porges, 2011; Porges & Dana, 2018). Many of the relational foundations of reflection are established at the bodily level.

Clearly, there are no simple answers here. With telehealth, we lose opportunities for in-person *human* contact and close observation in relationship-based practices (home visiting, infant mental health practice, psychotherapy). Yet telehealth remains the very best option for many families and practitioners. The shift to online practice also mirrors a larger societal shift toward online rather than in-person communication, a shift that has the potential to fundamentally alter our sense of ourselves and of others (Turkle, 2015). Emerging data point us toward the middle ground, finding a balance between in-person and virtual work. Practitioners working with families and young children anecdotally report that relationships that had already begun in person were easier to sustain once interventions moved online. In these instances, it seemed to be easier to engage families (and particularly children) when the in-person relationship had already been established. This leads us to believe that—when working with parents and their young children—at least some in-person contact will help solidify the therapeutic alliance in critical ways. Even with families who prefer to work remotely, a hybrid model might be preferable. One of our research collaborators, Maggie Holland, is currently testing the hypothesis that those home-visited families in NFP who had met their home visitors in person at the start of the intervention would do better across a range of outcomes than those who had never had in-person contact. We eagerly await these findings. In the meantime, practitioners across a range of disciplines are in the midst of a giant natural experiment that continuously tests their flexibility, openness, and resilience.

Embracing Complexity

In closing, we return to Sally Provence's wonderful words, "Embrace complexity." As is surely apparent to any reader of this book, the paths we have drawn over the last 372 pages are not straightforward and simple. None of what ails the families we work with has developed overnight, and none can be resolved easily. This makes our work difficult. But the rewards that come—to them and to us—from embracing complexity, taking the time and the space to understand, make meaning, and create coherence, are enormous. Deep change comes slowly, with reversals and ruptures a part of the process. In today's world, time is so often a rarity and a luxury. But if we are to heal wounds that are painful and profound, if we are to share knowledge and build foundations, we need time and we need our humanity, in all its richness and promise.

Appendix

The Pregnancy Interview

Arietta Slade

This interview is an adaptation of the Pregnancy Interview (Slade, Grunebaum, Huganir, & Reeves, 1987).

INSTRUCTIONS TO INTERVIEWERS

A. Before Mother Arrives

If the mother has agreed to be recorded, make sure all the materials are ready and that the equipment works. Remember to try and make the mother comfortable while you set up the equipment. If you anticipate interruptions, it would be a good idea to let the mother know you may turn the recorder off in these instances, and then turn it back on when the interruption has been addressed.

B. Introducing the Interview

Begin by endeavoring to put the mother at ease; the tone, from the outset, should be friendly and relaxed. Describe the basic features of the interview: It is aimed at learning about the woman's experience of pregnancy and some of her expectations about the child and about motherhood, it takes roughly an hour to complete, it has just over 20 questions.

Describe the interview in a conversational tone. The aim here is to give the mother an idea of the kinds of questions she will be asked, doing so in a relaxed

From Slade (2003). *The Pregnancy Interview* [Unpublished manuscript]. Yale Child Study Center. Reprinted by permission.

manner. Assure her there are no "right" or "wrong" answers—that you are interested in her thoughts and feelings about what parenting is like for her. Do not go overboard here. If she seems comfortable with the kind of introduction you are providing, do not feel you have to provide more information. Remind her that she is free to refuse to answer any question (although we do not expect she will want to).

After you have introduced and described the interview, ask mothers if they have any questions or concerns about the interview before you get started. Be sure to encourage mothers to ask any questions they wish then or during the interview if something should occur to them. Truly pause and genuinely ask for and wait for questions from the interviewee and listen for any concerns.

C. The Interview—General Comments

Begin by letting the mother know you will be asking a series of already pre-pared questions that have to be asked in a particular order. Let her know that you know that the nature of this format may mean that she will get asked about something you will have already discussed, but that there are methodological reasons for following the same order with each mother, and you hope she will bear with any redundancies. By the same token, let her that know the questions may sometimes seem irrelevant or foreign to her.

D. Administering the Interview

Ask questions exactly as they are written, except in situations where the same probe is asked repeatedly and you want to rephrase it slightly so that the interview sounds natural. You want to sound natural and conversational, but you do need to be consistent with the interview. So be careful when you reword that you don't change the meaning, and try to do this as little as possible. Of course there are times when mothers ask for a clarification or may actually not understand the question, in which case you will obviously have to rephrase the question. Just be careful not to change the meaning or elaborate the meaning of the question when you do so. Reliability (i.e., the comparability of inter-views across interviewers) depends upon interviewers' adopting similar styles of interviewing and on their adherence to the questions and probes as written. It is fine to contextualize or to use preambles appropriate to the mother (e.g., "*I know we talked about this before, but . . .* "). These kinds of remarks help the mother get to the question while leaving the questions themselves standard-ized.

A number of the questions have probes aimed at eliciting specific feelings, episodic memories, and reflective functioning. If the mother answers these questions without your having to probe, that is fine, but these probes must be asked if the mother does not answer them spontaneously. Probing adequately is probably the most important element of interview administration. The failure to probe as indicated can make it very difficult to score the interview.

You should have the interview nearly memorized, so that you are not glued to the materials and can maintain eye contact with the mother and insert comments and probes in an entirely natural manner. This is really important, because you are asking about difficult and complex issues, and the mother should feel that you are available and interested. This is essentially a semistructured interview, and it should be conducted in such a way as to make the mother maximally comfortable and responsive. These are difficult questions that touch upon powerful emotional issues; the more relaxed and unthreatened the mother feels, the more likely she is to be open and forthcoming.

It is very important to conduct the interview in such a way as not to interfere with the mother's particular style of responding. You need to let her know you hear her without saying too much or leading her on. For instance, some mothers are very guarded and limited in their responses. It is critical not to push such individuals too much; this will make them angry and even less forthcoming. Also, if you try too hard to get them to open up, you are intervening in a way that will affect their natural patterns of responsiveness. Some mothers are more vague and disorganized; it is very important to avoid the temptation to try to organize them. It is not your job to get them to make sense (which you won't be able to do anyway); it is your job to create a receptive atmosphere, so that they will communicate to you as fully as they're able. Just keep in mind that your job is to hear them as they are.

The most common interviewer errors are to probe too much or too little, either of which can make coding very difficult. Probing too much can arise for a variety of reasons, but the two most common are (1) getting enmeshed with a mother and trying to sort out a chaotic story, and (2) conducting a "clinical" interview, probing for unconscious material and the like. The first problem, enmeshment, is relatively easy to recognize because the interview goes on too long, and the interviewer finds themselves drowning in details and continually trying to get things straight. At this point, less probing is more. The tendency of clinicians to turn the PI into a true clinical interview also leads to too much probing. In clinical interviewing, we are working with the individual to get them to articulate diffuse, complex, and sometimes hidden meanings. In that sense, we are not after "meaning" on the PI. Do not supply words for her, do not say things like "*What I think you really mean to say is . . .*"; do not summarize, for example, "*When I think about all this together, I wonder whether. . . .*" Keep your clinical voice silent; this does not mean you shouldn't listen clinically, but it does mean you keep that line of thinking to yourself. You are really just trying to hear the story the way the mother tells it. Probes are meant to clarify the story, not reveal its other layers.

Probing too little usually occurs when a participant is herself defended and resistant in some way and subtly puts the interviewer off. In these circumstances, the interviewer often feels like they are being intrusive, bothering the participant, and that the kindest thing they can do is finish the interview fast. You certainly don't want to bug the participant any more than you have to, but if you find yourself rushing and uncomfortable, try to slow down and stick to the interview. If it is really difficult, probe selectively. In these cases, it is better to probe generally (*"Can you tell me more?"*) than to probe feelings (*"And how did that make you feel?"*). Probing too little also occurs when the interviewer does not follow up simple, unelaborated answers. For instance, if a mother gives a sparse answer (which often happens when participants are not especially comfortable with language and verbal communication), you can feel very free to ask her to tell you more, to invite her to flesh out the story. One-sentence answers are very difficult, if not impossible, to code. But some participants really need permission and encouragement to express themselves in this context, in which case you want to do the things you do with any person who is hesitant—encourage her and convey your interest in questions and full nonverbal engagement. Do not hesitate, ever, to ask questions that answer questions you have about an actual life event; any lack of clarity you feel is going to be just as vexing to the person coding the interview. Remember to always try to read your participant and adjust yourself to her comfort level to the extent that you get scorable and developed answers. Remember, too, that most mothers start off slowly and that your encouragement at a slow beginning will reinforce their warming up to the task.

E. Debriefing the Mother after the Interview

After the interview is completed, again inquire whether the mother has any questions about the interview or any other concerns that may have arisen during the course of the interview. Be sure to encourage the mother to raise even the slightest concern, and give her a way to reach you if she has any questions or feelings that she would like to discuss with you in the weeks after the meeting with you. This rarely happens, but sometimes mothers do have very strong feelings during the course of the interview, and they should be given a way to process these feelings with you if need be.

PREGNANCY INTERVIEW

Preamble

This interview is about the feelings you've been having during your pregnancy, about your baby and about yourself as an expectant mother. It has just over twenty questions, and usually takes about an hour—give or take—to finish. Before we get started, could you tell me just a little bit about the circumstances of your pregnancy, where you're living, who you're living with, what's happening with the father of the baby, are you working or going to school, etc. (Try to sensitively get a little sense of the mother's relationship to the father of the baby, etc., just so that a context is established for the interview. This section shouldn't take more than three minutes—it is just to get background and to have a little warmup.)

OK, thanks. That helps me get oriented. So, to start, now that you're in your _____ week of pregnancy . . . and you're how old?

1. What changes have you made in how active you are . . . for example, in what you eat, and how much you exercise?

   Have there been any changes in how you are sleeping?

   How do you feel about doing these things differently?

2. Can you remember the moment you found out that you were pregnant? (*Pause to let her think.*) Tell me about that moment. How did you feel? Why do you think you reacted that way?

3. Can you remember the father of the baby's reaction when he found out you were pregnant? (*Pause.*) Describe that moment to me. How did you feel about his reaction? Why do you think he reacted that way?

4. Can you remember what your family's reaction was when you told them? (*Pause.*) Describe that moment to me. How did you feel about their reaction? Why do you think they reacted that way?

5. Pregnancy is usually a pretty complicated time in terms of feelings and ups and downs. Let's start with your good feelings. What are some of the good feelings you've had during your pregnancy? (*If she is able to name feelings, probe for two of them, one at a time.*) Think of a time when you felt _____. Can you tell me about that time? Why do you think you felt _____?

6. Have you had any hard or difficult feelings during your pregnancy? (*If she can name feelings, probe for two of them, one at a time.*) Think of a time when you felt _____. Can you tell me about that time? Why do you think you felt _____?

   Have you had any worries about the baby? Think of a time when you felt _____. Can you tell me about that time? Why do you think you felt _____? (*Probe if she can't talk about negative feelings. If she can't come up with any negative feelings, probe for the following: Have you had any worries about the baby, or about how you'll manage once the baby's here, in terms of money, where to live, getting help with the baby, etc.? Does she know how she's going to manage financially, where she'll live, how she'll get help? Is she planning for it?*)

   What do you do when you have these feelings?

   Is there anyone you can talk to about the feelings that bother you during pregnancy?

   What makes it helpful to talk to that person?

7. When would you say you first really believed there was a baby growing inside of you?

Can you remember that moment? Tell me about that moment. How did you feel?

8. Would you say you have a relationship with the baby now?

(If she says yes:) Can you think of two words to describe that relationship? What makes you say the relationship is _____? (*Probe for both.*)

Do you have a nickname/special name for the baby?

9. Do you know the sex of the baby?

If yes: How do you feel about it?

If no: Do you have a preference or feelings either way?

10. What do you try to give the baby now?

How do you feel about taking care of those needs?

11. What will your baby need from you after it's born?

How will you feel taking care of those needs?

12. Take a minute to imagine your child in the future. What kind of person do you imagine your baby's going to be? What's the idea or picture that comes to mind? (*Pause.*) Why do you think ____ comes to mind?

13. When you think of the first six months of your baby's life, what do you imagine you'll be the happiest? (*If necessary: Why do you think that is going to be the happiest time?*)

14. When you think of the first six months of your baby's life, when do you imagine will be the hardest time? (*If necessary: Why do you think that is going to be the hardest time?*)

15. Who's going to help you take care of the baby after it's born?

Do you plan to go back to work/school? (And how easy/hard would that be for you?) If you are, who will be caring for the baby?

16. Since you've been pregnant, what has your relationship with your mother been like? (*Again, keep in mind that if mother uses any general descriptors, like "better," probe for that and examples.*)

17. In what ways do you imagine you will be like your mother as a parent?

In what ways do you imagine you'll be different?

18. Since you've been pregnant, what has your relationship with your father been like? (*Again, keep in mind that if mother uses any general descriptors, like "better," probe for that and examples.*)

19. In what ways do you imagine you will be like your father as a parent?

In what ways do you imagine you'll be different?

20. Are there things that you're afraid you'll do as a parent? Perhaps things your parents did to you that you're afraid you'll do, too?

21. How has your relationship with the father of the baby been affected by the pregnancy?

22. How do you expect him to be involved with the baby?

23. OK, we're almost done! If you had to think of five years from now and your child is five years old, and you had three wishes for your child, what would they be?

24. Is there anything else about what it's been like to be pregnant that you'd like to add?

Thank you very much!

Appendix

The Parent Development Interview—
Short Version (2004)

Arietta Slade, J. Lawrence Aber, Brenda Berger,
Ivan Bresgi, and Merryle Kaplan

This interview is an adaptation of the Parent Development Interview (Aber et al., 1985).

INSTRUCTIONS TO INTERVIEWERS

These instructions refer to the use of the PDI-R in a research setting. Obviously, if the interview is to be given in a clinical setting, the procedures will be modified somewhat, although the basic instructions should remain unchanged.

A. Before Parent Arrives

It is very important that the parent know that the interview will be conducted without the child present, so that other arrangements are made for the child. When the parent arrives, make sure all the materials are ready and that the equipment works (seems obvious, but it is surprising how often data are lost to equipment failures!).

Reprinted from Slade et al. (2004). Parent Development Interview–Revised [Unpublished manuscript]. Yale Child Study Center. Reprinted by permission.

B. Introducing the Interview

Begin by endeavoring to put the parent at ease; the tone, from the outset, should be friendly and relaxed. Describe the basic features of the interview: It is 1–1½ hours in length, it has 30 questions, covering a number of themes: parent's view of child and of their relationship with child; their view of themselves as a parent, their view of the emotional upheavals and joys inherent in parenting, their notion of the ways they have changed as a parent over the course of their child's life. You should also let them know that you will be asking them about some of their own childhood experiences as well.

Describe the interview in a conversational tone. The aim here is to give them an idea of the kinds of questions they will be asked, doing so in a relaxed manner. Assure them there are no "right" or "wrong" answers—that you are interested in their thoughts and feelings about what parenting is like for them Do not go overboard here. If they seem comfortable with the kind of introduction you are providing, do not feel you have to provide more information. Remind them they are free to refuse to answer any question (although we do not expect they will want to).

After you have introduced and described the interview, ask parents if they have any questions or concerns about the interview before you get started. Be sure to encourage parents to ask any questions they wish then or during the interview if something should occur to them.

Truly pause and genuinely ask for and wait for questions from interviewee and listen for any concerns.

C. The Interview—General Comments

Begin by letting the parent know you will be asking a series of already prepared questions which have to be asked in a particular order. Let them know that you know that the nature of this format may mean that they get asked about something you will have already discussed, but that there are methodological reasons for following the same order with each parent, and you hope they will bear with any redundancies. By the same token, let them know that the questions may sometimes seem irrelevant or foreign to them.

Let them know that because the interview is a long one, there may be times when you, the interviewer, will feel it necessary to speed them up. This kind of warning lets them know that if you speed up it is not for lack of interest and also lets them know in a subtle way that there are limits on how long their answers can be (i.e., not to go on and on for the first few questions when there will be many more).

Introduce new sections. When you tell the parent about the interview at the outset, you will be indicating that the interview has a number of sections. During the interview, introduce each section with comments such as "Now we're going to shift gears," or "Now we're going to turn to the next section." If you wish, you may describe in a word or two what the section is exploring, but it is probably best to stay with the general kinds of comments indicated above.

D. Administering the Interview

Ask questions as they are written, except in situations where the same probe is asked repeatedly and you want to rephrase it slightly so that the interview sounds natural. On the questions that ask the parents to provide a memory or an example for an adjective (#A1 and #B1), you can rephrase the question so as to make sure they understand the meaning (e.g., "You said your child was loving; can you think of a time that would illustrate that? Can you think of a time when she was loving?"). You want to sound natural and conversational, but you do need to be consistent with the interview. So be careful when you reword that you don't change the meaning, and try to do this as little as possible. Reliability (i.e., the comparability of interviews across interviewers) depends upon interviewers' adopting similar styles of interviewing and on their adherence to the questions and probes as written. It is fine to contextualize or to use preambles appropriate to the parent (e.g., "I know we talked about this before, but . . ."). These kinds of remarks help the parent get to the question while leaving the questions themselves standardized. But also do avoid sounding like a robot reading the questions!

Standard probes must be asked. In other words, if it says "Probe if necessary," you need only probe if the question has not been answered, in which case you say something like, "Tell me more about it" or "How did your child feel?" The areas to be probed are indicated on the interview itself. Any probe instructions that are not followed by the proviso "if necessary" must be asked.

Obviously, learn the child's name right away. The interview should be conducted in a conversational tone; you should have the interview nearly memorized, so that you are not glued to the materials and can maintain eye contact with the parent and insert comments and probes, in a natural manner. This is really important, because we are asking about difficult and complex issues, and the parent should feel that you are available and interested. This is essentially a semistructured interview, and it should be conducted in such a way as to make the parent maximally comfortable and responsive. These are difficult questions that touch upon powerful emotional issues; the more relaxed and unthreatened the parent feels, the more likely they are to be open and forthcoming.

It is very important to conduct the interview in such a way as not to interfere with the parent's particular style of responding. You need to let them know you hear them without saying too much or leading them on. For instance, some parents are very guarded and limited in their responses. It is critical not to push such individuals too much; this will make them angry and even less forthcoming. Also, if you try too hard to get them to open up, you are intervening in a way that will affect their natural patterns of responsiveness. With parents who are vague and disorganized, it is very important to avoid the temptation to try to organize them. It is not your job to get them to make sense (which you won't be able to do anyway); it is your job to create a receptive atmosphere, so that they will communicate to you as fully as they are able. Just keep in mind that your job is to hear them as they are.

The most common interviewer errors are to probe too much or too little, either of which can make coding very difficult. Probing too much can arise for a variety of reasons, but the two most common are (1) getting enmeshed with a parent and trying to sort out a chaotic story, and (2) conducting a "clinical" interview, probing for unconscious material and the like. The first problem, enmeshment, is relatively easy to recognize because the interview goes on too long, and the interviewer finds him- or herself drowning in details and continually trying to get things straight. At this point, less probing is more. The tendency of clinicians to turn the PDI into a true clinical interview also leads to too much probing. In clinical interviewing, we are working with the individual to get them to articulate diffuse, complex, and sometimes hidden meanings. We are not after "meaning" in that sense on the PDI. Do not supply words for them, do not say things like "What I think you really mean to say is . . ."; do not summarize, for example, "When I think about all this together, I wonder whether. . . . " Keep your clinical voice silent; this does not mean you shouldn't listen clinically, but it does mean you keep that line of thinking to yourself. You are really just trying to hear the story the way they tell it. Probes are meant to clarify the story, not reveal its other layers.

Probing too little usually occurs when a participant is defended and resistant in some way and subtly puts the interviewer off. In these circumstances, the interviewer often feels like they are being intrusive, bothering the participant, and that the kindest thing they can do is finish the interview fast. You certainly don't want to bug the participant any more than you have to, but if you find yourself rushing and uncomfortable, try to slow down and stick to the interview. If it is really difficult, probe selectively. In these cases, it is better to probe generally ("Can you tell me more?") than to probe feelings ("And how did that make you feel?"). Probing too little also occurs when the interviewer does not follow up simple, unelaborated answers. For instance, if a mother gives a sparse answer (which often happens when participants are not especially comfortable with language and verbal communication), you can feel very free to ask them to tell you more, to invite them to flesh out the story. One-sentence answers are very difficult, if not impossible, to code. But some participants really need permission and encouragement to express themselves in this context, in which case you want to do the things you do with any person who is hesitant—encourage them and convey your interest in questions and full nonverbal engagement. Do not hesitate, ever, to ask questions that answer questions you have about an actual life event; any lack of clarity you feel is going to be just as vexing to the person coding the interview. Remember to always try to read your participants and adjust yourself to their comfort level to the extent that you get scorable and developed answers. Remember, too, that most parents start off slowly and that your encouragement at a slow beginning will reinforce their warming up to the task.

E. Debriefing the Parent after the Interview

After the interview is completed, again inquire whether the parent has any questions about the interview or any other concerns that may have arisen during the course of the interview. Be sure to encourage the parent to raise even the slightest concern, and give them a way to reach you if they have any questions or feelings that they would like to discuss with you in the weeks after their meeting with you. This rarely happens, but sometimes parents do have very strong feelings during the course of the interview, and they should be given a way to process these feelings with you if need be.

PARENT DEVELOPMENT INTERVIEW—SHORT VERSION

A. View of the Child

Today we're going to be talking about you and your child. We'll begin by talking about your child and your relationship, and then a little about your own experience as a child. Let's just start off by your telling me a little bit about your family—who lives in your family? How many children do you have? What are their ages? (Here you want to know how many children there are and their ages, including those living outside the home and parents or other adults living in the home. If it is an atypical rearing situation such as foster care, ask for the history of foster placements, who primary caregivers have been, etc.; likewise, if there appears to be a history of divorce or multiple moves, get some of the detail of that just to create a context for understanding the interview.)

1. I'd like to begin by getting a sense of the kind of person your child is, so could you get us started by choosing three adjectives that describe your child? (Pause while they list adjectives.) Now let's go back over each adjective. Does an incident or memory come to mind with respect to _____? (Go through and get a specific memory for each adjective.)

2. In an average week, what would you describe as his or her favorite things to do, his or her favorite times?

3. And the times or things he or she has most trouble with?

4. What do you like most about your child?

5. What do you like least about your child?

B. View of the Relationship

1. I'd like you to choose three adjectives that you feel reflect the relationship between you and (your child). (Pause while they list adjectives.) Now let's go back over each adjective. Does an incident or memory come to mind with respect to _____? (Go through and get a specific memory for each adjective.)

2. Describe a time in the last week when you and (your child) really "clicked." (Probe if necessary: Can you tell me more about the incident? How did you feel? How do you think (your child) felt?)

3. Now, describe a time in the last week when you and (your child) really weren't "clicking." (Probe if necessary: Can you tell me more about the incident? How did you feel? How do you think (your child) felt?)

4. How do you think your relationship with your child is affecting his or her development or personality?

C. Affective Experience of Parenting

1. Can you describe yourself as a parent?

2. What gives you the most joy in being a parent?

3. What gives you the most pain or difficulty in being a parent?

4. When you worry about (your child), what do you find yourself worrying most about?

5. How has having your child changed you?

6. Tell me about a time in the last week or two when you felt really angry as a parent. (Probe, if necessary: What kinds of situations make you feel this way? How do you handle your angry feelings?)

   6a. What kind of effect do these feelings have on your child?

7. Tell me about a time in the last week or two when you felt really guilty as a parent. (Probe, if necessary: What kinds of situations make you feel this way? How do you handle your guilty feelings?)

   7a. What kind of effect do these feelings have on your child?

8. Tell me about a time in the last week or two when you felt you really needed someone to take care of you. (Probe, if necessary: What kinds of situations make you feel this way? How do you handle your needy feelings?)

   8a. What kind of effect do these feelings have on (your child?)

9. Tell me about a time in the last week or two when you felt frightened as a parent. (Probe, if necessary: Can you tell me a little bit more about the situation? How did you handle your fearful feelings?)

   9a. What kind of effect do these feelings have on (your child?)

10. Tell me about a time in the last week or two when you have felt deeply moved or touched as a parent.

   10a. What kind of effect do these feelings have on (your child?)

11. When your child is upset, what does he or she do? How does that make you feel? What do you do?

12. Does (your child) ever feel rejected?

D. Parent's Family History

Now I'd like to ask you a few questions about your own parents, and about how your childhood experiences might have affected your feelings about parenting.

1. How do you think your experiences being parented affect your experience of being a parent now?
2. How do you want to be like and unlike your mother as a parent?
3. How about your father?
4. How are you like and unlike your mother as a parent?
5. How about your father?

E. Separation/Loss

1. Now, I'd like you to think of a time you and your child weren't together, when you were separated. Can you describe it to me? (Probe: What kind of effect did it have on the child? What kind of effect did it have on you? Note: If the parent describes something other than a recent—that is, within 1 year—separation, repeat the question asking for a more recent incident.)
2. Has there ever been a time in your child's life when you felt as if you were losing him or her just a little bit? What did that feel like for you?
3. Is there anyone very important to you who (your child) doesn't know but who you wish he or she was close to?
4. Do you think there are experiences in your child's life that you feel have been a setback for him or her?

F. Looking Behind, Looking Ahead

1. Your child is [age] already, and you're an experienced parent (modify as appropriate). If you had the experience to do all over again, what would you change? What wouldn't you change?

   Anything else you'd like to add?

   Thank you very much!

References

Aber, J. L., Slade, A., Berger, B., Bresgi, I., & Kaplan, M. (1985). *The Parent Development Interview* [Unpublished manuscript]. Barnard College.

Ahnert, L., Gunnar, M. R., Lamb, M. E., & Barthel, M. (2004). Transition to child care: Associations with infant–mother attachment, infant negative emotion, and cortisol elevations. *Child Development, 75*(3), 639–650.

Ainsworth, M. D. S. (1967). *Infancy in Uganda.* Johns Hopkins University Press.

Ainsworth, M. D. S., Blehar, M. C., Waters, E., & Wall, S. (1978). *Patterns of attachment: A psychological study of the strange situation.* Erlbaum.

Ainsworth, M. D. S., & Marvin, E. (1995). Interview with Mary Ainsworth. In E. Waters, B. E. Vaughn, G. Posada, & K. Kondo-Ikemura (Eds.), Caregiving, cultural, and cognitive perspectives on secure base behavior and working models: New growing points of attachment theory and research. *Monographs of the Society for Research in Child Development, 60,* 2–21.

Ainsworth, M. D. S., & Wittig, B. A. (1965). Attachment and exploratory behavior of one-year-olds in a strange situation. In B. M. Foss (Ed.), *Determinants of infant behavior* (Vol. 4, pp. 111–136). Methuen.

Allen, J. G. (2012). *Restoring mentalizing in attachment relationships: Treating trauma with plain old therapy.* American Psychiatric Association.

Allen, J. G. (2013). *Mentalizing in the development and treatment of attachment trauma.* Karnac Books.

Allen, J. G. (2022). *Trusting in psychotherapy.* American Psychiatric Association.

Allen, J. G., Fonagy, P., & Bateman, A. W. (2008). *Mentalizing in clinical practice.* American Psychiatric Association.

Alvarez, M. (2021, March 5). Symbolic play using telehealth: A brief case study during the COVID-19 pandemic. *Perspectives in Infant Mental Health.* Retrieved from *https://perspectives.waimh.org/2021/03/05/symbolic-play-using-telehealth-a-brief-case-study-during-the-covid-19-pandemic* .

American Psychiatric Association. (2022). *Diagnostic and statistical manual of mental disorders* (5th ed., text rev.). Author.

Ammerman, R. T., Shenk, C. E., Teeters, A. R., Noll, J. G., Putnam, F. W., & Van Ginkel, J. B. (2013). Multiple mediation of trauma and parenting stress in mothers in home visiting. *Infant Mental Health Journal, 34*(3), 234–241.

Ammerman, R. T., Stevens, J., Putnam, F. W., Altaye, M., Hulsmann, J. E., Lehmkuhl, H. D., . . . Van Ginkel, J. B. (2006). Predictors of early engagement in home visitation. *Journal of Family Violence, 21*(2), 105–115.

Anis, L., Perez, G., Benzies, K. M., Ewashen, C., Hart, M. H., & Letourneau, N. (2020). Convergent validity of three measures of reflective function: Parent Development Interview, Parental Reflective Function Questionnaire, and Reflective Function Questionnaire. *Frontiers in Psychology, 11*, Article 574719.

Badenoch, B. (2017). *The heart of trauma: Healing the embodied brain in the context of relationships.* Norton.

Bailey, Z. D., Krieger, N., Agenor, M., Graves, J., Linos, N., & Bassett, M. T. (2017). Structural racism and health inequities in the USA: Evidence and interventions. *Lancet, 389*, 1453–1463.

Bakermans-Kranenburg, M. J., & van IJzendoorn, M. H. (2009). The first 10,000 Adult Attachment Interviews: Distributions of adult attachment representations in clinical and non-clinical groups. *Attachment and Human Development, 11*(3), 223–263.

Bakermans-Kranenburg, M. J., & van IJzendoorn, M. H. (2016). Attachment, parenting, and genetics. In J. Cassidy & P. R. Shaver (Eds.), *Handbook of attachment: Theory, research, and clinical applications* (3rd ed., pp. 155–179). Guilford Press.

Bakermans-Kranenburg, M. J., van IJzendoorn, M. H., & Kroonenberg, P. M. (2004). Differences in attachment security between African-American and white children: Ethnicity or socio-economic status? *Infant Behavior and Development, 27*(3), 417–433.

Baldini, L. L., Parker, S. C., Nelson, B. W., & Siegel, D. J. (2014). The clinician as neuroarchitect: The importance of mindfulness and presence in clinical practice. *Clinical Social Work Journal, 42*(3), 218–227.

Banyard, V. L., Williams, L. M., & Siegel, J. A. (2001). The long-term mental health consequences of child sexual abuse: An exploratory study of the impact of multiple traumas in a sample of women. *Journal of Traumatic Stress, 14*, 697–715.

Banyard, V. L., Williams, L. M., & Siegel, J. A. (2003). The impact of complex trauma and depression on parenting: An exploration of mediating risk and protective factors. *Child Maltreatment, 8*(4), 334–349.

Barlow, J., Sleed, M., & Midgley, N. (2021). Enhancing parental reflective functioning through early dyadic interventions: A systematic review and meta-analysis. *Infant Mental Health Journal, 42*(1), 21–34.

Bashshur, R. L., Shannon, G. W., Bashshur, N., & Yellowlees, P. M. (2016). The empirical evidence for telemedicine interventions in mental disorders. *Telemedicine Journal and e-Health, 22*, 87–113.

Basu, S., Rehkopf, D. H., Siddiqi, A., Glymour, M. M., & Kawachi, I. (2016).

Health behaviors, mental health, and health care utilization among single mothers after welfare reforms in the 1990s. *American Journal of Epidemiology, 183*(6), 531–538.

Bateman, A., & Fonagy, P. (2004). *Psychotherapy for borderline personality disorder: Mentalization-based treatment.* Oxford University Press.

Bateman, A., & Fonagy, P. (2009). Randomized controlled trial of outpatient mentalization-based treatment versus structured clinical management for borderline personality disorder. *American Journal of Psychiatry, 166*(12), 1355–1364.

Bateman, A., & Fonagy, P. (2016). *Mentalization-based treatment for personality disorders: A practical guide.* Oxford University Press.

Beebe, B., Jaffe, J., Markese, S., Buck, K., Chen, H., Cohen, P., . . . Feldstein, S. (2010). The origins of 12-month attachment: A microanalysis of 4-month mother–infant interaction. *Attachment and Human Development, 12*(1–2), 6–141.

Beebe, B., & Stern, D. N. (1977). Engagement–disengagement and early object experiences. In N. Freedman & S. Grand (Eds.), *Communicative structures and psychic structure: A psychoanalytic interpretation of communication* (pp. 35–55). Springer.

Belsky, J. (1997). Theory testing, effect-size evaluation, and differential susceptibility to rearing influence: The case of mothering and attachment. *Child Development, 68*(4), 598–600.

Belsky, J., Bakermans-Kranenburg, M. J., & van IJzendoorn, M. H. (2007). For better and for worse: Differential susceptibility to environmental influences. *Current Directions in Psychological Science, 16*(6), 300–304.

Belsky, J., & Pluess, M. (2009). Beyond diathesis stress: Differential susceptibility to environmental influences. *Psychological Bulletin, 135*(6), 885–908.

Belsky, J., & Rovine, M. (1987). Temperament and attachment security in the Strange Situation: An empirical rapprochement. *Child Development, 58*(3), 787–795.

Benbassat, N., & Priel, B. (2012). Parenting and adolescent adjustment: The role of parental reflective function. *Journal of Adolescence, 35*(1), 163–174.

Benedek, T. (1959). Parenthood as a developmental phase: A contribution to the libido theory. *Journal of the American Psychoanalytic Association, 7*(3), 389–417.

Benoit, D., & Parker, K. C. (1994). Stability and transmission of attachment across three generations. *Child Development, 65*(5), 1444–1456.

Berthelot, N., Ensink, K., Bernazzani, O., Normandin, L., Luyten, P., & Fonagy, P. (2015). Intergenerational transmission of attachment in abused and neglected mothers: The role of trauma-specific reflective functioning. *Infant Mental Health Journal, 36*(2), 200–212.

Berthelot, N., Lemieux, R., Garon-Bissonnette, J., Lacharité, C., & Muzik, M. (2019). The protective role of mentalizing: Reflective functioning as a mediator between child maltreatment, psychopathology and parental attitude in expecting parents. *Child Abuse and Neglect, 95,* Article 104065.

Bethell, C., Gombojav, N., Solloway, M., & Wissow, L. (2016). Adverse childhood experiences, resilience and mindfulness-based approaches: Common denominator issues for children with emotional, mental, or behavioral problems. *Child and Adolescent Psychiatric Clinics, 25*(2), 139–156.

Bethell, C., Jones, J., Gombojav, N., Linkenbach, J., & Sege, R. (2019). Positive childhood experiences and adult mental and relational health in a statewide sample: Associations across adverse childhood experiences levels. *JAMA Pediatrics, 173*(11), e193007.

Blanck, P., Stoffel, M., Bents, H., Ditzen, B., & Mander, J. (2019). Heart rate variability in individual psychotherapy: Associations with alliance and outcome. *Journal of Nervous and Mental Disease, 207*(6), 451–458.

Bleiberg, E. (2013). Mentalizing-based treatment with adolescents and families. *Child and Adolescent Psychiatric Clinics, 22*(2), 295–330.

Blevins, C. A., Weathers, F. W., Davis, M. T., Witte, T. K., & Domino, J. L. (2015). The Posttraumatic Stress Disorder Checklist for *DSM-5* (PCL-5): Development and initial psychometric evaluation. *Journal of Traumatic Stress, 28*, 489–498.

Bögels, S. M., Lehtonen, A., & Restifo, K. (2010). Mindful parenting in mental health care. *Mindfulness, 1*(2), 107–120.

Bokhorst, C. L., Bakermans-Kranenburg, M. J., Fearon, P. R. M., van IJzendoorn, M. H., Fonagy, P., & Schuengel, C. (2003). The importance of shared environment in mother–infant attachment security: A behavioral genetic study. *Child Development, 74*(6), 1769–1782.

Borelli, J. L., Cohen, C., Pettit, C., Normandin, L., Target, M., Fonagy, P., & Ensink, K. (2019). Maternal and child sexual abuse history: An intergenerational exploration of children's adjustment and maternal trauma-reflective functioning. *Frontiers in Psychology, 10*, Article 1062.

Borelli, J. L., St. John, H. K., Cho, E., & Suchman, N. E. (2016). Reflective functioning in parents of school-aged children. *American Journal of Orthopsychiatry, 86*(1), 24–36.

Boris, N. W., Larrieu, J. A., Zeanah, P. D., Nagle, G. A., Steier, A., & McNeill, P. (2006). The process and promise of mental health augmentation of nurse home-visiting programs: Data from the Louisiana Nurse–Family Partnership. *Infant Mental Health Journal, 27*(1), 26–40.

Bowlby, J. (1944). Forty-four juvenile thieves: Their characters and home-life. *International Journal of Psychoanalysis, 25*, 19–53.

Bowlby, J. (1969/1982). Attachment and loss: Retrospect and prospect. *American Journal of Orthopsychiatry, 52*(4), 664–687.

Bowlby, J. (1973). *Attachment and loss: Vol. 2. Separation.* Basic Books.

Bowlby, J. (1979). On knowing what you are not supposed to know and feeling what you are not supposed to feel. *Canadian Journal of Psychiatry, 24*(5), 403–408.

Bowlby, J. (1980). *Attachment and loss: Vol. 3. Loss, sadness and depression.* Basic Books.

Bowlby, J. (1988). *A secure base: Clinical applications of attachment theory.* Routledge.

Brazelton, T. B. (1984). *Neonatal Behavioral Assessment Scale* (2nd ed.). Lippincott.

Bretherton, I. (1985). Attachment theory: Retrospect and prospect. *Monographs of the Society for Research in Child Development, 50*(1–2), 3–35.

Bretherton, I., & Beeghly, M. (1982). Talking about internal states: The acquisition of an explicit theory of mind. *Developmental Psychology, 18*(6), 906–921.

Bronfman, E. T., Parsons, E., & Lyons-Ruth, K. (1992–2008). *Disrupted Maternal Behavior Instrument for Assessment and Classification (AMBIANCE): Manual for coding disrupted affective communication* [Unpublished manuscript]. Harvard University Medical School.

Brophy-Herb, H. E., Barlow, J., Foley, M., Lawler, J., & von Klitzing, K. (Eds.). (2022). A brief overview from the editors: Infant and early childhood mental health in the context of COVID-19 [Special issue]. *Infant Mental Health Journal, 43*, 5–7.

Brown, D. W., Anda, R. F., Edwards, V. J., Felitti, V. J., Dube, S. R., & Giles, W. H. (2007). Adverse childhood experiences and childhood autobiographical memory disturbance. *Child Abuse and Neglect, 31*(9), 961–969.

Brown, S. M., Doom, J. R., Lechuga-Peña, S., Watamura, S. E., & Koppels, T. (2020). Stress and parenting during the COVID-19 pandemic. *Child Abuse and Neglect, 110*, 104699.

Bruce, N. G., Manber, R., Shapiro, S. L., & Constantino, M. J. (2010). Psychotherapist mindfulness and the psychotherapy process. *Psychotherapy: Theory, Research, Practice, Training, 47*(1), 83–97.

Bublitz, M. H., Parade, S., & Stroud, L. R. (2014). The effects of childhood sexual abuse on cortisol trajectories in pregnancy are moderated by current family functioning. *Biological Psychology, 103*, 152–157.

Buchanan, N. T., Perez, M., Prinstein, M., & Thurston, I. (2021). Upending racism in psychological science: Strategies to change how our science is conducted, reported, reviewed, and disseminated. *American Psychologist, 76*(7), 1097–1112.

Bullinger, L. R., Marcus, S., Reuben, K., Whitaker, D., & Self-Brown, S. (2022). Evaluating child maltreatment and family violence risk during the COVID-19 pandemic: Using a telehealth home visiting program as a conduit to families. *Infant Mental Health Journal, 43*, 143–158.

Byun, S., Brumariu, L. E., & Lyons-Ruth, K. (2016). Disorganized attachment in young adulthood as a partial mediator of relations between severity of childhood abuse and dissociation. *Journal of Trauma and Dissociation, 17*(4), 460–479.

Camoirano, A. (2017). Mentalizing makes parenting work: A review about parental reflective functioning and clinical interventions to improve it. *Frontiers in Psychology, 8*, 14.

Campos, J., Barrett, K., Lamb, M., Goldsmith, H., & Sternberg, C., (1983). Socioemotional development. In M. Haith & J. Campos (Eds.), *Handbook of child psychology: Vol. 2. Infancy and developmental psychobiology* (pp. 783–916). Wiley.

Carlson, E. A. (1998). A prospective longitudinal study of attachment disorganization/disorientation. *Child Development, 69*(4), 1107–1128.

Cassidy, J. (1994). Emotion regulation: Influences of attachment relationships. *Monographs of the Society for Research in Child Development, 59*(2–3), 228–249.

Cassidy, J. (2016). The nature of the child's ties. In J. Cassidy & P. R. Shaver (Eds.),

Handbook of attachment: Theory, research, and clinical applications (3rd ed., pp. 3–24). Guilford Press.

Cassidy, J. (2021). In the service of protection from threat: Attachment and internal working models. In J. Simpson, L. Berlin, & R. Thompson (Eds.), *Attachment: The fundamental questions* (pp. 103–109). Guilford Press.

Cassidy, J., & Berlin, L. J. (1994). The insecure/ambivalent pattern of attachment: Theory and research. *Child Development, 65*(4), 971–991.

Cassidy, J., & Shaver, P. R. (Eds.). (1999). *Handbook of attachment: Theory, research, and clinical applications.* Guilford Press.

Cassidy, J., & Shaver, P. R. (Eds.). (2008). *Handbook of attachment: Theory, research, and clinical applications* (2nd ed.). Guilford Press.

Cassidy, J., & Shaver, P. R. (Eds.). (2016). *Handbook of attachment: Theory, research, and clinical applications* (3rd ed.). Guilford Press.

Cassidy, J., Woodhouse, S. S., Cooper, G., Hoffman, K., Powell, B., & Rodenberg, M. (2005). Examination of the precursors of infant attachment security: Implications for early intervention and intervention research. In L. J. Berlin, Y. Ziv, L. Amaya-Jackson, & M. T. Greenberg (Eds.), *Enhancing early attachments: Theory, research, intervention, and policy* (pp. 34–60). Guilford Press.

Cassidy, J., Woodhouse, S., Sherman, L., Stupica, B., & Lejuez, C. W. (2011). Enhancing infant attachment security: An examination of treatment efficacy and differential susceptibility. *Development and Psychopathology, 23*(1), 131–148.

Cassidy, J., Ziv, Y., Stupica, B., Sherman, L. J., Butler, H., Karfgin, A., . . . Powell, B. (2010). Enhancing attachment security in the infants of women in a jail-diversion program. *Attachment and Human Development, 12*(4), 333–353.

Chapman, M. (2021). *Reflecting on babies in the NICU: An exploration of parental reflective functioning in a quaternary neonatal intensive care unit* [Unpublished doctoral dissertation]. University of Melbourne.

Chapman, M., & Paul, C. (2016). Using the PDI in neonatal intensive care. *Infant Mental Health Journal, 37*(Suppl. 1), 356–357.

Chung, E. K., Mathew, L., Elo, I. T., Coyne, J. C., & Culhane, J. F. (2008). Depressive symptoms in disadvantaged women receiving prenatal care: The influence of adverse and positive childhood experiences. *Ambulatory Pediatrics, 8*(2), 109–116.

Cicchetti, D., & Garmezy, N. (1993). Prospects and promises in the study of resilience. *Development and Psychopathology, 5*(4), 497–502.

Cicchetti, D., Rogosch, F. A., & Toth, S. (2000). The efficacy of toddler–parent psychotherapy for fostering cognitive development in offspring of depressed mothers. *Journal of Abnormal Child Psychology, 28*, 135–148.

Cicchetti, D., Rogosch, F. A., & Toth, S. L. (2006). Fostering secure attachment in infants in maltreating families through preventive interventions. *Development and Psychopathology, 18*(3), 623–649.

Cicchetti, D., Rogosch, F. A., & Toth, S. L. (2011a). The effects of child maltreatment and polymorphisms of the serotonin transporter and dopamine D4 receptor genes on infant attachment and intervention efficacy. *Development and Psychopathology, 23*, 357–372.

Cicchetti, D., Rogosch, F. A., Toth, S. L., & Sturge-Apple, M. L. (2011b). Normalizing the development of cortisol regulation in maltreated infants through preventive interventions. *Development and Psychopathology, 23,* 789–800.

Cloitre, M., Hyland, P., Bisson, J. I., Brewin, C. R., Roberts, N. P., Karatzias, T., & Shevlin, M. (2019). ICD-11 posttraumatic stress disorder and complex posttraumatic stress disorder in the United States: A population-based study. *Journal of Traumatic Stress, 32,* 833–842.

Close, N. (2002). *Listening to children: Talking with children about difficult issues.* Allyn & Bacon.

Coard, S. I. (2022). Race, discrimination, and racism as "growing points" for consideration: Attachment theory and research with African American families. *Attachment and Human Development, 24*(3), 373–383.

Cohen, L. R., Hien, D. A., & Batchelder, S. (2008). The impact of cumulative maternal trauma and diagnosis on parenting behavior. *Child Maltreatment, 13*(1), 27–38.

Cohen, M. M., Jing, D., Yang, R. R., Tottenham, N., Lee, F. S., & Casey, B. J. (2013). Early-life stress has persistent effects on amygdala function and development in mice and humans. *Proceedings of the National Academy of Sciences of the USA, 110*(45), 18274–18278.

Cohen, N. J., Muir, E., & Lojkasek, M. (2003). The first couple: Using watch, wait, and wonder to change troubled infant–mother relationships. In S. M. Johnson & V. E. Whiffen (Eds.), *Attachment processes in couple and family therapy* (pp. 215–233). Guilford Press.

Coldwell, J., Pike, A., & Dunn, J. (2006). Household chaos: Links with parenting and child behaviour. *Journal of Child Psychology and Psychiatry, 47*(11), 1116–1122.

Colich, N. L., Rosen, M. L., Williams, E. S., & McLaughlin, K. A. (2020). Biological aging in childhood and adolescence following experiences of threat and deprivation: A systematic review and meta-analysis. *Psychological Bulletin, 146*(9), 721–764.

Condon, E. M. (2019). Maternal, infant, and early childhood home visiting: A call for a paradigm shift in states' approaches to funding. *Policy, Politics, and Nursing Practice, 20,* 28–40.

Condon, E. M., Holland, M. L., Slade, A., Redeker, N. S., Mayes, L. C., & Sadler, L. S. (2019a). Associations between maternal caregiving and child indicators of toxic stress among multiethnic, urban families. *Journal of Pediatric Health Care, 33*(4), 425–436.

Condon, E. M., Holland, M. L., Slade, A., Redeker, N. S., Mayes, L. C., & Sadler, L. S. (2019b). Associations between maternal experiences of discrimination and biomarkers of toxic stress in school-aged children. *Maternal and Child Health Journal, 23*(9), 1147–1151.

Condon, E. M., Londoño Tobón, A., Holland, M. L., Slade, A., Mayes, L., & Sadler, L. S. (2022). Examining mothers' childhood maltreatment history, parental reflective functioning, and the long-term effects of the *Minding the Baby*® home visiting intervention. *Child Maltreatment, 27*(3), 378–388.

Conger, R. D., & Elder, G. H., Jr. (Eds.). (1994). *Families in troubled times: Adapting to change in rural America.* Aldine de Gruyter.

Cook, A., Spinazzola, J., Ford, J., Lanktree, C., Blaustein, M., Cloitre, M., . . . van der Kolk, B. (2005). Complex trauma in children and adolescents. *Psychiatric Annals, 35*(5), 390–398.

Cooper, A., & Redfern, S. (2015). *Reflective parenting: A guide to understanding what's going on in your child's mind.* Routledge.

Courtois, C. A. (2004). Complex trauma, complex reactions: Assessment and treatment. *Psychotherapy: Theory, Research, Practice, Training, 41*(4), 412–425.

Cox, J. L., Holden, J. M., & Sagovsky, R. (1987). Detection of postnatal depression: Development of the 10-item Edinburgh Postnatal Depression Scale. *British Journal of Psychiatry, 150,* 782–786.

Crouch, E., Radcliff, E., Brown, M., & Hung, P. (2019). Exploring the association between parenting stress and a child's exposure to adverse childhood experiences (ACEs). *Children and Youth Services Review, 102,* 186–192.

Crumbley, A. H. (2009). *The relationship specificity of the reflective function: An empirical investigation* [Unpublished doctoral dissertation]. City University of New York.

Cyr, C., Euser, E. M., Bakermans-Kranenburg, M. J., & van IJzendoorn, M. H. (2010). Attachment security and disorganization in maltreating and high-risk families: A series of meta-analyses. *Development and Psychopathology, 22*(1), 87–108.

Cyr, G., Godbout, N., Cloitre, M., & Bélanger, C. (2022). Distinguishing among symptoms of posttraumatic stress disorder, complex posttraumatic stress disorder, and borderline personality disorder in a community sample of women. *Journal of Traumatic Stress, 35*(1), 186–196.

Davis, A. E., Saad, G., Williams, D., Wortham, W., Perry, D. F., Aron, E., . . . Biel, M. G. (2021, May 14). Clinician perspectives on adapting evidence-based mental health treatment for infants and toddlers during COVID-19. *Perspectives in Infant Mental Health.* Retrieved from *https://perspectives.waimh. org/2021/05/14/clinician-perspectives-on-adapting-evidence-based-mental-health-treatment-for-infants-and-toddlers-during-covid-19.*

de Marneffe, D. (2004). *Maternal desire: On children, love, and the inner life.* Little, Brown.

De Roo, M., Wong, G., Rempel, G. R., & Fraser, S. N. (2019). Advancing optimal development in children: Examining the construct validity of a parent reflective functioning questionnaire. *JMIR Pediatrics and Parenting, 2*(1), e11561.

De Wolff, M. S., & van IJzendoorn, M. H. (1997). Sensitivity and attachment: A meta-analysis on parental antecedents of infant attachment. *Child Development, 68*(4), 571–591.

Dexter, C. A., Wong, K., Stacks, A. M., Beeghly, M., & Barnett, D. (2013). Parenting and attachment among low-income African American and Caucasian preschoolers. *Journal of Family Psychology, 27*(4), 629–638.

Di Pellegrino, G., Fadiga, L., Fogassi, L., Gallese, V., & Rizzolatti, G. (1992). Understanding motor events: A neurophysiological study. *Experimental Brain Research, 91*(1), 176–180.

Donelan-McCall, N., & Olds, D. (2018). The nurse–family partnership: Theoretical and empirical foundations. In H. Steele & M. Steele (Eds.), *Handbook of attachment-based interventions* (pp. 79–103). Guilford Press.

Dozier, M. (1990). Attachment organization and treatment use for adults with serious psychopathological disorders. *Development and Psychopathology, 2*(1), 47–60.

Dozier, M. (2022). Introduction of Special Section of *Infant Mental Health Journal*: Meeting the needs of vulnerable infants and families during COVID-19: Moving to a telehealth approach for home visiting implementation and research. *Infant Mental Health Journal, 43*(1), 140–142.

Dunbar, A. S., Lozada, F. T., Ahn, L. H., & Leerkes, E. M. (2022). Mothers' preparation for bias and responses to children's distress predict positive adjustment among Black children: An attachment perspective. *Attachment and Human Development, 24*(3), 287–303.

Dunn, E. C., Soare, T. W., Zhu, Y., Simpkin, A. J., Suderman, M. J., Klengel, T., . . . Relton, C. L. (2019). Sensitive periods for the effect of childhood adversity on DNA methylation: Results from a prospective, longitudinal study. *Biological Psychiatry, 85*(10), 838–849.

Ekeland, A. G., Bowes, A., & Flottorp, S. (2010). Effectiveness of telemedicine: A systematic review of reviews. *International Journal of Medical Informatics, 79*, 736–771.

Ellis, B. J., Abrams, L. S., Masten, A. S., Sternberg, R. J., Tottenham, N., & Frankenhuis, W. E. (2022). Hidden talents in harsh environments. *Development and Psychopathology, 34*, 95–113.

Enav, Y., Erhard-Weiss, D., Golderberg, A., Knudston, M., Hardan, A. Y., & Gross, J. J. (2020). Contextual determinants of parental reflective functioning: Children with autism versus their typically developing siblings. *Autism, 24*, 1578–1582.

Ensink, K., Bégin, M., Normandin, L., & Fonagy, P. (2016). Maternal and child reflective functioning in the context of child sexual abuse: Pathways to depression and externalising difficulties. *European Journal of Psychotraumatology, 7*(1), 30611.

Ensink, K., Bégin, M., Normandin, L., & Fonagy, P. (2017a). Parental reflective functioning as a moderator of child internalizing difficulties in the context of child sexual abuse. *Psychiatry Research, 257*, 361–366.

Ensink, K., Berthelot, N., Bernazzani, O., Normandin, L., & Fonagy, P. (2014). Another step closer to measuring the ghosts in the nursery: Preliminary validation of the Trauma Reflective Functioning Scale. *Frontiers in Psychology, 5*, Article 1471.

Ensink, K., Leroux, A., Normandin, L., Biberdzic, M., & Fonagy, P. (2017b). Assessing reflective parenting in interaction with school-aged children. *Journal of Personality Assessment, 99*(6), 585–595.

Essex, M. J., Thomas Boyce, W., Hertzman, C., Lam, L. L., Armstrong, J. M., Neumann, S. M., & Kobor, M. S. (2013). Epigenetic vestiges of early developmental adversity: Childhood stress exposure and DNA methylation in adolescence. *Child Development, 84*(1), 58–75.

Esteves, K. C., Jones, C. W., Wade, M., Callerame, K., Smith, A. K., Theall, K. P., & Drury, S. S. (2020). Adverse childhood experiences: Implications for offspring telomere length and psychopathology. *American Journal of Psychiatry, 177*(1), 47–57.

Fearon, P., Target, M., Sargent, J., Williams, L. L., McGregor, J., Bleiberg, E., & Fonagy, P. (2006a). Short-term mentalization and relational therapy (SMART): An integrative family therapy for children and adolescents. In J. G. Allen & P. Fonagy (Eds.), *Handbook of mentalization-based treatment* (pp. 201–222). Wiley.

Fearon, R. M. P., van IJzendoorn, M. H., Fonagy, P., Bakermans-Kranenburg, M. J., Schuengel, C., & Bokhorst, C. L. (2006b). In search of shared and non-shared environmental factors in security of attachment: A behavior–genetic study of the association between sensitivity and attachment security. *Developmental Psychology, 42*(6), 1026–1040.

Feldman, R. (2015). The adaptive human parental brain: Implications for children's social development. *Trends in Neuroscience, 38*, 387–399.

Felitti, V. J., Anda, R. F., Nordenberg, D., Williamson, D. F., Spitz, A. M., Edwards, V., & Marks, J. S. (1998). Relationship of childhood abuse and household dysfunction to many of the leading causes of death in adults: The Adverse Childhood Experiences (ACE) Study. *American Journal of Preventive Medicine, 14*(4), 245–258.

Fenichel, E. (1992). *Learning through supervision and mentorship to support the development of infants, toddlers and their families: A source book.* ZERO TO THREE/National Center for Clinical Infant Programs.

Fernández-Álvarez, J., & Fernández-Álvarez, H. (2021). Videoconferencing psychotherapy during the pandemic: Exceptional times with enduring effects? *Frontiers in Psychology, 12*, 589536.

Field, T. (2018). Infant massage therapy research review. *Clinical Research in Pediatrics, 1*, 1–9.

Finger, B. (2006). *Exploring the intergenerational transmission of attachment disorganization* [Unpublished doctoral dissertation]. University of Chicago.

Finger, B., Byun, S., Melnick, S., & Lyons-Ruth, K. (2015). Hostile–helpless states of mind mediate relations between childhood abuse severity and personality disorder features. *Translational Developmental Psychiatry, 3*, 1–11.

Finkelhor, D. (2018). Screening for adverse childhood experiences (ACEs): Cautions and suggestions. *Child Abuse and Neglect, 85*, 174–179.

Fonagy, P. (1993). Psychoanalytic and empirical approaches to developmental psychopathology: Can they be usefully integrated? *Journal of the Royal Society of Medicine, 86*(10), 577–581.

Fonagy, P., & Allison, E. (2014). The role of mentalizing and epistemic trust in the therapeutic relationship. *Psychotherapy, 51*(3), 372–380.

Fonagy, P., Campbell, C., Constantinou, M., Higgitt, A., Allison, E., & Luyten, P. (2021). Culture and psychopathology: An attempt at reconsidering the role of social learning. *Development and Psychopathology, 34*(4), 1–16.

Fonagy, P., Gergely, G., Jurist, E. L., & Target, M. (2002). *Affect regulation, mentalization, and the development of the self.* Other Press.

Fonagy, P., Luyten, P., Allison, E., & Campbell, C. (2019). Mentalizing, epistemic trust and the phenomenology of psychotherapy. *Psychopathology, 52*(2), 94–103.

Fonagy, P., Rossouw, T., Sharp, C., Bateman, A., Allison, L., & Farrar, C. (2014). Mentalization-based treatment for adolescents with borderline traits. In C.

Sharp & J. L. Tackett (Eds.), *Handbook of borderline personality disorder in children and adolescents* (pp. 313–332). Springer.

Fonagy, P., Sleed, M., & Baradon, T. (2016). Randomized controlled trial of parent–infant psychotherapy for parents with mental health problems and young infants. *Infant Mental Health Journal, 37*(2), 97–114.

Fonagy, P., Steele, H., & Steele, M. (1991a). Maternal representations of attachment during pregnancy predict the organization of infant–mother attachment at one year of age. *Child Development, 62*(5), 891–905.

Fonagy, P., Steele, M., Steele, H., Leigh, T., Kennedy, R., Mattoon, G., & Target, M. (1995). Attachment, the reflective self, and borderline states: The predictive specificity of the Adult Attachment Interview and pathological emotional development. In S. Goldberg, R. Muir, & J. Kerr (Eds.), *Attachment theory: Social, developmental and clinical perspectives* (pp. 233–279). Analytic Press.

Fonagy, P., Steele, M., Steele, H., Moran, G. S., & Higgitt, A. C. (1991b). The capacity for understanding mental states: The reflective self in parent and child and its significance for security of attachment. *Infant Mental Health Journal, 12*(3), 201–218.

Fonagy, P., & Target, M. (1995). Understanding the violent patient: The use of the body and the role of the father. *International Journal of Psychoanalysis, 76*(3), 487–501.

Fonagy, P., & Target, M. (1996). Playing with reality: I. Theory of mind and the normal development of psychic reality. *International Journal of Psychoanalysis, 77*(2), 217–233.

Fonagy, P., & Target, M. (1997). Attachment and reflective function: Their role in self-organization. *Development and Psychopathology, 9*(4), 679–700.

Fonagy, P., & Target, M. (1998). Mentalization and the changing aims of child psychoanalysis. *Psychoanalytic Dialogues, 8*, 87–114.

Fonagy, P., Target, M., Steele, H., & Steele, M. (1998). *Reflective-functioning manual, version 5.0, for application to Adult Attachment Interviews*. University College London.

Fraiberg, S. (1980). *Clinical studies in infant mental health: The first year of life*. Basic Books.

Fraiberg, S., Adelson, E., & Shapiro, V. (1975). Ghosts in the nursery: A psychoanalytic approach to the problems of impaired infant–mother relationships. *Journal of American Academy of Child Psychiatry, 14*(3), 387–421.

Frankl, V. (1985). *Man's search for meaning*. Beacon Press. (Original work published 1946)

Frigerio, A., Constantino, E., Ceppi, E., & Barone, L. (2013). Adult Attachment Interviews of women from low-risk, poverty, and maltreatment risk samples: Comparisons between the hostile/helpless and traditional AAI coding systems. *Attachment and Human Development, 15*(4), 424–442.

Gaensbauer, T. J. (1982). Regulation of emotional expression in infants from two contrasting caretaking environments. *Journal of the American Academy of Child Psychiatry, 21*(2), 163–170.

Gallotti, M., & Frith, C. D. (2013). Social cognition in the we-mode. *Trends in Cognitive Sciences, 17*(4), 160–165.

Garmezy, N. (1974). The study of competence in children at risk for severe psycho-pathology. In E. J. Anthony & C. Koupernik (Eds.), *The child in his family: Children at psychiatric risk* (Vol. 3, pp. 77–97). Wiley.

Garner, A. S. (2013). Home visiting and the biology of toxic stress: Opportunities to address early childhood adversity. *Pediatrics, 132*(Suppl. 2), S65–S73.

Geller, S. M., & Porges, S. W. (2014). Therapeutic presence: Neurophysiological mechanisms mediating feeling safe in therapeutic relationships. *Journal of Psychotherapy Integration, 24*(3), 178–192.

George, C., Kaplan, N., & Main, M. (1984/1988/1996). *Adult Attachment Interview* [Unpublished manuscript]. University of California, Berkeley.

George, C., & Solomon, J. (1996). Representational models of relationships: Links between caregiving and attachment. *Infant Mental Health Journal, 17*(3), 198–216.

George, C., & Solomon, J. (1999). Attachment and caregiving: The caregiving behavioral system. In J. Cassidy & P. R. Shaver (Eds.), *Handbook of attachment: Theory, research, and clinical applications* (pp. 649–670). Guilford Press.

George, C., & Solomon, J. (2008). The caregiving system: A behavioral systems approach to parenting. In J. Cassidy & P. R. Shaver (Eds.), *Handbook of attachment: Theory, research, and clinical applications* (2nd ed., pp. 833–856). Guilford Press.

Gergely, G., & Watson, J. S. (1996). The social biofeedback theory of parental affect-mirroring: The development of emotional self-awareness and self-control in infancy. *International Journal of Psychoanalysis, 77*(6), 1181–1212.

Ghosh Ippen, C. M. (2019). Wounds from the past: Integrating historical trauma into a multicultural infant mental health framework. In C. H. Zeanah (Ed.), *Handbook of infant mental health* (4th ed., pp. 134–153). Guilford Press.

Ghosh Ippen, C. M., & Lewis, M. (2011). They just don't get it: A diversity-informed approach to understanding engagement. In J. D. Osofsky (Ed.), *Clinical work with traumatized young children* (pp. 31–52). Guilford Press.

Giesbrecht, G. F., Letourneau, N., & Campbell, T. S. (2017). Sexually dimorphic and interactive effects of prenatal maternal cortisol and psychological distress on infant cortisol reactivity. *Development and Psychopathology, 29*(3), 805–818.

Gilkerson, L. (2004). Reflective supervision in infant–family programs: Adding clinical process to nonclinical settings. *Infant Mental Health Journal, 25*(5), 424–439.

Gilkerson, L., & Imberger, J. (2016, November). Strengthening reflective capacity in skilled home visitors. *ZERO TO THREE*, 46–52.

Gilliam, W. S., Maupin, A. N., & Reyes, C. R. (2016). Early childhood mental health consultation: Results of a statewide random-controlled evaluation. *Journal of the American Academy of Child and Adolescent Psychiatry, 55*(9), 754–761.

Gold, C. M. (2011). *Keeping your child in mind: Overcoming defiance, tantrums, and other everyday behavior problems by seeing the world through your child's eyes*. Da Capo Lifelong Books.

Gonzalez, A., & MacMillan, H. L. (2008). Preventing child maltreatment: An evidence-based update. *Journal of Postgraduate Medicine, 54*(4), 280–286.

Gray, A. E. (2018). Roots, rhythm, reciprocity: Polyvagal-informed dance movement therapy for survivors of trauma. In D. A. Dana & P. W. Porges (Eds.), *Clinical applications of the polyvagal theory: The emergence of polyvagal-informed therapies* (pp. 207–226). Norton.

Grienenberger, J., Denham, W., & Reynolds, D. (2015). Reflective and mindful parenting: A new relational model of assessment, prevention, and early intervention. In P. Luyten, L. C. Mayes, P. Fonagy, M. Target, & S. J. Blatt (Eds.), *Handbook of psychodynamic approaches to psychopathology* (pp. 445–468). Guilford Press.

Grienenberger, J., Kelly, K., & Slade, A. (2005). Maternal reflective functioning, mother–infant affective communication, and infant attachment: Exploring the link between mental states and observed caregiving behavior in the intergenerational transmission of attachment. *Attachment and Human Development, 7*(3), 299–311.

Grigorenko, E. L., Cicchetti, D., Monk, C., Spicer, J., & Champagne, F. A. (2012). Linking prenatal maternal adversity to developmental outcomes in infants: The role of epigenetic pathways. *Development and Psychopathology, 24*(4), 1361–1376.

Grossmann, K., Grossmann, K., & Keppler, A. (2005). Universal and culture-specific aspects of human behavior: The case of attachment. In W. Friedlmeier, P. Chakkarath, & B. Schwartz (Eds.), *Culture and human development: The importance of cross-cultural research for the social sciences* (pp. 71–91). Psychology Press.

Grossmann, K., Grossmann, K. E., Spangler, G., Suess, G., & Unzner, L. (1985). Maternal sensitivity and newborns' orientation responses as related to quality of attachment in northern Germany. *Monographs of the Society for Research in Child Development, 50*(1–2), 233–256.

Grossmann, K. E., Grossmann, K., & Waters, E. (Eds.). (2006). *Attachment from infancy to adulthood: The major longitudinal studies.* Guilford Press.

Gunnar, M. R., Brodersen, L., Nachmias, M., Buss, K., & Rigatuso, J. (1996). Stress reactivity and attachment security. *Developmental Psychobiology, 29*(3), 191–204.

Gunnar, M. R., & Hostinar, C. E. (2015). The social buffering of the hypothalamic–pituitary–adrenocortical axis in humans: Developmental and experiential determinants. *Social Neuroscience, 10*(5), 479–488.

Haft, W. L., & Slade, A. (1989). Affect attunement and maternal attachment: A pilot study. *Infant Mental Health Journal, 10*(3), 157–172.

Håkansson, U., Söderström, K., Watten, R., Skårderud, F., & Øie, M. G. (2018a). Parental reflective functioning and executive functioning in mothers with substance use disorder. *Attachment and Human Development, 20*(2), 181–207.

Håkansson, U., Watten, R., Söderström, K., Skårderud, F., & Øie, M. G. (2018b). Adverse and adaptive childhood experiences are associated with parental reflective functioning in mothers with substance use disorder. *Child Abuse and Neglect, 81*, 259–273.

Hall, W. J., Chapman, M. V., Lee, K. M., Merino, Y. M., Thomas, T. W., Payne, B.

K., . . . Coyne-Beasley, T. (2015). Implicit racial/ethnic bias among health care professionals and its influence on health care outcomes: A systematic review. *American Journal of Public Health, 105*(12), e60–e76.

Harlow, H. F. (1958). The nature of love. *American Psychologist, 13*(12), 673–685.

Hart, A. (2017). From multicultural competence to radical openness: A psychoanalytic engagement of otherness. *American Psychoanalyst, 51*, 12–27.

Hautamäki, A., Hautamäki, L., Neuvonen, L., & Maliniemi-Piispanen, S. (2010). Transmission of attachment across three generations. *European Journal of Developmental Psychology, 7*(5), 618–634.

Heffron, M. C. (2005). Reflective supervision in infant, toddler, and preschool work. In K. M. Finello (Ed.), *Handbook of training and practice in infant and preschool mental health* (pp. 114–136). California School of Professional Psychology.

Heffron, M. C., & Murch, T. (2010). *Reflective supervision and leadership in infant and early childhood programs.* ZERO TO THREE.

Heffron, M. C., Reynolds, D., & Talbot, B. (2016). Reflecting together: Reflective functioning as a focus for deepening group supervision. *Infant Mental Health Journal, 37*(6), 628–639.

Heim, C., Young, L. J., Newport, D. J., Mletzko, T., Miller, A. H., & Nemeroff, C. B. (2009). Lower CSF oxytocin concentrations in women with a history of childhood abuse. *Molecular Psychiatry, 14*(10), 954–958.

Henderson, V., & Nite, G. (1978). *Principles and practice of nursing.* Macmillan.

Herman, J. L. (1992a). *Trauma and recovery.* Basic Books/Hachette Book Group.

Herman, J. L. (1992b). Complex PTSD: A syndrome in survivors of prolonged and repeated trauma. *Journal of Traumatic Stress, 5*(3), 377–391.

Hesse, E., & Main, M. (1999). Second-generation effects of unresolved trauma in non-maltreating parents: Dissociated, frightened, and threatening parental behavior. *Psychoanalytic Inquiry, 19*(4), 481–540.

Hesse, E., & Main, M. (2000). Disorganized infant, child, and adult attachment: Collapse in behavioral and attentional strategies. *Journal of the American Psychoanalytic Association, 48*, 1097–1127.

Hillis, S. D., Anda, R. F., Dube, S. R., Felitti, V. J., Marchbanks, P. A., Macaluso, M., & Marks, J. S. (2010). The protective effect of family strengths in childhood against adolescent pregnancy and its long-term psychosocial consequences. *Permanente Journal, 14*(3), 18–27.

Hogg, B., Gardoki-Souto, I, Valente-Gómez, A., Rosa, A., R., Fortea, F., Radua, J., . . . Moreno-Alcázar, A. (2022). Psychological trauma as a transdiagnostic risk factor for mental disorder: An umbrella meta-analysis. *European Archives of Psychiatry and Clinical Neuroscience.*

Hoehl, S., Wiese, L., & Striano, T. (2008). Young infants' neural processing of objects is affected by eye gaze direction and emotional expression. *PloS ONE, 3*(6), e2389.

Hoekzema, E., Barba-Müller, E., Pozzobon, C., Picado, M., Lucco, F., García-García, D., . . . Vilarroya, O. (2017). Pregnancy leads to long-lasting changes in human brain structure. *Nature Neuroscience, 20*(2), 287–296.

Hoekzema, E., Tamnes, C. K., Berns, P., Barba-Müller, E., Pozzobon, C., Picado,

M., . . . Carmona, S. (2020). Becoming a mother entails anatomical changes in the ventral striatum of the human brain that facilitate its responsiveness to offspring cues. *Psychoneuroendocrinology, 112,* 104507.

Hofer, M. A. (2006). Psychobiological roots of early attachment. *Current Directions in Psychological Science, 15,* 84–88.

Hoffman, K., Cooper, G., & Powell, B. (2017). *Raising a secure child: How Circle of Security parenting can help you nurture your child's attachment, emotional resilience, and freedom to explore.* Guilford Press.

Hoffman, K. T., Marvin, R. S., Cooper, G., & Powell, B. (2006). Changing toddlers' and preschoolers' attachment classifications: The Circle of Security intervention. *Journal of Consulting and Clinical Psychology, 74*(6), 1017–1026.

Holmes, D. E., Hart, A., Powell, D. R., & Stoute, B. (2023). The Holmes' commission's journey toward racial equality in American psychoanalysis: Reflection and hope. *American Psychoanalyst, 57,* 1–7.

Holmes, J. (2010). *Exploring in security: Towards an attachment-informed psychoanalytic psychotherapy.* Routledge/Taylor & Francis Group.

Holmes, J. (2014). *John Bowlby and attachment theory* (2nd ed.). Routledge.

Holmes, J., & Slade, A. (2018). *Attachment in therapeutic practice.* SAGE.

Hostinar, C. E., Johnson, A. E., & Gunnar, M. R. (2015). Parent support is less effective in buffering cortisol stress reactivity for adolescents compared to children. *Developmental Science, 18*(2), 281–297.

Hostinar, C. E., Sullivan, R. M., & Gunnar, M. R. (2014). Psychobiological mechanisms underlying the social buffering of the hypothalamic–pituitary–adrenocortical axis: A review of animal models and human studies across development. *Psychological Bulletin, 140*(1), 256–282.

Hrdy, S. B. (2009). *Mothers and others.* Harvard University Press.

Huber, A., McMahon, C. A., & Sweller, N. (2015). Efficacy of the 20-week COS Intervention: Changes in caregiver reflective functioning, representations, and child attachment in an Australian clinical sample. *Infant Mental Health Journal, 36*(6), 556–574.

Hughes, K., Bellis, M. A., Hardcastle, K. A., Sethi, D., Butchart, A., Mikton, C., . . . Dunne, M. P. (2017). The effect of multiple adverse childhood experiences on health: A systematic review and meta-analysis. *Lancet Public Health, 2*(8), e356–e366.

Hughes, M., & Cossar, J. (2016). The relationship between maternal childhood emotional abuse/neglect and parenting outcomes: A systematic review. *Child Abuse Review, 25*(1), 31–45.

Huth-Bocks, A. C., Muzik, M., Beeghly, M., Earls, L., & Stacks, A. M. (2014). Secure base scripts are associated with maternal parenting behavior across contexts and reflective functioning among trauma-exposed mothers. *Attachment and Human Development, 16*(6), 535–556.

Hyland, P., Karatzias, T., Shevlin, M., & Cloitre, M. (2019). Examining the discriminant validity of complex posttraumatic stress disorder and borderline personality disorder symptoms: Results from a United Kingdom population sample. *Journal of Traumatic Stress, 32*(6), 855–863.

Ilardi, M. (2010). *Maternal mentalization and child psychosocial adaptation for children with learning and behavioral disorders* [Unpublished doctoral dissertation]. City University of New York.

International Council of Nurses. (2002). Nursing definitions. Retrieved from *www.icn.ch/nursing-policy/nursing-definitions*.

Isosävi, S., Diab, S. Y., Qouta, S., Kangaslampi, S., Sleed, M., Kankaanpää, S., . . . Punamäki, R. L. (2020). Caregiving representations in war conditions: Associations with maternal trauma, mental health, and mother–infant interaction. *Infant Mental Health Journal, 41*(2), 246–263.

Jacobs, H. (1861). *Incidents in the life of a slave girl.* Thayer & Eldridge.

James, W. (1890). *The principles of psychology* (Vol. 2). Holt.

Jessee, A. (2020). Associations between maternal reflective functioning, parenting beliefs, nurturing, and preschoolers' emotion understanding. *Journal of Child and Family Studies, 29*(11), 3020–3028.

Jones, D., Greenberg, M., & Crowley, M. (2015). Early social–emotional functioning and public health: The relationship between kindergarten social competence and future wellness. *American Journal of Public Health, 105*, 2283–2290.

Julian, M. M., Rosenblum, K. L., Doom, J. R., Leung, C. Y., Lumeng, J. C., Cruz, M. G., . . . Miller, A. L. (2018). Oxytocin and parenting behavior among impoverished mothers with low vs. high early life stress. *Archives of Women's Mental Health, 21*(3), 375–382.

Kabat-Zinn, J. (1994). *Wherever you go, there you are: Mindfulness meditation in everyday life.* Hachette Books.

Kabat-Zinn, J., & Kabat-Zinn, M. (1997). *Everyday blessings: The inner work of mindful parenting.* Little, Brown.

Kagan, J. (1995). On attachment. *Harvard Review of Psychiatry, 3*(2), 104–106.

Kamerman, S. B., & Kahn, A. J. (1993). Home health visiting in Europe. *The Future of Children, 3*(3), 39–52.

Kendi, I. X. (2019). *How to be an antiracist.* One World.

Khoury, J. E., Pechtel, P., Andersen, C. M., Teicher, M. H., & Lyons-Ruth, K. (2019). Relations among maternal withdrawal in infancy, borderline features, suicidality/self-injury, and adult hippocampal volume: A 30-year longitudinal study. *Behavioural Brain Research, 374*, 1121–1139.

Kim, P., Strathearn, L., & Swain, J. E. (2016). The maternal brain and its plasticity in humans. *Hormones and Behavior, 77*, 113–123.

Kirsch, P., Esslinger, C., Chen, Q., Mier, D., Lis, S., Siddhanti, S., . . . Meyer-Lindenberg, A. (2005). Oxytocin modulates neural circuitry for social cognition and fear in humans. *Journal of Neuroscience, 25*(49), 11489–11493.

Kitzman, H., Olds, D. L., Henderson, C. R., Hanks, C., Cole, R., Tatelbaum, R., . . . Engelhardt, K. (1997). Effect of prenatal and infancy home visitation by nurses on pregnancy outcomes, childhood injuries, and repeated childbearing. *JAMA, 278*, 644–652.

Kolomeyer, E., Renk, K., Cunningham, A., Lowell, A., & Khan, M. (2016). Mothers' adverse childhood experiences and negative parenting behaviors: Connecting mothers' difficult pasts to present parenting behavior via reflective functioning. *ZERO TO THREE, 37*(1), 5–12.

Koren-Karie, N., Oppenheim, D., Dolev, S., Sher, E., & Etzion-Carasso, A. (2002). Mothers' insightfulness regarding their infants' internal experience. *Developmental Psychology, 38*(4), 534–542.

Krink, S., Muehlhan, C., Luyten, P., Romer, G., & Ramsauer, B. (2018). Parental reflective functioning affects sensitivity to distress in mothers with postpartum depression. *Journal of Child and Family Studies, 27*(5), 1671–1681.

Lange, B. C., Callinan, L. S., & Smith, M. V. (2019). Adverse childhood experiences and their relation to parenting stress and parenting practices. *Community Mental Health Journal, 55*(4), 651–662.

LeDoux, J. (1996). *The emotional brain: The mysterious underpinnings of emotional life.* Simon & Schuster.

Leroux, J., Terradas, M. M., & Grenier, C. (2017). Mothers' prementalizing psychic functioning and reactive attachment disorder: Two clinical cases. *Journal of Infant, Child, and Adolescent Psychotherapy, 16*(1), 60–72.

Letourneau, N., Dewey, D., Kaplan, B. J., Ntanda, H., Novick, J., Thomas, J. C., . . . APrON Study Team. (2019). Intergenerational transmission of adverse childhood experiences via maternal depression and anxiety and moderation by child sex. *Journal of Developmental Origins of Health and Disease, 10*(1), 88–99.

Levy, D. W. (2004). *The impact of prenatal cocaine use on maternal reflective functioning* [Unpublished doctoral dissertation]. City University of New York.

Li, Z., He, Y., Wang, D., Tang, J., & Chen, X. (2017). Association between childhood trauma and accelerated telomere erosion in adulthood: A meta-analytic study. *Journal of Psychiatric Research, 93*, 64–71.

Lieberman, A. F. (1983). Infant–parent psychotherapy during pregnancy. In S. Provence (Ed.), *Infants and parents: Clinical case reports* (pp. 84–141). International Universities Press.

Lieberman, A. F. (2004). Traumatic stress and quality of attachment: Reality and internalization in disorders of infant mental health. *Infant Mental Health Journal, 25*, 336–351.

Lieberman, A. F., & Blos, P. (1980). Make way for baby. In S. Fraiberg (Ed.), *Clinical studies in infant mental health: The first year of life* (pp. 242–259). Basic Books.

Lieberman, A. F., Diaz, M. A., Castro, G., & Bucio, G. O. (2020). *Make room for baby: Perinatal child–parent psychotherapy to repair trauma and promote attachment.* Guilford Press.

Lieberman, A. F., Ghosh Ippen, C., & Van Horn, P. (2006). Child–parent psychotherapy: 6-month follow-up of a randomized controlled trial. *Journal of the American Academy of Child and Adolescent Psychiatry, 45*, 913–918.

Lieberman, A. F., Ghosh Ippen, C., & Van Horn, P. (2015). *"Don't hit my mommy!": A manual for child–parent psychotherapy with young children exposed to violence and other trauma* (2nd ed.). ZERO TO THREE.

Lieberman, A. F., Padrón, E., Van Horn, P., & Harris, W. W. (2005a). Angels in the nursery: The intergenerational transmission of benevolent parental influences. *Infant Mental Health Journal, 26*(6), 504–520.

Lieberman, A. F., & Pawl, J. H. (1993). Infant–parent psychotherapy. In C. H.

Zeanah, Jr. (Ed.), *Handbook of infant mental health* (pp. 427–442). Guilford Press.

Lieberman, A. F., & Van Horn, P. (2005). *"Don't hit my mommy!": A manual for child–parent psychotherapy with young children exposed to violence and other trauma.* ZERO TO THREE.

Lieberman, A. F., & Van Horn, P. (2008). *Psychotherapy with infants and young children: Repairing the effects of stress and trauma on early attachment.* Guilford Press.

Lieberman, A. F., Van Horn, P., & Ghosh Ippen, C. (2005b). Toward evidence-based treatment: Child–parent psychotherapy with preschoolers exposed to marital violence. *Journal of the American Academy of Child and Adolescent Psychiatry, 44*(12), 1241–1248.

Lieberman, A. F., Weston, D. R., & Pawl, J. H. (1991). Preventive intervention and outcome with anxiously attached dyads. *Child Development, 62*(1), 199–209.

Lo, C. K. M., & Wong, S. Y. (2022). The effectiveness of parenting programs in regard to improving parental reflective functioning: A meta-analysis. *Attachment and Human Development, 24*(1), 76–92.

Loman, M. M., & Gunnar, M. R. (2010). Early experience and the development of stress reactivity and regulation in children. *Neuroscience and Biobehavioral Reviews, 34*(6), 867–876.

Lomanowska, A. M., Boivin, M., Hertzman, C., & Fleming, A. S. (2017). Parenting begets parenting: A neurobiological perspective on early adversity and the transmission of parenting styles across generations. *Neuroscience, 342,* 120–139.

Londoño Tobón, A., Condon, E., Sadler, L. S., Holland, M. L., Mayes, L. C., & Slade, A. (2022). School age effects of Minding the Baby—an attachment-based home-visiting intervention—on parenting and child behaviors. *Development and Psychopathology, 34*(1), 55–67.

Londoño Tobón, A., Condon, E., Slade, A., Holland, M. L., Mayes, L. C., & Sadler, L. S. (2023). Participation in an attachment-based home visiting program is associated with lower child salivary C-reactive protein levels at follow-up. *Journal of Behavioral and Developmental Pediatrics.*

Londoño Tobón, A., Newport, D. J., & Nemeroff, C. B. (2018). The role of oxytocin in early life adversity and later psychopathology: A review of preclinical and clinical studies. *Current Treatment Options in Psychiatry, 5*(4), 401–415.

Longhi, E., Murray, L., Wellsted, D., Hunter, R., MacKenzie, K., Taylor-Colls, S., & Fearon, P. (2019). *Minding the Baby (MTB) home-visiting programme for vulnerable young mothers: Results of a randomized controlled trial in the UK.* NSPCC Learning.

Lozada, F. T., Riley, T. N., Catherine, E., & Brown, D. W. (2022). Black emotions matter: Understanding the impact of racial oppression on black youth's emotional development. *Journal of Research on Adolescence, 32*(1), 13–33.

Luijk, M. P. C. M., Saridjan, N., Tharner, A., van IJzendoorn, M. H., Bakermans-Kranenburg, M. J., . . . Tiemeier, H. (2010a). Attachment, depression, and cortisol: Deviant patterns in insecure–resistant and disorganized infants. *Developmental Psychobiology, 52*(5), 441–452.

Luijk, M. P. C. M., Velders, F. P., Tharner, A., van IJzendoorn, M. H., Bakermans-Kranenburg, M. J., Jaddoe, V. W. V., . . . Tiemeier, H. (2010b). FKBP5 and resistant attachment predict cortisol reactivity in infants: Gene–environment interaction. *Psychoneuroendocrinology, 35*(10), 1454–1461.

Luthar, S. S., Cicchetti, D., & Becker, B. (2000). The construct of resilience: A critical evaluation and guidelines for future work. *Child Development, 71*(3), 543–562.

Luyten, P., & Fonagy, P. (2015). The neurobiology of mentalizing. *Personality Disorders: Theory, Research, and Treatment, 6*(4), 366–379.

Luyten, P., Mayes, L. C., Nijssens, L., & Fonagy, P. (2017). The Parental Reflective Functioning Questionnaire: Development and preliminary validation. *PLOS ONE, 12*(5), Article e0176218.

Luyten, P., Mayes, L. C., Sadler, L., Fonagy, P., Nicholls, S., Crowley, M., & Slade, A. (2009). *The Parental Reflective Functioning Questionnaire–1 (PRFQ-1)* [Unpublished manuscript]. University of Leuven.

Luyten, P., Nijssens, L., Fonagy, P., & Mayes, L. C. (2020). Parental reflective functioning: Theory, research, and clinical applications. *Psychoanalytic Study of the Child, 70*(1), 174–199.

Lyons-Ruth, K., Bronfman, E., & Atwood, G. (1999a). A relational diathesis model of hostile–helpless states of mind: Expressions in mother–infant interaction. In J. Solomon & C. George (Eds.), *Attachment disorganization* (pp. 33–69). Guilford Press.

Lyons-Ruth, K., Bronfman, E., & Parsons, E. (1999b). Maternal frightened, frightening, or atypical behavior and disorganized infant attachment patterns. *Monographs of the Society for Research in Child Development, 64*(3), 67–96.

Lyons-Ruth, K., Bureau, J. F., Holmes, B., Easterbrooks, A., & Brooks, N. H. (2013). Borderline symptoms and suicidality/self-injury in late adolescence: Prospectively observed relationship correlates in infancy and childhood. *Psychiatry Research, 206*(2–3), 273–281.

Lyons-Ruth, K., & Jacobvitz, D. (2016). Attachment disorganization from infancy to adulthood: Neurobiological correlates, parenting contexts, and pathways to disorder. In J. Cassidy & P. R. Shaver (Eds.), *Handbook of attachment: Theory, research, and clinical applications* (3rd ed., pp. 667–695). Guilford Press.

Lyons-Ruth, K., Melnick, S., Patrick, M., & Hobson, R. P. (2007). A controlled study of hostile–helpless states of mind among borderline and dysthymic women. *Attachment and Human Development, 9*(1), 1–16.

Lyons-Ruth, K., Pechtel, P., Yoon, S. A., Anderson, C. M., & Teicher, M. H. (2016). Disorganized attachment in infancy predicts greater amygdala volume in adulthood. *Behavioural Brain Research, 308*, 83–93.

Lyons-Ruth, K., Yellin, C., Melnick, S., & Atwood, G. (2005). Expanding the concept of unresolved mental states: Hostile/helpless states of mind on the Adult Attachment Interview are associated with disrupted mother–infant communication and infant disorganization. *Development and Psychopathology, 17*(1), 1–23.

Madigan, S., Bakermans-Kranenburg, M. J., van IJzendoorn, M. H., Moran, G., Pederson, D. R., & Benoit, D. (2006). Unresolved states of mind, anomalous parental behavior, and disorganized attachment: A review and meta-analysis of a transmission gap. *Attachment and Human Development, 8*(2), 89–111.

Madigan, S., Cyr, C., Eirich, R., Fearon, R. P., Ly, A., Rash, C., . . . Alink, L. R. (2019). Testing the cycle of maltreatment hypothesis: Meta-analytic evidence of the intergenerational transmission of child maltreatment. *Development and Psychopathology, 31*(1), 23–51.

Madigan, S., Wade, M., Plamondon, A., Maguire, J. L., & Jenkins, J. M. (2017). Maternal adverse childhood experience and infant health: Biomedical and psychosocial risks as intermediary mechanisms. *Journal of Pediatrics, 187,* 282–289.

Magesh, S., John, D., Li, W. T., Li, Y., Mattingly, A., Jain, S., . . . Ongkeko, W. (2021). Disparities in COVID-19 outcomes by race, ethnicity, and socioeconomic status: A systematic review and meta-analysis. *JAMA Network Open, 4*(11), e2134147.

Maguire-Jack, K., Lanier, P., & Lombardi, B. (2020). Investigating racial differences in clusters of adverse childhood experiences. *American Journal of Orthopsychiatry, 90*(1), 106–114.

Main, M. (1981). Avoidance in the service of proximity: A working paper. In K. Immelman, G. Barlow, L. Petrinovitch, & M. Main (Eds.), *Behavioral development: The Bielefeld interdisciplinary project* (pp. 651–669). Cambridge University Press.

Main, M. (1991). Metacognitive knowledge, metacognitive monitoring, and singular (coherent) vs. multiple (incoherent) models of attachment. In C. M. Parkes, J. Stevenson-Hinde, & P. Marris (Eds.), *Attachment across the life cycle* (pp. 127–159). Tavistock/Routledge.

Main, M. (2000). The organized categories of infant, child, and adult attachment: Flexible vs. inflexible attention under attachment-related stress. *Journal of the American Psychoanalytic Association, 48*(4), 1055–1096.

Main, M., & Hesse, E. (1990). Parents' unresolved traumatic experiences are related to infant disorganized attachment status: Is frightened and/or frightening parental behavior the linking mechanism? In M. Greenberg, D. Cicchetti, & E. M. Cummings (Eds.), *Attachment in the preschool years: Theory, research and intervention* (pp. 161–184). University of Chicago Press.

Main, M., Kaplan, N., & Cassidy, J. (1985). Security in infancy, childhood, and adulthood: A move to the level of representation. *Monographs of the Society for Research in Child Development, 50*(1–2), 66–104.

Main, M., & Solomon, J. (1986). Discovery of an insecure–disorganized/disoriented attachment pattern. In T. B. Brazelton & M. W. Yogman (Eds.), *Affective development in infancy* (pp. 95–124). Ablex.

Main, M., & Solomon, J. (1990). Procedures for identifying infants as disorganized/disoriented during the Ainsworth Strange Situation. In M. T. Greenberg, D. Cicchetti, & E. M. Cummings (Eds.), *Attachment in the preschool years: Theory, research, and intervention* (pp. 121–160). University of Chicago Press.

Malchiodi, C. A. (2020). *Trauma and expressive arts therapy: Brain, body, and imagination in the healing process.* Guilford Press.

Marchesseault, C., Close, N., Sadler, L., Simpson, T., Slade, A., & Webb, D. (2020). *Minding the Baby home visiting (MTB-HV) replication operations manual for implementing agencies.* Yale University.

Marchesseault, C., Close, N., Sadler, L., Simpson, T., Slade, A., & Webb, D. (2019). *Minding the Baby home visiting (MTB-HV) replication planning guide: Implementation considerations.* Yale University.

Martínez-García, M., Paternina-Die, M., Barba-Müller, E., Martín de Blas, D., Beumala, L., Cortizo, R., . . . Carmona, S. (2021). Do pregnancy-induced brain changes reverse? The brain of a mother six years after parturition. *Brain Sciences, 11*(2), 168.

Masten, A. S. (2014). *Ordinary magic: Resilience in development.* Guilford Press.

Masten, A. S., & Cicchetti, D. (2016). Resilience in development: Progress and transformation. *Developmental Psychopathology, 6*(4), 1–63.

Masten, A. S., Narayan, A. J., Silverman, W. K., & Osofsky, J. D. (2015). Children in war and disaster. In R. Lerner (Ed.), *Handbook of child psychology and developmental science: Vol. 4. Ecological settings and processes* (7th ed., pp. 1–42). Wiley.

Mayers, H. (2021, February 19). When the screen becomes a playground: A dyadic therapy program's transition to telehealth during COVID-19. *Perspectives in Infant Mental Health.* Retrieved from *https://perspectives.waimh.org/2021/02/19/when-the-screen-becomes-a-playground-a-dyadic-therapy-programs-transition-to-telehealth-during-covid-19.*

Mayes, L. C. (2006). Arousal regulation, emotional flexibility, medial amygdala function, and the impact of early experience: Comments on the paper of Lewis et al. *Annals of the New York Academy of Sciences, 1094*(1), 178–192.

Mazzeschi, C., Buratta, L., Cavallina, C., Ghignoni, R., Margheriti, M., & Pazzagli, C. (2019). Parental reflective functioning in mothers and fathers of children with ADHD: Issues regarding assessment and implications for intervention. *Frontiers in Public Health, 7*, 263.

McCann, I. L., & Pearlman, L. A. (1990). Vicarious traumatization: A framework for understanding the psychological effects of working with victims. *Journal of Traumatic Stress, 3*, 131–149.

McDonnell, C. G., & Valentino, K. (2016). Intergenerational effects of childhood trauma: Evaluating pathways among maternal ACEs, perinatal depressive symptoms, and infant outcomes. *Child Maltreatment, 21*(4), 317–326.

McEwen, B. S. (2000). Allostasis and allostatic load: Implications for neuropsychopharmacology. *Neuropsychopharmacology, 22*(2), 108–124.

McEwen, B. S. (2017). Neurobiological and systemic effects of chronic stress. *Chronic Stress, 1*, 1–11.

McEwen, B. S. (2020). Hormones and behavior and the integration of brain–body science. *Hormones and Behavior, 119*, 104619.

McLaughlin, K. A., & Sheridan, M. A. (2016). Beyond cumulative risk: A dimensional approach to childhood adversity. *Current Directions in Psychological Science, 25*(4), 239–245.

McLaughlin, K. A., Sheridan, M. A., Gold, A. L., Duys, A., Lambert, H. K., Peverill, M., . . . Pine, D. S. (2016). Maltreatment exposure, brain structure, and fear conditioning in children and adolescents. *Neuropsychopharmacology, 41*(8), 1956–1964.

McLaughlin, K. A., Sheridan, M. A., & Lambert, H. K. (2014). Childhood adversity and neural development: Deprivation and threat as distinct dimensions of early experience. *Neuroscience and Biobehavioral Reviews, 47,* 578–591.

McLaughlin, K. A., Sheridan, M. A., & Nelson, C. A. (2017). Neglect as a violation of species-expectant experience: Neurodevelopmental consequences. *Biological Psychiatry, 82*(7), 462–471.

McLoyd, V. C. (1990). The impact of economic hardship on Black families and children: Psychological distress, parenting, and socioemotional development. *Child Development, 61*(2), 311–346.

Meins, E., Fernyhough, C., Fradley, E., & Tuckey, M. (2001). Rethinking maternal sensitivity: Mothers' comments on infants' mental processes predict security of attachment at 12 months. *Journal of Child Psychology and Psychiatry and Allied Disciplines, 42,* 637–648.

Menashe-Grinberg, A., Shneor, S., Meiri, G., & Atzaba-Poria, N. (2022). Improving the parent–child relationship and child adjustment through parental reflective functioning group intervention. *Attachment and Human Development, 24*(2), 208–228.

Merino, Y., Adams, L., & Hall, W. J. (2018). Implicit bias and mental health professionals: Priorities and directions for research. *Psychiatric Services, 269,* 723–725.

Merrick, M. T., Ford, D. C., Ports, K. A., & Guinn, A. S. (2018). Prevalence of adverse childhood experiences from the 2011–2014 behavioral risk factor surveillance system in 23 states. *JAMA Pediatrics, 172*(11), 1038–1044.

Mesman, J., van IJzendoorn, M. H., & Bakermans-Kranenburg, M. J. (2012). Unequal in opportunity, equal in process: Parental sensitivity promotes positive child development in ethnic minority families. *Child Development Perspectives, 6*(3), 239–250.

Mesman, J., van IJzendoorn, M. H., & Sagi-Schwartz, A. (2016). Cross-cultural patterns of attachment. In J. Cassidy & P. R. Shaver (Eds.), *Handbook of attachment: Theory, research, and clinical applications* (3rd ed., pp. 852–877). Guilford Press.

Michigan Association for Infant Mental Health (MI-AIMH). (2017). *Competency Guidelines for Endorsement for Culturally Sensitive, Relationship-Focused Practice Promoting Infant and Early Childhood Mental Health®.* Author.

Midgley, N., Ensink, K., Lindqvist, K., Malberg, N., & Muller, N. (2017). *Mentalization-based treatment for children: A time-limited approach.* American Psychological Association.

Miles, T. (2021). *All that she carried: The journey of Ashley's sack, a Black family keepsake.* Random House.

Milot, T., Lorent, A., St-Laurent, D., Bernier, A., Tarabulsy, G., Lemelin, J. P., & Ethier, L. S. (2014). Hostile–helpless state of mind as further evidence of adult disorganized states of mind in neglecting families. *Child Abuse and Neglect, 38*(8), 1351–1357.

Mitchell, S. (1988). *Relational concepts in psychoanalysis: An integration.* Harvard University Press.

Miyake, K., Chen, S.-J., & Campos, J. J. (1985). Infant temperament, mother's mode of interaction, and attachment in Japan: An interim report. *Monographs of the Society for Research in Child Development, 50*(1–2), 276–297.

Murry, V. M., Butler-Barnes, S. T., Mayo-Gamble, T. L., & Inniss-Thompson, M. N. (2018). Excavating new constructs for family stress theories in the context of everyday life experiences of Black American families. *Journal of Family Theory and Review, 10*(2), 384–405.

Murry, V. M., Gonzalez, C. M., Hanebutt, R. A., Bulgin, D., Coates, E. E., Inniss-Thompson, M. N., . . . Cortez, M. B. (2022). Longitudinal study of the cascading effects of racial discrimination on attachment processes and adjustment among African American youth. *Attachment and Human Development, 24*(3), 322–338.

Muzik, M., McGinnis, E. W., Bocknek, E., Morelen, D., Rosenblum, K. L., Liberzon, O., . . . Abelson, J. L. (2016). PTSD symptoms across pregnancy and early postpartum among women with lifetime PTSD diagnosis. *Depression and Anxiety, 33*, 584–591.

Nachmias, M., Gunnar, M., Mangelsdorf, S., Parritz, R. H., & Buss, K. (1996). Behavioral inhibition and stress reactivity: The moderating role of attachment security. *Child Development, 67*(2), 508–522.

Narayan, A. J., Ghosh Ippen, C., Harris, W. W., & Lieberman, A. F. (2017). Assessing angels in the nursery: A pilot study of childhood memories of benevolent caregiving as protective influences. *Infant Mental Health Journal, 38*(4), 461–474.

Narayan, A. J., Ghosh Ippen, C., Harris, W. W., & Lieberman, A. F. (2019). Protective factors that buffer against the intergenerational transmission of trauma from mothers to young children: A replication study of angels in the nursery. *Development and Psychopathology, 31*(1), 173–187.

Narayan, A. J., Lieberman, A. F., & Masten, A. S. (2021). Intergenerational transmission and prevention of adverse childhood experiences (ACEs). *Clinical Psychology Review, 85*, 101997.

Narayan, A. J., Rivera, L. M., Bernstein, R. E., Harris, W. W., & Lieberman, A. F. (2018). Positive childhood experiences predict less psychopathology and stress in pregnant women with childhood adversity: A pilot study of the benevolent childhood experiences (BCEs) scale. *Child Abuse and Neglect, 78*, 19–30.

National Alliance on Mental Illness (2023). Retrieved from *https://nami.org/About-Mental-Illness.*

National Scientific Council on the Developing Child. (2012). The science of neglect: The persistent absence of responsive care disrupts the developing brain (Working Paper #12). Retrieved from *https://developingchild.harvard.edu/resources.*

National Scientific Council on the Developing Child. (2020). Connecting the brain to the rest of the body: Early childhood development and lifelong health are deeply intertwined (Working Paper #15). Retrieved from *https://developingchild.harvard.edu/resources.*

Nerlander, L. M., Callaghan, W. M., Smith, R. A., & Barfield, W. D. (2015). Short interpregnancy interval associated with preterm birth in U.S. adolescents. *Maternal and Child Health Journal, 19*(4), 850–858.

Nijssens, L., Vliegen, N., & Luyten, P. (2020). The mediating role of parental reflective functioning in child social–emotional development. *Journal of Child and Family Studies, 29*(8), 2342–2354.

Olds, D. L. (2002). Prenatal and infancy home visiting by nurses: From randomized trials to community replication. *Prevention Science, 3*(3), 153–172.

Olds, D. L. (2006). The nurse–family partnership: An evidence-based preventive intervention. *Infant Mental Health Journal, 27*(1), 5–25.

Olds, D. L., Robinson, J., O'Brien, R., Luckey, D. W., Pettitt, L. M., Henderson, C. R., . . . Talmi, A. (2002). Home visiting by paraprofessionals and by nurses: A randomized, controlled trial. *Pediatrics, 110*(3), 486–496.

Olds, D. L., Sadler, L., & Kitzman, H. (2007). Programs for parents of infants and toddlers: Recent evidence from randomized trials. *Journal of Child Psychology and Psychiatry, 48*(3–4), 355–391.

Olds, S. (1984). *The dead and the living: Poems* (Vol. 12). Knopf.

Oliveira, P., & Fearon, P. (2019). The biological bases of attachment. *Adoption and Fostering, 43*(3), 274–293.

Oppenheim, D., & Koren-Karie, N. (2013). The insightfulness assessment: Measuring the internal processes underlying maternal sensitivity. *Attachment and Human Development, 15*, 545–561.

Ordway, M. R., Sadler, L. S., Dixon, J., Close, N., Mayes, L., & Slade, A. (2014). Lasting effects of an interdisciplinary home visiting program on child behavior: Preliminary follow-up results of a randomized trial. *Journal of Pediatric Nursing, 29*(1), 3–13.

Ordway, M. R., Sadler, L. S., Holland, M. L., Slade, A., Close, N., & Mayes, L. C. (2018). A home visiting parenting program and child obesity: A randomized trial. *Pediatrics, 141*(2), e20171076.

Ordway, M. R., Webb, D., Sadler, L. S., & Slade, A. (2015). Parental reflective functioning: An approach to enhancing parent–child relationships in pediatric primary care. *Journal of Pediatric Health Care, 29*, 325–334.

O'Rourke, P. (2011). The significance of reflective supervision for infant mental health work. *Infant Mental Health Journal, 32*, 165–173.

Osofsky, J. D. (2009). Perspectives on helping traumatized infants, young children, and their families. *Infant Mental Health Journal, 30*(6), 673–677.

Osofsky, J. D., & Lieberman, A. F. (2011). A call for integrating a mental health perspective into systems of care for abused and neglected infants and young children. *American Psychologist, 66*(2), 120–128.

Pajulo, M., Pyykkönen, N., Kalland, M., Sinkkonen, J., Helenius, H., Punamäki, R. L., & Suchman, N. (2012). Substance-abusing mothers in residential treatment with their babies: Importance of pre-and postnatal maternal reflective functioning. *Infant Mental Health Journal, 33*(1), 70–81.

Pajulo, M., Tolvanen, M., Karlsson, L., Halme-Chowdhury, E., Öst, C., Luyten, P., . . . Karlsson, H. (2015). The Prenatal Parental Reflective Functioning Questionnaire: Exploring factor structure and construct validity of a new measure in the Finn Brain Birth Cohort pilot study. *Infant Mental Health Journal, 36*(4), 399–414.

Pajulo, M., Tolvanen, M., Pyykkönen, N., Karlsson, L., Mayes, L., & Karlsson, H. (2018). Exploring parental mentalization in postnatal phase with a self-report questionnaire (PRFQ): Factor structure, gender differences and association with sociodemographic factors. The Finn brain birth cohort study. *Psychiatry Research, 262,* 431–439.

Pally, R. (2017). *The reflective parent: How to do less and relate more with your kids.* Norton.

Panksepp, J. (2004). *Affective neuroscience: The foundations of human and animal emotions.* Oxford University Press.

Paris, R., Herriott, M., Holt, M., & Gould, K. (2015). Differential responsiveness to a parenting intervention for mothers in substance abuse treatment. *Child Abuse and Neglect, 50,* 206–217.

Parisa, B., Reza, N., Afsaneh, R., & Sarieh, P. (2016). Cultural safety: An evolutionary concept analysis. *Holistic Nursing Practice, 30,* 33–38.

Parlakian, R. (2001). *Look, listen, and learn: Reflective supervision and relationship-based work.* ZERO TO THREE.

Pawl, J., & St. John, M. (1988). *How you are is as important as what you do . . . in making a positive difference for infants, toddlers and their families.* Zero to Three.

Pawluski, J. L., Hoekzema, E., Leuner, B., & Lonstein, J. S. (2022). Less can be more: Fine tuning the maternal brain. *Neuroscience and Biobehavioral Reviews, 133,* Article 104475.

Pazzagli, C., Delvecchio, E., Raspa, V., Mazzeschi, C., & Luyten, P. (2018). The Parental Reflective Functioning Questionnaire in mothers and fathers of school-aged children. *Journal of Child and Family Studies, 27*(1), 80–90.

Pazzagli, C., Germani, A., Buratta, L., Luyten, P., & Mazzeschi, C. (2019). Childhood obesity and parental reflective functioning: Is there a relation? *International Journal of Clinical and Health Psychology, 19*(3), 209–217.

Pearlman, L. A., & Saakvitne, K. W. (1995). *Trauma and the therapist: Countertransference and vicarious traumatization in psychotherapy with incest survivors.* Norton.

Peters, M. F., & Massey, G. (1983). Mundane extreme environmental stress in family stress theories: The case of black families in white America. *Marriage and Family Review, 6*(1–2), 193–218.

Pine, F. (1985). *Developmental theory and clinical process.* Yale University Press.

Pixley, M. M. (2015). *Singing motherhood: First time mothers' experiences singing to their infants* [Unpublished doctoral dissertation]. City University of New York.

Plant, D. T., Jones, F. W., Pariante, C. M., & Pawlby, S. (2017). Association between maternal childhood trauma and offspring childhood psychopathology: Mediation analysis from the ALSPAC cohort. *British Journal of Psychiatry, 211*(3), 144–150.

Plomin, R. (2013). Child development and molecular genetics: 14 years later. *Child Development, 84*(1), 104–120.

Porges, S. W. (2003). Social engagement and attachment: A phylogenetic perspective. *Annals of the New York Academy of Sciences, 1008*(1), 31–47.

Porges, S. W. (2004). Neuroception: A subconscious system for detecting threats and safety. *ZERO TO THREE, 24*(5), 19–24.

Porges, S. W. (2011). *The polyvagal theory: Neurophysiological foundations of emotions, attachment, communication, and self-regulation.* Norton.

Porges, S. W., & Dana, D. A. (2018). *Clinical applications of the polyvagal theory: The emergence of polyvagal-informed therapies.* Norton.

Powell, B., Cooper, G., Hoffman, K., & Marvin, B. (2013). *The Circle of Security intervention: Enhancing attachment in early parent–child relationships.* Guilford Press.

Poznansky, O. (2010). *Stability and change in maternal reflective functioning in early childhood* [Unpublished doctoral dissertation]. City University of New York.

Putnam, K. T., Harris, W. W., & Putnam, F. W. (2013). Synergistic childhood adversities and complex adult psychopathology. *Journal of Traumatic Stress, 26,* 435–442.

Regan, A. K., Ball, S. J., Warren, J. L., Malacova, E., Padula, A., Marston, C., . . . Pereira, G. (2019). A population-based matched-sibling analysis estimating the associations between first interpregnancy interval and birth outcomes. *American Journal of Epidemiology, 188*(1), 9–16.

Ridout, K. K., Levandowski, M., Ridout, S. J., Gantz, L., Goonan, K., Palermo, D., . . . Tyrka, A. R. (2018). Early life adversity and telomere length: A meta-analysis. *Molecular Psychiatry, 23*(4), 858–871.

Roben, C. K. P., Kipp, E., Schein, S. S., Costello, A. H., & Dozier, M. (2022). Transitioning to telehealth due to COVID-19: Maintaining model fidelity in a home visiting program for parents of vulnerable infants. *Infant Mental Health Journal, 43,* 173–184.

Roberts, S. O., Bareket-Shavit, C., Dollins, F. A., Goldie, P. D., & Mortenson, E. (2020). Racial inequality in psychological research: Trends of the past and recommendations for the future. *Perspectives on Psychological Science, 15*(6), 1295–1309.

Roney, L., Knapik, K., Eaves, T., Neitlich, J., & LaPointe, K. (2021). An interprofessional approach to family-centered child-protective services referral: A case report. *Journal of Trauma Nursing, 28,* 401–405.

Rostad, W. L., & Whitaker, D. J. (2016). The association between reflective functioning and parent–child relationship quality. *Journal of Child and Family Studies, 25*(7), 2164–2177.

Rutherford, H. J., Booth, C. R., Luyten, P., Bridgett, D. J., & Mayes, L. C. (2015). Investigating the association between parental reflective functioning and distress tolerance in motherhood. *Infant Behavior and Development, 40,* 54–63.

Rutherford, H. J., Byrne, S. P., Crowley, M. J., Bornstein, J., Bridgett, D. J., & Mayes, L. C. (2018). Executive functioning predicts reflective functioning in mothers. *Journal of Child and Family Studies, 27*(3), 944–952.

Rutherford, H. J., Maupin, A. N., Landi, N., Potenza, M. N., & Mayes, L. C. (2017). Parental reflective functioning and the neural correlates of processing infant affective cues. *Social Neuroscience, 12*(5), 519–529.

Rutter, M. (1985). Resilience in the face of adversity: Protective factors and resistance to psychiatric disorders. *British Journal of Psychiatry, 147*(6), 598–611.

Rybińska, A., Best, D., Goodman, W. B., Bai, Y., & Dodge, K. A. (2022).

Transitioning to virtual interaction during the COVID-19 pandemic: Impact on implementation of the Family Connects postpartum home visiting program activity. *Infant Mental Health Journal, 43*(1), 159–172.

Saakvitne, K. W. (2002). Shared trauma: The therapist's increased vulnerability. *Psychoanalytic Dialogues, 12,* 443–449.

Saakvitne, K. W., Gamble, S., Pearlman, L. A., & Lev, B. T. (2000). *Risking connection: A training curriculum for working with survivors of childhood abuse.* Sidran Press.

Sacks, V., & Murphey, D. (2018, February). The prevalence of adverse childhood experiences, nationally, by state, and by race or ethnicity. *Child Trends.* Retrieved from *www.childtrends.org/publications/prevalence-adverse-childhood-experiences-nationally-state-race-ethnicity.*

Sadler, L. S., Anderson, S. A., & Sabatelli, R. (2001). Parental competence among African American adolescent mothers and grandmothers. *Journal of Pediatric Nursing, 16,* 217–233.

Sadler, L. S., & Clemmens, D. A. (2004). Ambivalent grandmothers raising teen daughters and their babies. *Journal of Family Nursing, 10,* 211–232.

Sadler, L. S., Novick, G., & Meadows-Oliver, M. (2016). "Having a baby changes everything": Reflective functioning in pregnant adolescents. *Journal of Pediatric Nursing, 31*(3), S219–S231.

Sadler, L. S., Slade, A., Close, N., Webb, D., Simpson, T., Fennie, K., & Mayes, L. C. (2013). Minding the Baby: Enhancing reflectiveness to improve early health and relationship outcomes in an interdisciplinary home-visiting program. *Infant Mental Health Journal, 34,* 391–405.

Sadler, L. S., Slade, A., & Mayes, L. C. (2006). *Minding the Baby®: A mentalization based parenting program.* In J. G. Allen & P. Fonagy (Eds.), *Handbook of mentalization-based treatment* (pp. 271–288). Wiley.

Sagi, A., van IJzendoorn, M. H., Scharf, M., Joels, T., Koren-Karie, N., Mayseless, O., & Aviezer, O. (1997). Ecological constraints for intergenerational transmission of attachment. *International Journal of Behavioral Development, 20*(2), 287–299.

San Cristobal, P., Santelices, M. P., & Miranda Fuenzalida, D. A. (2017). Manifestation of trauma: The effect of early traumatic experiences and adult attachment on parental reflective functioning. *Frontiers in Psychology, 8,* 449.

Sander, L. W. (1962). Issues in early mother–child interaction. *Journal of the American Academy of Child Psychiatry, 1,* 141–166.

Saraiya, T. C., Fitzpatrick, S., Zumberg-Smith, K., Lopez-Castro, T., Back, S. E., & Hien, D. A. (2021). Social-emotional profiles of PTSD, complex PTSD, and borderline personality disorder among racially and ethnically diverse young adults: A latent class analysis. *Journal of Traumatic Stress, 34,* 56–68.

Savage, L. É., Tarabulsy, G. M., Pearson, J., Collin-Vézina, D., & Gagné, L. M. (2019). Maternal history of childhood maltreatment and later parenting behavior: A meta-analysis. *Development and Psychopathology, 31*(1), 9–21.

Schafer, R. (1958). How was this story told? *Journal of Projective Techniques, 22,* 181–210.

Schechter, D. S., Coates, S. W., Kaminer, T., Coots, T., Zeanah, C. H., Jr., Davies, M., . . . McCaw, J. E. (2008). Distorted maternal mental representations and atypical behavior in a clinical sample of violence-exposed mothers and their toddlers. *Journal of Trauma and Dissociation, 9*(2), 123–147.

Schechter, D. S., Coots, T., Zeanah, C. H., Davies, M., Coates, S. W., Trabka, K. A., . . . Myers, M. M. (2005). Maternal mental representations of the child in an inner-city clinical sample: Violence-related posttraumatic stress and reflective functioning. *Attachment and Human Development, 7*(3), 313–331.

Scheeringa, M. S., & Zeanah, C. H. (2001). A relational perspective on PTSD in early childhood. *Journal of Traumatic Stress, 14*(4), 799–815.

Schuengel, C., Bakermans-Kranenburg, M. J., & van IJzendoorn, M. H. (1999). Frightening maternal behavior linking unresolved loss and disorganized infant attachment. *Journal of Consulting and Clinical Psychology, 67*(1), 54–63.

Schultheis, A. M., Mayes, L. C., & Rutherford, H. J. (2019). Associations between emotion regulation and parental reflective functioning. *Journal of Child and Family Studies, 28*(4), 1094–1104.

Schwartz, J. A., Wright, E. M., & Valgardson, B. A. (2019). Adverse childhood experiences and deleterious outcomes in adulthood: A consideration of the simultaneous role of genetic and environmental influences in two independent samples from the United States. *Child Abuse and Neglect, 88*, 420–431.

Seuss, Dr. [Theodor Seuss Geisel]. (1954). *Horton hears a who.* Random House.

Shai, D., & Belsky, J. (2011). When words just won't do: Introducing parental embodied mentalizing. *Child Development Perspectives, 5*(3), 173–180.

Shai, D., & Belsky, J. (2017). Parental embodied mentalizing: How the nonverbal dance between parents and infants predicts children's socio-emotional functioning. *Attachment and Human Development, 19*(2), 191–219.

Shai, D., Dollberg, D., & Szepsenwol, O. (2017). The importance of parental verbal and embodied mentalizing in shaping parental experiences of stress and coparenting. *Infant Behavior and Development, 49*, 87–96.

Shai, D., & Meins, E. (2018). Parental embodied mentalizing and its relation to mind-mindedness, sensitivity, and attachment security. *Infancy, 23*(6), 857–872.

Shapiro, J. (2008). Walking a mile in their patients' shoes: Empathy and othering in medical students' education. *Philosophy, Ethics, and Humanities in Medicine, 3*(1), 10.

Shapiro, S. L., Astin, J. A., Bishop, S. R., & Cordova, M. (2005). Mindfulness-based stress reduction for health care professionals: Results from a randomized trial. *International Journal of Stress Management, 12*(2), 164–176.

Shonkoff, J. P., Garner, A. S., Siegel, B. S., Dobbins, M. I., Earls, M. F., McGuinn, L., . . . Committee on Psychosocial Aspects of Child and Family Health and Committee on Early Childhood, Adoption, and Dependent Care. (2012). The lifelong effects of early childhood adversity and toxic stress. *Pediatrics, 129*(1), e232–e246.

Shonkoff, J. P., Slopen, N., & Williams, D. R. (2021). Early childhood adversity, toxic stress, and the impacts of racism on the foundations of health. *Annual Review of Public Health, 42*, 115–134.

Siegel, D. J. (2007). *The mindful brain: Reflection and attunement in the cultivation of well-being.* Norton.

Simkin, P. (1992). Overcoming the legacy of childhood sexual abuse: The role of caregivers and childbirth educators. *Birth, 19*(4), 224–225.

Simkin, P., & Klaus, P. (2004). *When survivors give birth: Understanding and healing the effects of early sexual abuse on childbearing women.* Classic Day.

Simpson, T. E., Robinson, J. L., & Brown, E. (2018). Is reflective supervision enough?: An exploration of workforce perspectives. *Infant Mental Health Journal, 39*(4), 478–488.

Slade, A. (2000). The development and organization of attachment: Implications for psychoanalysis. *Journal of the American Psychoanalytic Association, 48*(4), 1147–1174.

Slade, A. (2002). Keeping the baby in mind. *ZERO TO THREE, 6*, 10–15.

Slade, A. (2003). *The Pregnancy Interview* [Unpublished manuscript]. Yale University, Yale Child Study Center.

Slade, A. (2005). Parental reflective functioning: An introduction. *Attachment and Human Development, 7*(3), 269–281.

Slade, A. (2007). Reflective parenting programs: Theory and development. *Psychoanalytic Inquiry, 26*(4), 640–657.

Slade, A. (2014). Imagining fear: Attachment, threat, and psychic experience. *Psychoanalytic Dialogues, 24*, 253–266.

Slade, A. (2017). *The pregnancy interview for fathers* [Unpublished manuscript]. Yale University, Yale Child Study Center.

Slade, A. (2020, April). We're all on the frontlines: Parenting children with complex needs during COVID-19 [FAR Fund Lecture]. Retrieved from *https:// farfund.org/resources.*

Slade, A., Aber, J. L., Berger, B., Bresgi, I., & Kaplan, M. (2004a). *Parent Development Interview—Revised* [Unpublished manuscript]. Yale University, Yale Child Study Center.

Slade, A., Bernbach, E., Grienenberger, J., Levy, D., & Locker, A. (2004b). *Manual for scoring reflective functioning on the Parent Development Interview* [Unpublished manuscript]. Yale University.

Slade, A., & Cohen, L. J. (1996). The process of parenting and the remembrance of things past. *Infant Mental Health Journal, 17*(3), 217–238.

Slade, A., Grienenberger, J., Bernbach, E., Levy, D., & Locker, A. (2005). Maternal reflective functioning, attachment, and the transmission gap: A preliminary study. *Attachment and Human Development, 7*(3), 283–298.

Slade, A., Grunebaum, L., Reeves, M., & Ross, A. (1987). *The pregnancy interview* [Unpublished manuscript]. City College of New York, Doctoral Program in Clinical Psychology.

Slade, A., Holland, M. L., Ordway, M. R., Carlson, E. A., Jeon, S., Close, N., . . . Sadler, L. S. (2019). Minding the Baby: Enhancing parental reflective functioning and infant attachment in an attachment-based, interdisciplinary home visiting program. *Development and Psychopathology, 32*(1), 123–137.

Slade, A., & Holmes, J. (Eds.). (2013). *Attachment theory.* SAGE.

Slade, A., Patterson, M., & Miller, M. (2004c). *Addendum to Reflective Functioning Scoring Manual for use with the Pregnancy Interview* [Unpublished manuscript]. Yale University, Yale Child Study Center.

Slade, A., & Sadler, L. S. (2013). Minding the Baby: Complex trauma and home visiting. *International Journal of Birth and Parent Education, 1,* 50–53.

Slade, A., & Sadler, L. (2019). Pregnancy and infant mental health. In C. H. Zeanah (Ed.), *Handbook of infant mental health* (4th ed., pp. 25–40). Guilford Press.

Slade, A., Sadler, L., Close, N., Fitzpatrick, S. E., Simpson, T. E., & Webb, D. (2017a). Minding the Baby: The impact of threat on the mother–baby and mother–clinician relationship. In S. Gojman-de-Millan, C. Herreman, & L. A. Sroufe (Eds.), *Attachment across clinical and cultural perspectives* (pp. 182–205). Routledge.

Slade, A., Sadler, L. S., Webb, D., Simpson, T., & Close, N. (2018). *Minding the Baby Home Visitation Program Treatment Manual: Intervention and training guide* (5th ed.). Yale University.

Slade, A., Simpson, T. E., Webb, D., Albertson, J., Close, N., & Sadler, L. (2017b). *Minding the Baby*: Developmental trauma and home visiting. In H. Steele & M. Steele (Eds.), *Handbook of attachment-based interventions* (pp. 151–173). Guilford Press.

Slade, A., & Sleed, M. (2023). *Parental reflective functioning on the Parent Development and Pregnancy Interviews: Assessments, correlations, and future directions.* Manuscript submitted for publication.

Sleed, M., Baradon, T., & Fonagy, P. (2013). New beginnings for mothers and babies in prison: A cluster randomized controlled trial. *Attachment and Human Development, 15,* 349–367.

Sleed, M., Isosävi, S., & Fonagy, P. (2021). The assessment of representational risk (ARR): Development and psychometric properties of a new coding system for assessing risk in the parent–infant relationship. *Infant Mental Health Journal, 42,* 525–545.

Sleed, M., Slade, A., & Fonagy, P. (2018). Reflective functioning on the Parent Development Interview: Validity and reliability in relation to socio-demographic factors. *Attachment and Human Development, 22*(3), 310–331.

Smaling, H. J., Huijbregts, S. C., Suurland, J., van der Heijden, K. B., Mesman, J., van Goozen, S. H., & Swaab, H. (2016a). Prenatal reflective functioning and accumulated risk as predictors of maternal interactive behavior during free play, the still-face paradigm, and two teaching tasks. *Infancy, 21*(6), 766–784.

Smaling, H. J., Huijbregts, S. C., Suurland, J., van der Heijden, K. B., van Goozen, S. H., & Swaab, H. (2015). Prenatal reflective functioning in primiparous women with a high-risk profile. *Infant Mental Health Journal, 36*(3), 251–261.

Smaling, H. A., Huijbregts, S. C. J., van der Heijden, K. B., Hay, D. F., van Goozen, S. H. M., & Swaab, H. (2017). Prenatal reflective functioning and development of aggression in infancy: The roles of maternal intrusiveness and sensitivity. *Journal of Abnormal Child Psychology, 45*(2), 237–248.

Smaling, H. J., Huijbregts, S. C. J., van der Heijden, K. B., van Goozen, S. H. M., & Swaab, H. (2016b). Maternal reflective functioning as a multidimensional construct: Differential associations with children's temperament and externalizing behavior. *Infant Behavior and Development, 44,* 263–274.

SmithBattle, L., Phengnum, W., & Punsuwun, S. (2020). Navigating a minefield:

Meta-synthesis of teen mothers' breastfeeding experience. *American Journal of Maternal Child Nursing, 45,* 45–54.

Solomon, J., & George, C. (1996). Defining the caregiving system: Toward a theory of caregiving. *Infant Mental Health Journal, 17*(3), 183–197.

Sorce, J. F., & Emde, R. N. (1981). Mother's presence is not enough: Effect of emotional availability on infant exploration. *Developmental Psychology, 17*(6), 737–745.

Squires, J., Bricker, D., & Twombly, E. (2002). *The ASQ:SE User's Guide for the Ages & Stages Questionnaires: Social-Emotional: A parent-completed, child-monitoring system for social-emotional behaviors.* Brookes.

Sroufe, L. A. (1985). Attachment classification from the perspective of infant–caregiver relationships and infant temperament. *Child Development, 56*(1), 1–14.

Sroufe, L. A., Egeland, B., Carlson, E., & Collins, W. A. (2005). Placing early attachment experiences in developmental context: The Minnesota Longitudinal Study. In K. E. Grossmann, K. Grossmann, & E. Waters (Eds.), *Attachment from infancy to adulthood: The major longitudinal studies* (pp. 48–70). Guilford Press.

Sroufe, L. A., & Waters, E. (1977). Heart rate as a convergent measure in clinical and developmental research. *Merrill-Palmer Quarterly, 23*(1), 3–27.

St. John, M. S., Thomas, K., & Noroña, C. R. (2013, June 15). Diversity-informed infant mental health tenets: Together in the struggle for social justice. *Perspectives in Infant Mental Health.* Rerieved from *https://perspectives.waimh. org/2013/06/15/zero-three-corner-diversity-informed-infant-mental-health-tenets-together-struggle-social-justice.*

Stacks, A. M., Barron, C. C., & Wong, K. (2019). Infant mental health home visiting in the context of an infant–toddler court team: Changes in parental responsiveness and reflective functioning. *Infant Mental Health Journal, 40*(4), 523–540.

Stacks, A. M., Muzik, M., Wong, K., Beeghly, M., Huth-Bocks, A., Irwin, J. L., & Rosenblum, K. L. (2014). Maternal reflective functioning among mothers with childhood maltreatment histories: Links to sensitive parenting and infant attachment security. *Attachment and Human Development, 16*(5), 515–533.

Stacks, A. M., Wong, K., & Dykehouse, T. (2013). Teacher reflective functioning: A preliminary study of measurement and self-reported teaching behavior. *Reflective Practice, 14,* 487–505.

Steele, H., Bate, J., Steele, M., Dube, S. R., Danskin, K., Knafo, H., . . . Murphy, A. (2016). Adverse childhood experiences, poverty, and parenting stress. *Canadian Journal of Behavioural Science, 48*(1), 32–38.

Steele, H., & Steele, M. (2008). On the origins of reflective functioning. In F. Busch (Ed.), *Mentalization: Theoretical considerations, research findings, and clinical implications* (pp. 133–158). Routledge.

Steele, H., & Steele, M. (Eds.). (2018). *Handbook of attachment-based interventions.* Guilford Press.

Steele, H., Steele, M., Bonuck, K., Meissner, P., & Murphy, A. (2018). Group attachment-based intervention: A multifamily trauma-informed intervention.

In H. Steele & M. Steele (Eds.), *Handbook of attachment-based interventions* (pp. 198–219). Guilford Press.

Steele, M., Hodges, J., Kaniuk, J., & Steele, H. (2009). Mental representation and change: Developing attachment relationships in an adoption context. *Psychoanalytic Inquiry, 30*(1), 25–40.

Steele, M., Kaniuk, J., Hodges, J., Asquith, K., Hillman, S., & Steele, H. (2008). Measuring mentalization across contexts: Links between representations of childhood and representations of parenting in an adoption sample. In E. L. Jurist, A. Slade, & S. Bergner (Eds.), *Mind to mind: Infant research, neuroscience, and psychoanalysis* (pp. 115–138). Other Press.

Steinberg, D., & Pianta, R. (2006). Maternal representations of relationships: Assessing multiple parenting dimensions. In O. Mayseless (Ed.), *Parenting representations: Theory, research, and clinical implications* (pp. 41–78). Cambridge University Press.

Stern, D. N. (1977). *The first relationship: Mother and infant.* Harvard University Press.

Stern, D. N. (1985). *The interpersonal world of the infant: A view from psychoanalysis and developmental psychology.* Basic Books.

Stern, J. A., Barbarin, O., & Cassidy, J. (Eds.). (2022a). Attachment perspectives on race, prejudice, and anti-racism. *Attachment and Human Development, 24*(3), 253–259.

Stern, J. A., Barbarin, O., & Cassidy, J. (2022b). Working toward anti-racist perspectives in attachment theory, research, and practice. *Attachment and Human Development, 24*(3), 392–422.

Stern, J. A., Jones, J. D., Nortey, B. M., Lejuez, C. W., & Cassidy, J. (2022c). Pathways linking attachment and depressive symptoms for Black and White adolescents: Do race and neighborhood racism matter? *Attachment and Human Development, 24*(3), 304–321.

Stevens, W. (1923). Thirteen ways of looking at a blackbird. In W. Stevens, *Harmonium.* Knopf.

Stob, V., Slade, A., Brotnow, L., Adnopoz, J., & Woolston, J. (2019). The Family Cycle: An activity to enhance parents' mentalization in children's mental health treatment. *Journal of Infant, Child, and Adolescent Psychotherapy, 18*(2), 103–119.

Stoute, B. (2017). Race and racism in psychoanalytic thought: The ghosts in our nursery. *American Psychoanalyst, 51*, 10–11.

Stover, C. S., & Kiselica, A. (2014). An initial examination of the association of reflective functioning to parenting of fathers. *Infant Mental Health Journal, 35*(5), 452–461.

Strathearn, L., Fonagy, P., Amico, J., & Montague, P. R. (2009). Adult attachment predicts maternal brain and oxytocin response to infant cues. *Neuropsychopharmacology, 34*(13), 2655–2666.

Striano, T., Stahl, D., Cleveland, A., & Hoehl, S. (2007). Sensitivity to triadic attention between 6 weeks and 3 months of age. *Infant Behavior and Development, 30*(3), 529–534.

Stronach, E. P., Toth, S. L., Rogosch, F., & Cicchetti, D. (2013). Preventive interventions and sustained attachment security in maltreated children. *Development and Psychopathology, 25*(4), 919–930.

Suchman, N., Berg, A., Abrahams, L., Abrahams, T., Adams, A., Cowley, B., . . . Cader-Mokoa, N. (2020). Mothering from the Inside Out: Adapting an evidence-based intervention for high-risk mothers in the Western Cape of South Africa. *Development and Psychopathology, 32*(1), 105–122.

Suchman, N. E., DeCoste, C., Borelli, J. L., & McMahon, T. J. (2018). Does improvement in maternal attachment representations predict greater maternal sensitivity, child attachment security and lower rates of relapse to substance use? A second test of Mothering from the Inside Out treatment mechanisms. *Journal of Substance Abuse Treatment, 85*, 21–30.

Suchman, N. E., DeCoste, C., Castiglioni, N., McMahon, T. J., Rounsaville, B., & Mayes, L. (2010). The Mothers and Toddlers Program, an attachment-based parenting intervention for substance using women: Post-treatment results from a randomized clinical pilot. *Attachment and Human Development, 12*(5), 483–504.

Suchman, N. E., DeCoste, C. L., McMahon, T. J., Dalton, R., Mayes, L. C., & Borelli, J. (2017). Mothering from the Inside Out: Results of a second randomized clinical trial testing a mentalization-based intervention for mothers in addiction treatment. *Development and Psychopathology, 29*(2), 617–636.

Suchman, N. E., DeCoste, C., McMahon, T. J., Rounsaville, B., & Mayes, L. (2011). The mothers and toddlers program, an attachment-based parenting intervention for substance-using women: Results at 6-week follow-up in a randomized clinical pilot. *Infant Mental Health Journal, 32*(4), 427–449.

Suchman, N. E., Decoste, C., Rosenberger, P., & McMahon, T. J. (2012). Attachment-based intervention for substance-using mothers: A preliminary test of the proposed mechanisms of change. *Infant Mental Health Journal, 33*(4), 360–371.

Suchman, N. E., Ordway, M. R., de Las Heras, L., & McMahon, T. J. (2016). Mothering from the Inside Out: Results of a pilot study testing a mentalization-based therapy for mothers enrolled in mental health services. *Attachment and Human Development, 18*(6), 596–617.

Sue, D. W. (2010). *Microaggressions in everyday life: Race, gender, and sexual orientation.* Wiley.

Sullivan, H. S. (1947). *Conceptions of modern psychiatry.* William Alanson White Psychiatric Foundation.

Talia, A., Daniel, S. I. F., Miller-Bottome, M., Brambilla, A., Miccoli, D., Safran, J. D., & Lingiardi, V. (2014). AAI predicts patients' in-session interpersonal behavior and discourse: A "move to the level of the relation" for attachment-informed psychotherapy research. *Attachment and Human Development, 16*(2), 192–209.

Terry, M., Finger, B., Lyons-Ruth, K., Sadler, L. S., & Slade, A. (2021). Hostile/helpless maternal representations in pregnancy and later child removal: A pilot study. *Infant Mental Health Journal, 42*(1), 60–73.

Tervalon, M., & Murray-Garcia, J. (1998). Cultural humility versus cultural competence: A critical distinction in defining physician training outcomes in multicultural education. *Journal of Health Care for the Poor and Underserved, 9*(2), 117–125.

Theede, A. (2018). Polyvagal theory affirms the importance of nursing. In S. W. Porges & D. Dana (Eds.), *Clinical applications of the polyvagal theory: The emergence of polyvagal-informed therapies* (pp. 149–167). Norton.

Thomas, J. C., Letourneau, N., Campbell, T. S., Giesbrecht, G. F., & APrON Study Team. (2018). Social buffering of the maternal and infant HPA axes: Mediation and moderation in the intergenerational transmission of adverse childhood experiences. *Development and Psychopathology, 30*(3), 921–939.

Toepfer, P., Heim, C., Entringer, S., Binder, E., Wadhwa, P., & Buss, C. (2017). Oxytocin pathways and the intergenerational transmission of maternal early life stress. *Neuroscience and Biobehavioral Reviews, 73*, 293–308.

Tomasik, J., & Fleming, C. (2015). *Lessons from the field: Promising interprofessional collaboration practices*. Robert Wood Johnson Foundation.

Tomlin, A. M., Weatherston, D. J., & Pavkov, T. (2014). Critical components of reflective supervision: Responses from expert supervisors in the field. *Infant Mental Health Journal, 35*(1), 70–80.

Tortora, S. (2005). *The dancing dialogue: Using the communicative power of movement with young children*. Redleaf Press.

Toth, S. L., Michl-Petzing, L. C., Guild, D., & Lieberman, A. F. (2018). Child–parent psychotherapy: Theoretical bases, clinical applications, and empirical support. In H. Steele & M. Steele (Eds.), *Handbook of attachment-based interventions* (pp. 296–317). Guilford Press.

Toth, S. L., Rogosch, F. A., Manly, J. T., & Cicchetti, D. (2006). The efficacy of toddler–parent psychotherapy to reorganize attachment in the young offspring of mothers with major depressive disorder: A randomized preventive trial. *Journal of Consulting and Clinical Psychology, 74*, 1006–1016.

Toth, S. L., Rogosch, F. A., Manly, J. T., Spagnola, M., & Cicchetti, D. (2002). The relative efficacy of two interventions in altering maltreated preschool children's representational models: Implications for attachment theory. *Development and Psychopathology, 14*, 877–908.

Tottenham, N., & Sheridan, M. A. (2010). A review of adversity, the amygdala and the hippocampus: A consideration of developmental timing. *Frontiers in Human Neuroscience, 3*, Article 68.

Trent, M., Dooley, D. G., Dougé, J., & Section on Adolescent Health, Council on Community Pediatrics, Committee on Adolescence. (2019). The impact of racism on child and adolescent health. *Pediatrics, 144*(2), e20191765.

Trevarthen, C. (1979). Communication and cooperation in early infancy: A description of primary intersubjectivity. In M. M. Bullowa (Ed.), *Before speech: The beginning of interpersonal communication* (pp. 321–349). Cambridge University Press.

Tronick, E. (2007). *The neurobehavioral and social-emotional development of infants and children*. Norton.

Tronick, E., & Gold, C. (2020). *The power of discord: Why the ups and downs of relationships are the secret to building intimacy, resilience, and trust*. Little, Brown.

Tso, W. W. Y., Wong, R. S., Tung, K. T. S., Rao, N., Fu, K. W., Yam, J. C. S., . . .

Lp, P. (2022). Vulnerability and resilience in children during the COVID-19 pandemic. *European Child and Adolescent Psychiatry, 31,* 151–176.

Turkle, S. (2015). *Reclaiming conversation: The power of talk in a digital age.* Penguin Press.

van den Boom, D. C. (1994). The influence of temperament and mothering on attachment and exploration: An experimental manipulation of sensitive responsiveness among lower-class mothers with irritable infants. *Child Development, 65*(5), 1457–1477.

van der Kolk, B. A. (1994). The body keeps the score: Memory and the evolving psychobiology of posttraumatic stress. *Harvard Review of Psychiatry, 1*(5), 253–265.

van der Kolk, B. (2014). *The body keeps the score: Mind, brain and body in the transformation of trauma.* Penguin Random House.

van der Kolk, B., Roth, S., Pelcovitz, D., Sunday, S., & Spinazzola, J. (2005). Disorders of extreme stress: The empirical foundation of a complex adaptation to trauma. *Journal of Traumatic Stress, 18,* 389–399.

Van Horn, P., Lieberman, A. F., & Harris, W. W. (2008). *The Angels in the Nursery interview* [Unpublished manuscript]. Department of Psychiatry, University of California, San Francisco.

van IJzendoorn, M. H. (1995). Adult attachment representations, parental responsiveness, and infant attachment: A meta-analysis on the predictive validity of the Adult Attachment Interview. *Psychological Bulletin, 117*(3), 387–403.

Vaughn, B. E., & Bost, K. K. (2016). Attachment and temperament as intersecting developmental products and interacting developmental contexts throughout infancy and childhood. In J. Cassidy & P. R. Shaver (Eds.), *Handbook of attachment: Theory, research, and clinical applications* (3rd ed., pp. 202–222). Guilford Press.

Verhage, M. L., Fearon, R. M. P., Schuengel, C., van IJzendoorn, M. H., Bakermans-Kranenburg, M. J., Madigan, S., . . . Brisch, K.-H. (2018). Examining ecological constraints on the intergenerational transmission of attachment via individual participant data meta-analysis. *Child Development, 89*(6), 2023–2037.

Verhage, M. L., Schuengel, C., Madigan, S., Fearon, R. M. P., Oosterman, M., Cassibba, R., . . . van IJzendoorn, M. H. (2016). Narrowing the transmission gap: A synthesis of three decades of research on intergenerational transmission of attachment. *Psychological Bulletin, 142*(4), 337–366.

Vreeswijk, C. M., Maas, A. J. B., & van Bakel, H. J. (2012). Parental representations: A systematic review of the working model of the child interview. *Infant Mental Health Journal, 33*(3), 314–328.

Vyas, A., Pillai, A. G., & Chattarji, S. (2004). Recovery after chronic stress fails to reverse amygdaloid neuronal hypertrophy and enhanced anxiety-like behavior. *Neuroscience, 128*(4), 667–673.

Vygotsky, L. S. (1980). *Mind in society: The development of higher psychological processes.* Harvard University Press.

Waddell, M. (1992). *Owl babies.* Candlewick Press.

Wampold, B. E., & Imel, Z. E. (2015). *The great psychotherapy debate: The evidence for what makes psychotherapy work* (2nd ed.). Routledge.

Ward, M. J., & Carlson, E. A. (1995). Associations among adult attachment representations, maternal sensitivity, and infant–mother attachment in a sample of adolescent mothers. *Child Development, 66*(1), 69–79.

Waters, E., Merrick, S., Treboux, D., Crowell, J., & Albersheim, L. (2000). Attachment security in infancy and early adulthood: A twenty-year longitudinal study. *Child Development, 71*(3), 684–689.

Watson, C. L., Harrison, M. E., Hennes, J. E., & Harris, M. M. (2016). Revealing "the space between": Creating an observation scale to understand infant mental health reflective supervision. *ZERO TO THREE, 37*(2), 14–21.

Weatherston, D., Kaplan-Esterin, M., & Goldberg, S. (2009). Strengthening and recognizing knowledge, skills, and reflective practice: The Michigan Association for Infant Mental Health Competency Guidelines and Endorsement process. *Infant Mental Health Journal, 30*(6), 648–663.

Weatherston, D. J., & Osofsky, J. D. (2009). Working within the context of relationships: Multidisciplinary, relational, and reflective practice, training, and supervision. *Infant Mental Health Journal, 30*(6), 573–578.

Webb, D., Simpson, T., Sadler, L. S., & Slade, A. (2019). *Minding the Baby Home Visitation Program clinician's quick reference guide* (2nd ed.). Yale University.

Werner, H., & Kaplan, B. (1963). *Symbol formation.* Erlbaum.

Winnicott, D. W. (1965). *The maturational processes and the facilitating environment.* Karnac Books.

Winnicott, D. W. (1967). Mirror-role of mother and family in child development. In P. Lomas (Ed.), *The predicament of the family: A psycho-analytical symposium* (pp. 26–33). Hogarth Press.

Winnicott, D. W. (1971). *Playing and reality.* Routledge.

Wong, K., Stacks, A. M., Rosenblum, K. L., & Muzik, M. (2017). Parental reflective functioning moderates the relationship between difficult temperament in infancy and behavior problems in toddlerhood. *Merrill–Palmer Quarterly, 63*(1), 54–76.

Woodhouse, S., Powell, B., Cooper, G., Hoffman, K., Cassidy, J. (2018). The Circle of Security intervention: Design, research, and implementation. In H. Steele & M. Steele (Eds.), *Handbook of attachment-based interventions* (pp. 50–78). Guilford Press.

Woodhouse, S. S., Scott, J. R., Hepworth, A. D., & Cassidy, J. (2020). Secure base provision: A new approach to examining links between maternal caregiving and infant attachment. *Child Development, 91*(1), e249–e265.

Wordsworth, W. (1807). My heart leaps up. In W. Wordsworth, *Poems, in two volumes.* Oxford University Press.

World Health Organization. (2019). *International statistical classification of diseases and related health problems* (11th ed.). Author.

Yang, J., Hou, C., Ma, N., Liu, J., Zhang, Y., Zhou, J., . . . Li, L. (2007). Enriched environment treatment restores impaired hippocampal synaptic plasticity and cognitive deficits induced by prenatal chronic stress. *Neurobiology of Learning and Memory, 87*(2), 257–263.

Yatziv, T., Kessler, Y., & Atzaba-Poria, N. (2020). When do mothers' executive functions contribute to their representations of their child's mind? A contextual view on parental reflective functioning and mind-mindedness. *Developmental Psychology, 56*(6), 1191–1206.

Young, A., Pierce, M. C., Kaczor, K., Lorenz, D. J., Hickey, S., Berger, S. P., . . . Thompson, R. (2018). Are negative/unrealistic parent descriptors of infant attributes associated with physical abuse? *Child Abuse and Neglect, 80,* 41–51.

Young, E. S., Doom, J. R., Farrell, A. K., Carlson, E. A., Englund, M. M., Miller, G. E., . . . Simpson, J. A. (2021). Life stress and cortisol reactivity: An exploratory analysis of the effects of stress exposure across life on HPA-axis functioning. *Development and Psychopathology, 33,* 301–312.

Zeanah, C. H. (Ed.). (2019). *Handbook of infant mental health* (4th ed.). Guilford Press.

Zeanah, C. H., Benoit, D., & Barton, M. (1986). *Working model of the child interview* [Unpublished manuscript]. Brown University.

Zeanah, C. H., Benoit, D., Hirshberg, L., Barton, M. L., & Regan, C. (1994). Mothers' representations of their infants are concordant with infant attachment classifications. *Developmental Issues in Psychiatry and Psychology, 1*(1), 1–14.

Zeanah, C. H., Carter, A. S., Cohen, J., Egger, H., Gleason, M. M., Keren, M., . . . Oser, C. (2016). Diagnostic classification of mental health and developmental disorders of infancy and early childhood DC:0–5: Selective reviews from a new nosology for early childhood psychopathology. *Infant Mental Health Journal, 37*(5), 471–475.

Zeegers, M. A., Colonessi, C., Stams, G., J., M., & Meins, E. (2017) Mind matters: A meta-analysis on parental mentalization and sensitivity as predictors of infant-parent attachment. *Psychological Bulletin, 143*(12), 1245–1272.

Index

Note. *f*, *t*, or *n* after a page number indicates a figure, a table, or a note.